Pharmacy
Case Studies

Pharmacy Case Studies

Edited by

Soraya Dhillon

MBE, BPharm(Hons), PhD, FRPharmS
Foundation Professor and Head of the School of Pharmacy
University of Hertfordshire
Hatfield, UK

and

Rebekah Raymond

BSc(Hons), DipPharmPrac, MRPharmS
Visiting Fellow, School of Pharmacy
University of Hertfordshire
Hatfield, UK

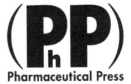

Pharmaceutical Press

Published by the Pharmaceutical Press
An imprint of RPS Publishing

1 Lambeth High Street, London SE1 7JN, UK

© Pharmaceutical Press 2009

(PP) is a trade mark of RPS Publishing
RPS Publishing is the publishing organisation
of the Royal Pharmaceutical Society of Great Britain

First published 2009

Typeset by Photoprint, Torquay, Devon
Printed in Great Britain by TJ International, Padstow, Cornwall

ISBN 978 0 85369 724 4

A catalogue record for this book is available from the British Library.

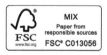

Contents

16   Paediatrics case studies   391
Stephen Tomlin

17   Care of older people case studies   409
Chris Cairns and Nina Barnett

Preface

Pharmacists and healthcare practitioners are required to demonstrate knowledge and understanding of the application of therapeutics in clinical practice. Pharmacists must ensure patient safety and achieve desired health outcomes through effective decision-making. The idea of designing these case studies was to meet the needs and challenges of a modern pharmacy undergraduate curriculum which integrates science and practice at the School of Pharmacy, University of Hertfordshire.

Case studies are increasingly used in pharmacy undergraduate as well as postgraduate education. The concept behind the design of these 'horizontal integration' case studies is to help students integrate the knowledge gained during their undergraduate and pre-registration study. The book provides case studies of increasing complexity, which tie in the strands of learning from across the pharmacy curriculum through Levels 1 to M. Although the cases are based on UK clinical practice, this book will be invaluable to practitioners who wish to develop their clinical skills.

Each chapter contains five case studies, increasing in complexity from those we would expect first-year students to complete (Level 1) through to cases designed for fourth-year/pre-registration students (Level M). The chapters have been designed to follow approximately the *British National Formulary* chapters for ease of use. Case study scenarios include both community and hospital pharmacy situations as suited to the disease and pharmaceutical care provision. In a number of cases, abbreviations have been used and the editors have taken the decision not to provide a glossary of terms as we felt this to be another learning opportunity.

This approach to teaching therapeutics has been implemented in the MPharm degree at the University of Hertfordshire and the students find this an exciting learning experience. Feedback from the students has been positive, with comments such as 'I learnt to think about different aspects of diseases from a professional role and from the patient's point of view' and 'it makes us link the knowledge we have gained in different subjects'.

Though primarily aimed at undergraduate pharmacy students and pre-registration pharmacists, we feel that this book will also be useful to qualified pharmacists as well as medical students, nurses and others with a professional interest in therapeutics. The book will also be of value to practitioners in other countries who wish to develop their pharmaceutical care skills. The editors are indebted to the chapter authors for providing clinical cases from their everyday practice.

Soraya Dhillon and Rebekah Raymond
January 2009

About the editors

Soraya Dhillon is a Foundation Professor and Head of The School of Pharmacy at the University of Hertfordshire. Professor Dhillon has extensive experience in Clinical Pharmacy and Clinical Pharmacokinetics and has held positions in Community and Hospital Pharmacy. She has published widely in the evaluation of clinical pharmacy services and education. She currently holds a non-executive role as Chairman of Luton & Dunstable Foundation Trust and has a particular interest in driving forward patient safety initiatives.

Rebekah Raymond has worked in community, hospital and academic pharmacy and is currently a visiting fellow at the School of Pharmacy, University of Hertfordshire. Rebekah graduated from De Montfort University in Leicester and later completed the Diploma in Pharmacy Practice at the University of London.

Contributors

Caroline Ashley, MSc, BPharm (Hons), MRPharmS
Lead Pharmacist Renal Services, Royal Free Hampstead NHS Trust, London

Nina L Barnett, MSc, MRPharmS
Consultant Pharmacist, Care of Older People, Northwick Park Hospital, Harrow PCT and East & South East England Specialist Pharmacy Services

Karen Baxter, BSc, MSc, MRPharmS
Editor, Pharmaceutical Press, RPS Publishing, London, UK

Narinder Bhalla, BSc (Hons), MSc, MRPharmS
Teacher Practitioner, School of Pharmacy, University of Hertfordshire and Lead Pharmacist, Clinical Governance, Cambridge University Hospitals NHS Foundation Trust

Chris Cairns, MSc, BSc, FRPharmS
Professor of Pharmacy Practice, Kingston University and Consultant Pharmacist, University Hospital Lewisham, London

Soraya Dhillon, MBE, BPharm (Hons), PhD, FRPharmS
Head of School of Pharmacy, University of Hertfordshire and Chairman Luton & Dunstable Hospital NHS Foundation Trust

Russell Foulsham, MSc, PhD, MRPharmS
Principal Lecturer, School of Pharmacy, University of Hertfordshire

Tracy Garnier, BSc (Hons), PhD, PgCert, MRPharmS
Principal Lecturer in Pharmaceutics, School of Pharmacy, University of Hertfordshire

Kieran Hand, PhD, MRPharmS
Consultant Pharmacist Anti-infectives, Southampton University Hospitals NHS Trust

Andrzej Kostrzewski, BSc, MSc, MMedEd, PhD, FHEA, MRPharmS
Senior Principal Academic/Pharmacist Manager in Clinical Development, Guy's Hospital, London and The School of Pharmacy, University of Hertfordshire

Niall McMullan, PhD
Senior Lecturer in Immunology, School of Life Sciences, University of Hertfordshire

Alka Mistry, BSc (Hons), DipClinPharm, MRPharmS
Principal Pharmacist Procurement, Directorate Pharmacist: Obs and Gynae, Lister and QEII Hospitals, East and North Herts NHS Trust

Gary Moss, BSc, MSc, PhD, PG Cert FHEA
Head of Pharmaceutics, School of Pharmacy, University of Hertfordshire

Sandeep Singh Nijjer, MPharm (Hons), MRPharmS
Clinical Lecturer, Department of Practice and Policy, The School of Pharmacy University of London

Nicola Parr, BPharm(Hons), MSc, MRPharmS
Senior Pharmacist, Addenbrooke's Hospital, Cambridge

Michael Powell, BPharm, MRPharmS, DipPharmPrac, AFCP
Senior Oncology Pharmacist, Pharmacy Department, Mount Vernon Hospital, Middlesex

Anita Rana, BSc (Hons), DipPharmPrac, MRPharmS
Pharmacy Team Manager, QEII Hospital, East and North Herts NHS Trust

Rebekah Raymond, BSc (Hons), DipPharmPrac, MRPharmS
Visting Fellow, School of Pharmacy, University of Hertfordshire

Rona Robinson, BPharm, MSc, MRPharmS
Teacher Practitioner, School of Pharmacy, University of Hertfordshire

Nader Siabi, BSc, MSc, MRPharmS
Independent Prescriber, School of Pharmacy, University of Hertfordshire

Fabrizio Schifano, MD, MRCPsych, Dip Clin Pharmacology
Chair in Clinical Pharmacology & Therapeutics, School of Pharmacy & Associate Dean, Postgraduate Medical School, University of Hertfordshire; Hon Consultant Psychiatrist

Mark Tomlin, BPharm, MSc, MRPharmS (IPresc)
Consultant Pharmacist, Critical Care, Southampton General Hospital

Steve Tomlin, BPharm, MRPharmS, ACPP
Consultant Pharmacist-Children's Services, Evelina Children's Hospital, Guy's & St Thomas' NHS Foundation Trust, London

Caron Weeks, BPharm (Hons), MRPharmS, DipPharmPrac
Lead pharmacist – Medicine, Southampton University Hospitals NHS Trust

1

Gastrointestinal case studies

Karen Baxter

Case study level 1 – Ulcerative colitis

Learning outcomes

Level 1 case study: You will be able to:

- describe the risk factors
- describe the disease
- describe the pharmacology of the drug
- outline the formulation, including drug molecule, excipients, etc. for the medicines
- summarise basic social pharmacy issues (e.g. opening containers, large labels).

Mrs Q is a 37-year-old woman who comes to your pharmacy with a prescription for Predsol enemas, one daily for four weeks. She tells you that she has recently been diagnosed with ulcerative colitis and that this is her first prescription for an enema. She says she would really rather have tablets but the doctor suggested that an enema would be more appropriate for her.

1a What is ulcerative colitis?
1b What is the aetiology (cause) of ulcerative colitis?
2a What sort of patient most commonly develops ulcerative colitis?
2b In what way does Mrs Q fit with this pattern?
3a What is the active ingredient of Predsol and what class of drugs does it come from?

3b   How do these drugs exert their action in conditions such as ulcerative colitis?
3c   What are the adverse effects of this type of drug?
3d   Why do you think Mrs Q has been prescribed an enema rather than tablets?
4a   What formulations of prednisolone are available which Mrs Q could self-administer?
4b   Describe the advantages and disadvantages of these formulations?
5a   What counselling points should you make to Mrs Q about how to use her enema?

General references

Joint Formulary Committee (2008) *British National Formulary 55*. London: British Medical Association and Royal Pharmaceutical Society of Great Britain, March.

Mpofu C and Ireland A (2006) Inflammatory bowel disease – the disease and its diagnosis. *Hospital Pharmacist* 13: 153–158.

Purvis J (1988) Enemas in ulcerative colitis. *Pharmaceutical Journal* 13 August: 208.

Predsol Retention Enema, Summary of Product Characteristics. Available at http://emc.medicines.org.uk/ [Accessed 7 July 2008].

Randall DM and Neil KE (2003) Inflammatory bowel disease. In: *Disease Management*. London: Pharmaceutical Press, pp. 135–138.

Case study level 2 – Constipation

Learning outcomes

Level 2 case study: You will be able to:

- interpret relevant lab and clinical data
- identify monitoring and referral criteria
- explain treatment choices
- describe goals of therapy, including monitoring and the role of the pharmacist/clinician
- describe issues – counselling points, adverse drug reactions, drug interactions, complementary/alternative therapies and lifestyle advice.

Scenario

Mr A is an 84-year-old man who is brought to your pharmacy by his wife to ask advice on his constipation. On discussion with him you establish that he has recently been experiencing back pain, which prevents him from getting about as much as he used to. The GP gave him some co-dydramol 10 days ago, and things are starting to improve. His wife says that she was given some little brown tablets when she was constipated, but they gave her stomach pains. She tried to get him to take them, but he won't. He thinks he should perhaps have something gentle, like a herbal medicine.

1a How is constipation defined?
1b Is it common?
2a Why do you think Mr A may have constipation?
2b What symptoms would prompt you to suggest that Mr A should go to his GP?
3a What sort of laxative do you think Mrs A has been taking? Explain your answer.
3b Is this sort of laxative suitable for Mr A? Explain your answer.
4a What lifestyle changes would you recommend Mr A should take? What counselling would you give him?
4b How would you assess the success of this action?
5   What would you suggest if your first recommendation fails?

General references

Anon (2004) The management of constipation. *MeReC Bulletin* 14: 21–24.
Greene RJ and Harris ND (2008) Constipation. In: *Pathology and Therapeutics for Pharmacists*. London: Pharmaceutical Press, pp. 125–129.
Joint Formulary Committee (2008) Laxatives. In: *British National Formulary* 55. London: British Medical Association and Royal Pharmaceutical Society of Great Britain, March, pp. 57–64.

Case study level 3 – Irritable bowel syndrome

Learning outcomes

Level 3 case study: You will be able to:

- interpret clinical signs and symptoms
- evaluate laboratory data
- evaluate treatment options
- state goals of therapy
- describe a pharmaceutical care plan to include advice to a clinician
- describe the prognosis and long-term complications
- describe the social pharmacy issues which could include supply (e.g. complex treatments at home, concordance and compliance) and lifestyle issues.

Scenario

Mrs P, a 32-year-old woman, comes to the dispensary asking to talk to a pharmacist. She has recently received a prescription for Colpermin from her GP. She says that they gave her terrible indigestion and so she has been taking Alu-Cap capsules, which have not worked terribly well. She has also decreased the number of Colpermin capsules she was taking. She wants to know if you can sell her anything stronger for the indigestion. She feels her problems are just getting worse and worse: first she had constipation, stomach cramps and bloating. Now she has indigestion as well, and her original symptoms are worse than ever. She didn't used to take any medicines and already she is on two, and she is seeing the hospital doctor in clinic this afternoon and fears she will be taking even more before long.

Questions

1   Mrs P has irritable bowel syndrome (IBS). What from her history is consistent with this?
2a   How would this diagnosis have been reached?
2b   What symptoms would require further investigation?
2c   What is her prognosis likely to be?
3   What lifestyle advice should she have been given?
4   Is there anything you should take into consideration when talking to Mrs P?
5   What advice can you give her about her current medication?
6   What particular difficulty is there with assessing the success of treatment in this type of patient?
7a   What other treatments are possible in patients with irritable bowel syndrome?
7b   Which would you recommend for Mrs P?
7c   What adverse effects are possible?

General references

Agrawal A and Whorwell PJ (2006) Irritable bowel syndrome: diagnosis and management. *British Medical Journal* 332: 280–283.

Anon (2000) Dietary advice tips: Irritable bowel syndrome. *Pharmaceutical Journal* 11 March: 397.

Colpermin, Summary of Product Characteristics. Available at http://emc.medicines.org. uk/ [Accessed 7 July 2008].

Joint Formulary Committee (2008) *British National Formulary 55*. London: British Medical Association and Royal Pharmaceutical Society of Great Britain, March.

Jones J, Boorman J, Cann P *et al.* (2000) British Society of Gastroenterology guidelines for the management of the irritable bowel syndrome. *Gut* 47(suppl 2): ii1–ii19.

Thomas L (2005) Current management options for irritable bowel syndrome. *Prescriber* 19 December: 13–20.

Case study level Ma – Duodenal ulcer

Learning outcomes

Level M case study: You will be able to:

- interpret clinical signs and symptoms
- evaluate laboratory data
- critically appraise treatment options
- state goals of therapy
- describe a pharmaceutical care plan to include advice to a clinician
- describe the prognosis and long-term complications
- describe the social pharmacy issues which could include supply (e.g. complex treatments at home, concordance and compliance) and lifestyle issues
- describe the monitoring of therapy.

Scenario

Mr B is a 57-year-old man who was admitted yesterday after starting to pass black stools. He has a two-day history of severe stomach pains and has suffered on and off with indigestion for some months. He is a life-long smoker, with mild chronic cardiac failure (CCF) for which he has been taking enalapril 5 mg twice daily for 2 years. He also recently started taking naproxen 500 mg twice daily for arthritis. Yesterday his haemoglobin was reported as 10.3 g/dL (range 12–18 g/dL), platelets 162×10^9/L (range $150–450 \times 10^9$/L), INR 1.1 (range 0.8–1.2) (ranges from Good Hope Hospital Biochemistry Department, available at http://www.goodhope.org.uk/departments/pathweb/refranges.htm) with U+Es and LFTs normal. He was mildly tachycardic (87 bpm) and had a slightly low blood pressure of 115/77 mmHg and was given 1.5 L of saline.

He has just returned from endoscopy this morning and has been newly diagnosed as having a bleeding duodenal ulcer. He has been written up for his usual medication for tomorrow if he is eating and drinking again.

Questions

1a What risk factors does Mr B have for a bleeding peptic ulcer?
1b Has his treatment so far been appropriate?
2   Should Mr B be given a proton pump inhibitor (PPI)? State your reasons. If yes, what would you recommend?
3   What is likely to be the next stage of treatment for Mr B?
4   What drugs should Mr B be discharged on?
5   What counselling would you give him?
6   What follow-up should Mr B have?

General references

Anon (2005) *H. pylori* eradication in NSAID-associated ulcers. *Drugs and Therapeutics Bulletin* 43: 37–40.
British Society of Gastroenterology Endoscopy Committee (2002) Non-variceal upper gastrointestinal haemorrhage: guidelines. *Gut* 51(Suppl IV): iv1–iv6. Available at http://www.bsg.org.uk/pdf_word_docs/nonvar3.pdf [Accessed 7 July 2008].
Enaganti S (2006) Peptic ulcer disease – the disease and non-drug treatment. *Hospital Pharmacist* 13: 239–244.
Greer D (2006) Peptic ulcer disease – pharmacological treatment. *Hospital Pharmacist* 13: 245–250.
National Institute for Health and Clinical Excellence (NICE) (2004) Dyspepsia: managing dyspepsia in adults in primary care. Available at http://www.nice.org.uk/page.aspx?o=CG017 [Accessed 7 July 2008].

Case study level Mb – Ulcerative colitis

Learning outcomes

Level M case study: You will be able to:

- interpret clinical signs and symptoms
- evaluate laboratory data
- critically appraise treatment options
- state goals of therapy
- describe a pharmaceutical care plan to include advice to a clinician
- describe the prognosis and long-term complications
- describe the social pharmacy issues which could include supply (e.g. complex treatments at home, concordance and compliance) and lifestyle issues
- describe the monitoring of therapy.

Mrs D has recently been admitted with an episode of acute severe ulcerative colitis. This is her third flare this year. This time she has a 5-day history of bloody diarrhoea with abdominal pain. On average she is opening her bowels seven times a day. She is currently taking mesalazine 800 mg three times daily and prednisolone 20 mg daily. Mrs D also has an elevated temperature of 38°C and a pulse rate of 92 bpm. She is due to have an abdominal X-ray and a stool culture.

Her biochemistry results are reported as:

Na^+	143 mmol/L	(range 133 to 145 mmol/L)
K^+	3.2 mmol/L	(range 3.3 to 5.1 mmol/L)
Creatinine	81 micromol/L	(range 44 to 80 micromol/L)
Urea	7.2 mmol/L	(range 1.7 to 8.3 mmol/L)
Albumin	28 g/L	(range 34 to 48 g/L)
Hb	10.4 g/dL	(range 11 to 16 g/L)
WCC	14×10^9/L	(range 3.5 to 11 x 10^9/L)
ESR	38 mm/h	(range 0 to 9 mm/h)
CRP	95 mg/L	(range less than 5 mg/L)

(Ranges from Good Hope Hospital Biochemistry Department, available at http://www.goodhope.org.uk/departments/pathweb/refranges.htm)

1a Why is she taking mesalazine?
1b What adverse effects should Mrs D be particularly aware of?
2a What signs and symptoms indicate that she needs to be admitted?
2b Why does she have a low potassium and a low albumin?
2c Why is she having an abdominal X-ray and stool cultures done?
3 How should this flare be managed?

Several days later you see Mrs D, who is distressed as she is not responding to treatment and she desperately wants to avoid surgery. The consultant has suggested that ciclosporin may be an option, and she asks to talk to you about it.

4 Why is surgery likely?
5a What is the evidence for the use of ciclosporin?
5b What should you discuss with her about the use of ciclosporin?
6 What dose of ciclosporin should she receive and how should it be given?

Mrs D is now very much recovered and is due to go home.

7a What drugs would you expect her to be discharged on?
7b What monitoring would you do?
7c What counselling should she be given?
7d What future treatment is she likely to receive?
8 Do antibacterials have a role in ulcerative colitis?

General references

Carter MJ, Lobo AJ, Travis SP *et al.* (2004) Guidelines for the management of inflamma-
    tory bowel disease in adults. *Gut* 53 (Suppl V): v1–v16. Available at: http://
    www.bsg.org.uk/pdf_word_docs/ibd.pdf [Accessed 7 July 2008].
Guslandi M (2005) Antibiotics for inflammatory bowel disease: do they work? *European
    Journal of Gastroenterology and Hepatology* 17: 145–147.
Mpofu C and Ireland A (2006) Inflammatory bowel disease – the disease and its diagno-
    sis. *Hospital Pharmacist* 13: 153–158.
Pham CQ, Efros Cb, Beradi RR (2006) Cyclosporine for severe ulcerative colitis. *Annals of
    Pharmacotherapy* 40: 96–101.
Sandimmun concentrate for infusion 50mg/ml, Summary of Product Characteristics.
    Available at http://emc.medicines.org.uk/ [Accessed 7 July 2008].
St Clair Jones A (2006) Inflammatory bowel disease – drug treatment and its implications.
    Hospital Pharmacist 13: 161–166.
Sweetman S (ed.) (2007) *Martindale: The Complete Drug Reference*, 35th edn. London:
    Pharmaceutical Press.

Answers

Case study level 1 – ulcerative colitis – see page 1

1a   What is ulcerative colitis?

Ulcerative colitis is an inflammatory disease of the lower gastrointestinal tract, which results in episodes of diarrhoea. There may also be extraintestinal symptoms, including anaemia, arthritis, dermatological problems and eye disorders.

1b   What is the aetiology (cause) of ulcerative colitis?

The exact causes are unclear, although there are several theories, which include genetic, environmental and microbial factors, possibly associated with an inappropriate immune response.

2a   What sort of patient most commonly develops ulcerative colitis?

Although anyone can develop ulcerative colitis it appears to be most common in developed countries, and the risk appears greater if a first-degree relative has the disease. Patients most commonly present at 20–40 years of age and some studies suggest that ulcerative colitis is slightly more common in women than men.

2b   In what way does Mrs Q fit with this pattern?

She is a woman of between 20 and 40 years of age.

3a What is the active ingredient of Predsol and what class of drugs does it come from?

Predsol contains prednisolone, a corticosteroid.

3b How do these drugs exert their action in conditions such as ulcerative colitis?

Corticosteroids have anti-inflammatory and immunosuppressive effects, which reduce the causes of the diarrhoea and thereby settle the disease.

3c What are the adverse effects of this type of drug?

The most significant adverse effect is adrenal suppression, which is most common with long-term, high-dose treatment (see *BNF* for definitions). Corticosteroids can also cause increased appetite, weight gain, insomnia, depression, osteoporosis, peptic ulceration and glucose intolerance, leading to diabetes. Immunosupression caused by this type of treatment can lead to an increased susceptibility to infection. Therefore patients taking corticosteroids (usually in high doses) should not be given live vaccines.

3d Why do you think Mrs Q has been prescribed an enema rather than tablets?

Although systemic absorption of the prednisolone from the enema probably does occur, especially when the colon is particularly inflamed, corticosteroids usually have less systemic effects when given this way. Furthermore, by giving an enema, the drug is being delivered directly to its site of action – remember that in ulcerative colitis the disease is confined to the lower gastrointestinal tract.

4a What formulations of prednisolone are available which Mrs Q could self-administer?

She could self-administer:

- tablets (either plain or enteric coated)
- suppositories
- foam enemas.

4b Describe the advantages and disadvantages of these formulations?

The tablets would be simple to use, but may have greater adverse effects. This is because they will enter the bloodstream in greater amounts by the oral route and have systemic effects. The higher the dose used the greater the potential for adverse effects. It is usually recommended that corticosteroids are used in the lowest possible dose for the shortest possible period of time.

The suppositories are also easier to use, but, because they only have a local action they are only suitable for localised disease (proctitis).

Foam enemas can be easier to retain than liquid enemas and do have a good spread into the colon, and so may be a possible alternative.

5a   What counselling points should you make to Mrs Q about how to use her enema?

- She should use the enema before bed to enhance retention.
- The enema should not be too cold as this can cause abdominal cramping. She could slightly warm the enema (e.g. in a cup of warm water) before administration.
- She should lie on her left side to facilitate the spread of the enema, with either her right leg, or both legs drawn up.
- The tip of the enema should be lubricated, with either K-Y jelly or petroleum jelly.
- She should gently insert the enema to about half the length of the tip using a gently twisting action. Deep breaths will help with this.
- She should gently and slowly (over 1–2 minutes) roll up the bag so as not to give the enema too quickly. This will aid retention.
- She should then roll on to her front and remain there for 3–5 minutes.

Case study level 2 – Constipation – see page 2

1a   How is constipation defined?

Constipation cannot solely be defined by bowel frequency, as this naturally varies in the population. Simply, constipation is defined as a decrease in the patient's normal pattern of defecation, although for research purposes other criteria are often considered (e.g. straining, hard stools).

1b   Is it common?

The incidence of constipation is hard to define, with rates in women stated to be 8.2% in one study and 52% in another. Constipation tends to be more common in women, and in the elderly.

2a   Why do you think Mr A may have constipation?

- Mr A is elderly. Although his age in itself does not cause constipation, factors such as decreased mobility and decreased dietary intake increase the prevalence of constipation in this group.
- Mr A has recently had back pain, which may have further decreased his mobility.
- Mr A has been taking dihydrocodeine (as part of co-dydramol), one of the adverse effects of which is constipation.

2b   What symptoms would prompt you to suggest that Mr A should go to his GP?

Blood in the stools, severe abdominal pain, unintentional weight loss, co-existing diarrhoea, persistent symptoms, tenesemus or failure of previous medication. These symptoms can point to more severe disorders such as impaction, or malignancy.

3a   What sort of laxative do you think Mrs A has been taking? Explain your answer.

From the description of the adverse effects, a stimulating laxative seems most likely, as they commonly cause abdominal cramps. Senna is a stimulant laxative and is available as brown tablets, and so this seems the most likely laxative.

3b   Is this sort of laxative suitable for Mr A? Explain your answer.

Yes. Although stimulant laxatives are often considered to be second line, it has been said that laxative choice is best based on symptoms, patients' preference, adverse effects and cost. In the case of Mr A the stimulant laxatives have the advantage of being fairly quick acting, and are often useful to counteract the effects of decreased bowel motility caused by opioid analgesics. They are also useful for occasional use.

Other types of laxative include the following:

- Bulk-forming laxatives (such as ispaghula husk), which work by increasing faecal mass, but they may take several days to become fully effective. They are of most use in those patients that pass small stools and have a diet lacking in fibre (but they should not replace dietary lifestyle measures)
- Faecal softeners (such as docusate, which is stimulating but which also has softening properties). These can be useful where passing stools may be uncomfortable e.g. with haemorrhoids
- Osmotic laxatives (such as lactulose) work by drawing fluid into the bowel and retaining the existing fluid. They may take several days to become fully effective and it is essential that fluid intake is maintained during their use.

4a   What lifestyle changes would you recommend Mr A should take? What counselling would you give him?

- Ensure that Mr A has none of the adverse effects that would lead to him being referred to his GP.
- Lifestyle measures may include increased dietary fibre, ensuring an adequate fluid intake, keeping as mobile as possible, etc.
- A laxative would seem appropriate at this stage as Mr A is elderly and it is likely that his constipation is drug-induced.
- Discuss the adverse effects his wife has experienced and explain that senna is in fact a herbal medicine and that herbal remedies may not necessarily be gentle.
- Discuss the benefits of senna (as above). He could try starting with one tablet to minimise the adverse effects. If he accepts this suggestion counsel him to take the tablets before bed (as they take 8–10 hours to work). If he is reluctant to try senna explain to him that lactulose is often insufficient alone in treating opioid-induced constipation, and may take 48 hours to work.

Bulk laxatives are really a more long-term solution. Bisacodyl may be an alternative stimulant laxative, but is likely to have similar adverse effects.

■   Also discuss his co-dydramol use – it may be short term, and encourage him to discuss the constipation with his GP (as an alternative analgesic may be appropriate).

4b   How would you assess the success of this action?

Ask Mr A to come back if he feels the laxative he has chosen has not worked. Ensure that the laxative has been taken in an adequate dose for a sufficient amount of time.

5   What would you suggest if your first recommendation fails?

Ensure that Mr A has been taking a reasonable dose for a reasonable period of time (several days would be needed to assess the efficacy of lactulose). Assuming Mr A has been taking the medication as recommended it would be prudent to refer him to his GP at this stage.

Case study level 3 – Irritable bowel syndrome – see page 3

1   Mrs P has irritable bowel syndrome. What from her history is consistent with this?

Patients with IBS commonly present with abdominal pain and altered bowel habits: constipation or diarrhoea. Bloating is common, and women are more affected than men. Presentation is often before the age of 45 years. Mrs P is a young female, with the typical symptoms of someone with constipation-predominant IBS. She is also taking peppermint oil, which is often prescribed in an attempt to relieve cramping.

2a   How would this diagnosis have been reached?

Mrs P is young, with a fairly typical presentation, and so a standard examination, associated with clinical suspicion is adequate for a diagnosis.

2b   What symptoms would require further investigation?

If Mrs P was over 45 years old and had a rapid onset of symptoms then she would be referred for further investigation. Symptoms likely to require further investigations include rectal bleeding, anaemia, weight loss, a family history of cancer or imflammatory bowel disease, or signs of an infection.

2c   What is her prognosis likely to be?

The prognosis can be very variable. IBS does not tend to develop into anything more sinister. However studies suggest that large numbers of patients will still have abdominal symptoms 5 years after diagnosis. Psychological symptoms, a long history of illness and previous abdominal surgery are all associated with a worse prognosis. If the IBS is linked to a stressful event, e.g. ongoing work-related stress, which is unremitting, the patient is highly likely to be resistant to treatment.

3   What lifestyle advice should she have been given?

A common first step in managing patients with IBS is to discuss lifestyle factors. Dietary changes and dietary fibre are likely to have been discussed, especially in patients presenting with constipation and bloating. Exclusion diets may have been tried, but these need to be under the guidance of a dietician.

4   Is there anything you should take into consideration when talking to Mrs P?

Patients with this disease often fear being labelled as psychologically disturbed. They often fear that their symptoms are symptomatic of a much more serious condition. It is important that the patient is listened to and given plenty of reassurance.

5   What advice can you give her about her current medication?

Peppermint oil commonly causes indigestion. It is likely that the aluminium hydroxide antacid taken by the patient is exacerbating the condition by breaking down the enteric coating of the capsules. It is recommended that patients suffering indigestion with peppermint oil stop taking the medication, and in Mrs P's case, as the capsules do not appear to be working very well, this seems a reasonable course of action. She would be best advised to discuss this at the clinic this afternoon, so that they are aware that the treatment was not successful. If she stops the peppermint oil she should not need to continue with the antacid, or any other indigestion remedy, which should reduce the amount of medication she needs to take.

6   What particular difficulty is there with assessing the success of treatment in this type of patient?

The placebo response to treatment is often very high – up to 47%, and so many treatments appear successful in the short term.

7a   What other treatments are possible in patients with irritable bowel syndrome?

Medical treatments of IBS are limited. Laxatives (particularly dietary fibre and bulking laxatives such as ispaghula) and antidiarrhoeals (loperamide and sometimes codeine) are prescribed to manage the symptoms of altered bowel habit. Colestyramine is of use in those with diarrhoea caused by bile salt malabsorption. Antispasmodics, particularly those with antimuscarinic actions (dicycloverine and hyoscine butylbromide) are useful in managing cramping. Low-dose tricyclic antidepressants have been shown to be of benefit, although use may be limited in some patients as they can cause constipation. They are of particular use when depression is a factor. Mebeverine, alverine and peppermint oil are also used.

Psychological treatments, such as relaxation and hypnotherapy are also of use, but due to limited NHS resources are saved for particularly resistant cases.

7b   Which would you recommend for Mrs P?

As Mrs P has been referred to a hospital clinic, it is likely that dietary measures have been tried. Therefore a bulking laxative such as ispaghula may be of benefit. As she suffers from cramping an antimuscarinic antispasmodic such as dicycloverine may be of benefit, although some caution is needed, as it may exacerbate her constipation.

7c   What adverse effects are possible?

Although dicycloverine has less marked antimuscarinic effects than other similar antispasmodics it still may lead to adverse effects such as dry mouth, dizziness, blurred vision and constipation. Fatigue, anorexia, nausea and vomiting, headache and dysuria (difficulty in urinating) are also possible.

Case study level Ma – Duodenal ulcer – see page 5

1a   What risk factors does Mr B have for a bleeding peptic ulcer?

The prevalence of peptic ulcers increases with age, as *Helicobacter pylori* infection rates increase with increasing age – Mr B is 57 years of age. Peptic ulcers are more common in smokers. Mr B is also taking an NSAID (non-steroidal anti-inflammatory drug), which is associated with ulceration.

1b   Has his treatment so far been appropriate?

The management of a bleeding ulcer is dictated by the severity of the bleed. Mr B is not particularly old, he is not shocked (pulse rate less than 100 bpm, systolic blood pressure over 100 mmHg), and active bleeding has not been reported. He had the appropriate fluid replacement (saline, a crystalloid). Blood was not needed as he did not have particular signs of hypovolaemic shock and his haemoglobin is above 10 g/dL. He had no risk factors to suggest that antibacterial prophylaxis was necessary before endoscopy. His enalapril and furosemide were temporarily stopped, and if his blood pressure, hydration state and renal function are normal it is reasonable to restart them tomorrow as planned. If not, his CCF should be reviewed. However, the naproxen should not be restarted.

2   Should Mr B be given a proton pump inhibitor (PPI)? State your reasons. If yes, what would you recommend?

The use of a PPI in this situation is not fully established. A Cochrane Review has suggested that the use of a PPI does not affect mortality in patients with a bleeding peptic ulcer. Mr B has clearly had a recent bleed, and in this situation the British Society of Gastroenterology guidelines suggest that he should be given an infusion of omeprazole, which may help prevent re-bleeding by stabilising the clotting process. However, this may also be achieved by giving oral omeprazole. Therefore it would have been advisable to start omeprazole 40 mg twice daily, by the oral route. High-dose omeprazole is usually given for 72 hours.

3   What is likely to be the next stage of treatment for Mr B?

Mr B needs a full-dose PPI (see below) for 4–8 weeks to heal his ulcer. Following this he should be tested for *H. pylori*, and if this test is positive he should have eradication treatment. Note that in patients already taking a PPI a two-week washout period is needed before a breath test or a stool antigen test is used.

4   What drugs should Mr B be discharged on?

He should be discharged with:

- enalapril 5 mg twice daily
- furosemide 40 mg daily
- omeprazole 20 mg twice daily (or other full-dose PPI).

If possible, his NSAID should be permanently stopped and therefore consideration will need to be given to managing his pain relief. A first option would be to try paracetamol with an opioid such as codeine. However, as he has rheumatoid arthritis it is unlikely that this will be adequate to control his symptoms. A selective COX-2 inhibitor (e.g. celecoxib) is unlikely to be suitable for Mr B as he has CCF. Therefore, after trying paracetamol/opioids it is likely that Mr B will need an NSAID. NSAIDs can be given during ulcer-healing, but they are best avoided if possible. If an NSAID proves to be necessary, the lowest dose of the safest NSAID (i.e. ibuprofen) should be given. When his treatment for ulcer healing is completed he should take a PPI (e.g. omeprazole 20 mg daily) for gastroprotection.

5   What counselling would you give him?

- Simple lifestyle advice – avoiding fatty foods, reducing weight where possible and giving up smoking.

- Discuss the use of NSAIDs. Ibuprofen is available without a prescription, and you should discuss the risks of using an NSAID without gastroprotection and the possibility of the inadvertent use of two NSAIDs if he is prescribed another NSAID in the future.
- Discuss his analgesia (as above).

6   What follow-up should Mr B have?

If Mr B is symptomatic following *H. pylori* eradication he should be re-tested for *H. pylori*, and if this test is positive he should be given a further course of eradication treatment, using a different antibacterial combination to the one given previously (regimens detailed in the *BNF*). He should also be reviewed annually and given advice on lifestyle and the management of any dyspeptic symptoms.

Case study level Mb – Ulcerative colitis – see page 6

1a   Why is she taking mesalazine?

Mesalazine is useful in maintaining remission in patients with ulcerative colitis.

1b   What adverse effects should Mrs D be particularly aware of?

Although significant adverse effects (such as Stevens Johnson syndrome, pancreatitis and agranulocytosis) are rare, all patients should be advised to report any unexplained symptoms such as bleeding, bruising, purpura (small areas of haemorrhage), sore throat, fever or malaise. These may be indicative of agranulocytosis and warrant urgent investigation.

2a   What signs and symptoms indicate that she needs to be admitted?

Her symptoms (more than six motions a day) suggest severe disease. The fact that she has an increased pulse rate and has a raised temperature suggest systemic disease, which requires urgent attention. The raised ESR and CRP are also markers of severe inflammation.

2b   Why does she have a low potassium and a low albumin?

Her low potassium is probably a result of the diarrhoea, although note that corticosteroids can also cause hypokalaemia. Her low albumin suggests that she has had longer term malabsorption; it is likely to take several weeks or longer to correct.

2c   Why is she having an abdominal X-ray and stool cultures done?

Stool cultures are to rule out an infective cause of the disease. The abdominal

X-ray is to exclude toxic dilation of the colon or bowel perforation, which would require urgent surgical attention.

3   How should this flare be managed?

- It is unlikely that she will be able to absorb any drugs by the oral route, so treatment will need to be given parenterally.
- Mesalazine has only been shown to be of benefit in mild to moderate flares of ulcerative colitis and so it can be stopped. It is unlikely to be absorbed.
- Her prednisolone should be replaced with full dose corticosteroid – most commonly intravenous hydrocortisone 100 mg four times daily to control the inflammation. Predsol enemas are often also given.
- She will also need deep vein thrombosis prophylaxis as she is at an increased risk of a thromboembolic event, and intravenous fluids, with potassium, to replace what she is losing with the diarrhoea.

4   Why is surgery likely?

Surgery is undertaken in patients not responding to medical treatments (or for the reasons mentioned previously). Surgery may also be used when patients have poorly controlled frequently relapsing disease. In ulcerative colitis surgery (a colectomy) offers the hope of a cure, by removing the diseased portion of the gastrointestinal tract. This contrasts with Crohn's disease, where surgery is undertaken for symptomatic relief. However, as Crohn's disease can affect the whole of the gastrointestinal tract it is not curative, and the disease often recurs in a different area following surgery.

5a   What is the evidence for the use of ciclosporin?

Several studies have been conducted, including some small randomised studies, to assess the use of ciclosporin in Crohn's disease. The evidence suggests that intravenous ciclosporin can induce disease remission in severe flares of ulcerative colitis that are unresponsive to corticosteroids. Oral ciclosporin has only been shown to be useful as a bridging treatment between intravenous ciclosporin and more long-term maintenance strategies.

5b   What should you discuss with her about the use of ciclosporin?

- Reason for using ciclosporin: Ciclosporin is used to suppress the immune system and therefore the disease activity, and has a rapid onset of action. Discuss its other uses and explain that this is an unlicensed but not uncommon treatment for patients in her situation (relapsing unresponsive disease). Although it may avoid the need for surgery in some patients it doesn't always work and surgery may still be needed.
- How the ciclosporin will be given: Initially the ciclosporin will be given through a drip. If it is successful in controlling the disease she will be given oral treatment, which you can come back to discuss.

- Possible adverse effects: Ciclosporin has many adverse effects. It would be prudent to discuss the most significant effects and offer to return when she has had the opportunity to read through a patient information leaflet.
- Discuss altered electrolyte levels (e.g. potassium, which is important for the heart). This will be monitored with blood tests.
- Increases in blood pressure are quite common, and these may be treated with blood pressure tablets, or by stopping the medicine.
- Other common adverse effects include tingling, most often in the hands and feet, cramps and muscle pains. Women may find that their periods alter.
- Kidney problems are a severe adverse effect. Problems tend to be more common with high doses, and blood levels of the drug will be monitored to ensure that they are within an acceptable range. Blood tests will also monitor kidney function.

6   What dose of ciclosporin should she receive and how should it be given?

The usual dose is 2–4 mg/kg/day (British Society of Gastroenterology guidelines recommend the lower dose). It is given as an infusion over 2–6 hours diluted in glucose 5% or sodium chloride 0.9%. Note that ciclosporin diluted in sodium chloride 0.9% is only stable for 8 hours. Some PVC giving sets are incompatible with ciclosporin and so a special giving set may need to be used with the infusion.

7a   What drugs would you expect her to be discharged on?

- Ciclosporin 6–8 mg/kg per day (target blood level 100–200 ng/mL).
- Prednisolone 40–60 mg daily, with a reducing course over several weeks (regimens vary, but reductions should not be more than 10 mg and will need to be smaller and slower towards the tail end of treatment. As Mrs D was previously taking prednisolone 10 mg daily, dosage reductions from this point down will need to be very gradual. Many patients end up taking long-term steroids.
- Co-trimoxazole 960 mg three times weekly as pneumocystis pneumonia prophylaxis. Local policy and dosing regimens vary and not all patients will necessarily receive this drug or dose.
- Mesalazine 800 mg three times daily.

7b   What monitoring would you do?

- Ciclosporin levels – although a therapeutic range has not been defined it is usual to aim for levels of between 100 and 200 ng/mL.
- U+Es – ciclosporin can cause hyperkalaemia and renal impairment.
- Full blood count.
- Blood pressure.

The British Society of Gastroenterology recommends that measurements are taken at baseline, after one and two weeks, and then monthly.

7c   What counselling should she be given?

Mrs D should be given the following advice:

- As ciclosporin is a powerful immunosuppressant you will be more susceptible to infection. You will be given an antibiotic three times a week to prevent some serious infections.
- If you are to have vaccines it is important you say that you are on ciclosporin as some should not be given to patients taking ciclosporin as they can result in infections.
- There is very little experience of using ciclosporin in pregnancy. Discuss any plans for pregnancy with your doctor.
- Let doctors, dentists, nurses and pharmacists know that you are taking this medicine. It may affect their choice of treatment. Note that ibuprofen is a general sale list medicine and so can be freely purchased. This can interact with ciclosporin and so should generally be avoided without further medical advice.
- Monitoring: Regular blood tests will be needed to guard against adverse effects. It is important to keep to the recommended schedule. Ciclosporin levels need to be taken before your first dose of the day (trough level). Therefore on some days (usually once a month) you will be asked not to take your ciclosporin until the blood has been taken. Once the blood has been taken the dose is taken as normal.

7d   What future treatment is she likely to receive?

Ciclosporin will be tailed off as azathioprine (1.5–2.5 mg/kg per day) is slowly started. The ciclosporin will be continued for 3–6 months to allow the azathioprine time to start working – a full effect may take three months. Co-trimoxazole will probably be stopped when ciclosporin is stopped. She is likely to continue aminosalicylates, and patients often remain on corticosteroids.

8   Do antibacterials have a role in ulcerative colitis?

Potentially, although controlled evidence for their use is sparse and more study is needed. Patients with pouchitis (which may occur following some surgical procedures for ulcerative colitis) may have significant clinical improvement following the use of metronidazole. Ciprofloxacin is also useful for pouchitis, and concurrent use with metronidazole appears to be superior to either antibacterial alone. Ciprofloxacin alone may also be of potential use for disease control in ulcerative colitis, but data in the absence of other standard treatments are lacking. Antibacterials tend to be of more use in Crohn's disease.

2

Cardiovascular case studies

Narinder Bhalla

Case study level 1 – Angina

Learning outcomes

Level 1 case study: You will be able to:

- describe the risk factors
- describe the disease
- describe the pharmacology of the drug
- outline the formulations available, including drug molecule, excipients, etc. for the medicines
- summarise basic social pharmacy issues (e.g. opening containers, large labels).

Scenario

Mr AG, a 57-year-old taxi driver of Indian origin, attends your community pharmacy with a new prescription for: glyceryl trinitrate (GTN) spray 400 micrograms – one or two puffs as required. You dispense this item and speak with him and he tells you that his GP thinks he has angina and has asked him to use the spray the next time he gets any minor chest pain or tightness. You counsel Mr AG on the correct use of the spray.

Mr AG returns a few days later complaining of a headache following the use of the spray. He is reluctant to use the spray again. He asks your advice on managing his headache. He also smokes about five cigarettes a week and asks if he should now stop.

1a   What is angina?
1b   What typical symptoms could a patient with angina present with?
2a   What are the risk factors for developing angina?
2b   What, if any, risk factors does Mr AG have for developing stable angina?
3a   What group of drugs does GTN spray belong to?
3b   What are the side-effects of GTN spray?
3c   How would you counsel Mr AG on the use of his spray?
3d   What other formulations of GTN are available? List their advantages and disadvantages.
4   Mr AG's headache may be caused by his use of GTN spray. What can you recommend to him to help manage his headache?
5   What advice would you give Mr AG in relation to his smoking?

General references

Clinical Knowledge Summaries (2003) Angina. Available: http://www.prodigy.nhs.uk/angina [Accessed 23/10/06].
Joint Formulary Committee (2008) *British National Formulary* 55. London: British Medical Association and Royal Pharmaceutical Society of Great Britain, March.
Nitrolingual Pump Spray, Summary of Product Characteristics. Available at http://emc.medicines.org.uk/ [Accessed 3 July 2008].

Case study level 2 – Hypertension

Learning outcomes

Level 2 case study: You will be able to:

- interpret relevant lab and clinical data
- identify monitoring and referral criteria
- explain treatment choices
- describe goals of therapy, including monitoring and the role of the pharmacist/clinician
- describe issues – counselling points, adverse drug reactions, drug interactions, complementary/alternative therapies and lifestyle advice.

You are a hospital pharmacist visiting your regular general medical ward to review patients and provide pharmaceutical advice. Mr HA is a 50-year-old accountant who was admitted 2 days ago to hospital following a blackout whilst watching a football match with his son. His preliminary examination reveals bruising to his left arm and upper thigh for which he has been prescribed paracetamol 1 g four times daily and as required ibuprofen 400 mg three times a day.

His past medical history indicates that that he is on no medication and seemed to be a reasonably fit man for his age with no existing diagnosed medical conditions. On examination he is slightly overweight at 81 kg, he smokes 20 cigarettes per day and drinks approximately 30 units of alcohol per week. His blood pressure on admission was 165/80 mmHg with a heart rate of 90 beats per minute. This degree of raised blood pressure and heart rate has been maintained over the last 48 hours. He is subsequently diagnosed as having hypertension.

Questions

1   What is hypertension?
2   What are the appropriate treatment targets for this patient's blood pressure?
3   Besides blood pressure, what other advice and treatment does this patient require to ensure his risk of a cardiovascular event is reduced? Give clear reasons for your advice and explain the risks associated with not taking this advice.
4   What are the main classes of drug used to treat hypertension?
5   Which class of drug would be appropriate first-line treatment for Mr HA? How would this treatment choice be affected if the patient had been of Afro-Caribbean origin?
6   For one of the classes of drugs mentioned in question 4 indicate the following:

   ■   a drug from that class
   ■   a suitable starting dose and frequency
   ■   the maximum dose for hypertension
   ■   three contraindications
   ■   three common side-effects.

7   In view of Mr HA's age he requires cardiovascular risk assessment. How would you assess this patient's cardiovascular risks?

References

British Cardiac Society, British Hypertension Society, Diabetes UK, HEART UK, Primary Care Cardiovascular Society and The Stroke Association (2005) JBS 2: Joint British Societies' guidelines on prevention of cardiovascular disease in clinical practice. *Heart* 91: v1–v52.
Clinical Knowledge Summaries (2007) Hypertension. Available at http://www.prodigy. nhs.uk/hypertension [Accessed 3 July 2008].
National Audit Office (NAO) (2001) *Tackling Obesity in England*. London: HMSO.

Available from http://www.nao.org.uk/publications/nao_reports/00-01/0001220. pdf [Accessed 3 July 2008].

NICE (National Institute for Health and Clinical Excellence) (2006). Hypertension – management of hypertension in adults in primary care. Available at http://www.nice. org.uk/download.aspx?o=cg034NICEguideline [Accessed 3 July 2008].

North of England Hypertension Guideline Development Group (2006) Essential hypertension: managing adult patients in primary care. Centre for Health Services Research, University of Newcastle upon Tyne. Available at http://www.nice.org.uk/ nicemedia/pdf/CG18background. pdf [Accessed 3 July 2008].

General references

Joint Formulary Committee (2008) *British National Formulary* 55. London: British Medical Association and Royal Pharmaceutical Society of Great Britain, March.

National Prescribing Centre (NPC) (2002) MeReC Briefing – Lifestyle measures to reduce cardiovascular risk. Available at http://www.npc.co.uk/MeReC_Briefings/2002/ briefing_no_19.pdf [Accessed 3 July 2008].

Case study level 3 – Atrial fibrillation

Learning outcomes

Level 3 case study: You will be able to:

- interpret clinical signs and symptoms
- evaluate laboratory data
- evaluate treatment options
- state goals of therapy
- describe a pharmaceutical care plan to include advice to a clinician
- describe the prognosis and long-term complications
- describe the social pharmacy issues which could include supply (e.g. complex treatments at home, concordance and compliance) and lifestyle issues.

Scenario

Mr John Jones (61 years) is admitted to the emergency assessment unit at his local hospital complaining of palpitations, breathlessness and dizziness. He has a 5-day history of some dizziness and palpitations. In the last 24 hours he complained additionally of shortness of breath. He collapsed at home and was then admitted to hospital via the emergency department.

He experienced similar symptoms two months ago but did not seek medical advice at that time and seemed to recover quickly. On examination and review by the admitting doctor the following information is obtained:

Previous medical history

Hypertension (diagnosed 5 years ago), no previous history of cardiovascular disease. The patient is a regular cigarette smoker (>20 per day) and drinks approximately 20 units of alcohol per week.

Drug history

No known allergies. Mr Jones had been prescribed lisinopril tablets 20 mg once daily but was poorly compliant with treatment.

Signs and symptoms on examination

- Blood pressure 100/70 mmHg
- Heart rate 175 bpm, irregular
- Respiratory rate 25 breaths per minute
- No basal crackles in the lungs.

Diagnosis

Atrial fibrillation.

Relevant test results

Full blood counts, liver function tests, electrolytes and renal function were all normal at admission and throughout the admission to discharge.

Mr Jones is subsequently transferred to the cardiology ward where his continuing atrial fibrillation is later confirmed as persistent atrial fibrillation. As the ward clinical pharmacist, you are responsible for daily review of drug charts and advice to medical and nursing staff on all aspects of drug treatment for patients on the ward.

Questions

1   What is atrial fibrillation?
2   What are the most common signs and symptoms exhibited by patients with atrial fibrillation? Indicate which of these signs and symptoms the patient is exhibiting.

3   What are the two options in terms of treatment strategy that may be employed to manage atrial fibrillation? Indicate what would be the most appropriate strategy that you could recommend to the doctor managing this patient and why you think this is the case.

4   Assuming a rate control strategy is to be used what class of drug should be the first-line treatment for this patient? If the first-line drug was contraindicated what class of drug could be used as alternative treatment?

5   What patient parameters should be monitored to assess therapy with the usual first-line treatment and what is an appropriate treatment target for such parameters?

6   What are the two options in terms of antithrombotic prophylaxis in this patient and what are the potential side-effects of each? State which of these is the most appropriate for this patient and why.

7   Assuming the patient is to be discharged on a beta-blocker and aspirin, what counselling does he require?

General references

Clinical Knowledge Summaries (2007) Atrial fibrillation. Available at http://www.prodigy. nhs.uk/atrial_fibrillation [Accessed 3 July 2008].

Joint Formulary Committee (2008) *British National Formulary* 55. London: British Medical Association and Royal Pharmaceutical Society of Great Britain, March.

Kumar P and Clark M (Eds) (2004) *Kumar and Clark's Clinical Medicine*, 5th edn. London: Saunders Ltd.

NICE (National Institute for Health and Clinical Excellence) (2006) Atrial fibrillation. Available at http://www.nice.org.uk/page.aspx?o=cg036quickrefguide [Accessed 3 July 2008].

Case study level Ma – Heart failure

Learning outcomes

Level M case study: You will be able to:

- interpret clinical signs and symptoms
- evaluate laboratory data
- critically appraise treatment options
- state goals of therapy
- describe a pharmaceutical care plan to include advice to a clinician
- describe the prognosis and long-term complications
- describe the social pharmacy issues which could include supply (e.g. complex treatments at home, concordance and compliance) and lifestyle issues.

Scenario

Mr AB is a 67-year-old man who was admitted to the emergency department complaining of increasing shortness of breath. He has woken on each of the last two nights, struggling for breath. On arrival at hospital and on subsequent examination and review by the admitting doctor the following information is obtained:

History of presenting complaint

Shortness of breath and tiredness increasing over the last two months. Is able to walk approximately 20 metres.

Past medical history

- Ischaemic heart disease over 10 years
- Myocardial infarction 1 year ago
- Hypertension (10 years).

Social history

The patient is a regular cigarette smoker (>30 per day) and drinks approximately 35 units of alcohol per week.

Family history

No family history of cardiovascular disease.

Drug history on admission

No known allergies. Prescribed drugs are listed in Table Q2.1.

Signs and symptoms on examination

Patient was pale on examination.

- Temperature 36.8°C
- Blood pressure 105/60 mmHg
- Heart rate 90 bpm, irregular
- Swelling of ankles (SOA) – pitting to the knees
- JVP +4 cm
- Weight 97 kg (usually 85 kg)
- CXR – cardiomegaly
- Basal crackles in both lungs
- ECG – normal.

Table Q2.1 Drugs prescribed for Mr AB

Drug name	Form	Strength	Dose	Frequency	Comments
Bisoprolol	Tablets	5 mg	One	Daily	Takes regularly
Aspirin	Dispersible tablets	75 mg	One	Daily	Takes regularly
Isosorbide mononitrate	MR tablets	60 mg	One	Daily	Takes regularly
Glyceryl trinitrate	Spray	400 micrograms	One or two puffs pain	As required for chest	

Biochemistry results at admission

Na$^+$	132 mmol/L (135–145 mmol/L)
K$^+$	4.3 mmol/L (3.5–5.0 mmol/L)
Urea	17 mmol/L (0–7.5 mmol/L)
Creatinine	169 micromol/L (35–125 micromol/L)
Total cholesterol	3.9 mmol/L (<4 mmol/L)
Blood glucose	4.4 mmol/L (4–10 mmol/L)
Bilirubin	12 micromol/L (0–17 micromol/L)
ALT	30 units/L (0–50 units/L)
Alk phos	65 units/L (30–135 units/L)

Thyroid function tests were also taken and have all returned as being within a normal range. A full blood count found all parameters were normal and within range.

Diagnosis

A preliminary diagnosis of acute heart failure is made.

Questions

1 What signs and symptoms experienced by this patient indicate that he has heart failure? Does he have right- or left-sided heart failure or both? Explain your answer.
2 What system is used to classify heart failure according to severity of symptoms?
3a What drug treatment should be initiated for the immediate management of the oedema associated with the acute heart failure?
3b What parameters should be monitored to ensure the effectiveness of the drug treatment for oedema and to minimise toxicity?
4 What are the overall aims of drug treatment in acute heart failure?

5a   The patient's symptoms stabilise over the initial 24 hours. What other class of drug treatment should now be initiated at this stage for management of chronic heart failure? Indicate a drug, starting dose and any parameters that need monitoring.

5b   What side-effect can occur when first initiating the treatment above and how can this side-effect be minimised?

6   What is the role of beta-blockers in heart failure? Summarise the clinical trial evidence to date.

7   What advice should be given to the patient at discharge with regard to lifestyle issues?

General references

Joint Formulary Committee (2008) *British National Formulary* 55. London: British Medical Association and Royal Pharmaceutical Society of Great Britain, March.

MTRAC (2004a) Summary sheet for Bisoprolol (Cardicor) – for the treatment of chronic heart failure. Available at http://www.keele.ac.uk/depts/mm/MTRAC/ProductInfo/summaries/B/BISOPROLOL%202.pdf [Updated March 2004; accessed 28 October 2006].

MTRAC (2004b) Summary sheet for Carvedilol (Eucardic) – for the treatment of chronic heart failure. Available at http://www.keele.ac.uk/depts/mm/MTRAC/ProductInfo/summaries/C/CARVEDILOL2.pdf [Updated March 2004; accessed 28 October 2006].

National Prescribing Centre. Lifestyle measures to reduce cardiovascular risk. MeReC Briefing No. 19, September 2002. Available at http://www.npc.co.uk/MeReC_Briefings/2002/briefing_no_19.pdf [Accessed 3 July 2008].

NICE (National Institute for Health and Clinical Excellence) (2003) Chronic heart failure: management of chronic heart failure in adults in primary and secondary care. Available at http://www.nice.org.uk/nicemedia/pdf/CG5NICEguideline.pdf [Accessed 3 July 2008].

Case study level Mb – Myocardial infarction

Learning outcomes

Level M case study: You will be able to:

- interpret clinical signs and symptoms
- evaluate laboratory data
- critically appraise treatment options
- state goals of therapy
- describe a pharmaceutical care plan to include advice to a clinician
- describe the prognosis and long-term complications
- describe the social pharmacy issues which could include supply (e.g. complex treatments at home, concordance and compliance) and lifestyle issues
- describe the monitoring of therapy.

Scenario

Mr FG is a 69-year-old retired school teacher who was admitted to the emergency department complaining of severe chest pain after climbing stairs at his daughter's house. In the ambulance he is administered aspirin 300 mg. On arrival at hospital and subsequent examination and review by the admitting doctor the following information is obtained.

Previous medical history

Hypertension (10 years). Type 2 diabetes mellitus (recently diagnosed, currently diet controlled). The patient is a regular cigarette smoker (>40 per day) and drinks approximately 10 units of alcohol per week. He has osteoarthritis of the knee.

Family history

Father died following a myocardial infarction at 60 years of age. No maternal history of cardiovascular disease.

Drug history

Allergies: Trimethoprim. Mr FG has been taking diclofenac MR tablets 75 mg (twice daily) and nifedipine (Adalat Retard) MR tablets 20 mg (twice daily). Both were stopped on admission.

Signs and symptoms on examination

- Temperature 36.4°C
- Blood pressure 160/80 mmHg
- Heart rate 75 bpm, regular
- Respiratory rate 15 breaths per minute
- No basal crackles in the lungs.

An ECG taken immediately on arrival reveals ST elevation of 3 mm in the inferior leads.

Diagnosis

A preliminary diagnosis of myocardial infarction is made.

Relevant test results

Full blood counts, liver function tests, electrolytes and renal function, CXR, total cholesterol, full blood count and blood glucose were taken at admission.

Questions

1   What further diagnostic and biochemical tests should be ordered to help confirm the diagnosis?
2   What is myocardial infarction and what are the classic symptoms?

Initial treatment

About 45 minutes after the onset of chest pain the patient received the following treatment in the emergency department:

- heparin 5000 units stat
- reteplase 10 units i.v. bolus followed by a further 10 unit i.v. bolus after 30 minutes
- diamorphine 2.5 mg IV stat
- metoclopramide 10 mg stat.

A sliding scale insulin infusion of Actrapid 50 units made up to 50 mL with sodium chloride 0.9% was initiated and titrated against blood glucose.

3   Explain the mechanism of action of thrombolytics such as reteplase in acute myocardial infarction.

The patient is subsequently transferred 2 hours later to the coronary care unit as he is pain-free. As the ward clinical pharmacist, you are responsible for daily review of drug charts and advice to medical and nursing staff on all aspects of drug treatment for patients on the ward.

The following tests taken at admission are reported:

Na^+	134 mmol/L (135–145 mmol/L)
K^+	4.3 mmol/L (3.5–4.0 mmol/L)
Urea	5.2 mmol/L (0–7.5 mmol/L)
Creatinine	81 micromol/L (35–125 micromol/L)
Total cholesterol	5.9 mmol/L (<4 mmol/L)
Blood glucose	4.4 mmol/L (4–10 mmol/L)

4   Following the initial dose of heparin (5000 units stat), what dose of heparin should be administered by i.v. infusion and for how long?

5   What classes of drugs should be initiated as standard secondary prevention treatment following acute myocardial infarction in this patient?

6   For each of the classes of drug to be initiated as secondary prevention state (a) a suitable drug choice and (b) a starting dose. Indicate what clinical trial evidence and national guidelines support the use of the drugs that you have mentioned.

7   As this patient has type 2 diabetes mellitus: (a) Which drug/drug class mentioned above as standard secondary prevention may cause problems in this patient? (b) What problems may be experienced in the use of this drug/drug class in a patient with type 2 diabetes mellitus? (c) What alternative drug could you recommend?

8a   If this patient is initiated on a statin as cholesterol-lowering treatment, when should the total cholesterol next be checked following drug initiation?

8b   What counselling should the patient receive regarding the side-effects of statins?

9   Mr FG experiences a chest infection 4 days post admission and is prescribed amoxicillin 500 mg three times daily and erythromycin 500 mg four times daily. What problems may this cause with this patient's statin therapy and what advice would you give in order to avoid this problem occurring?

References

Cholesterol Treatment Trialists' (CTT) Collaborators (2005) Efficacy and safety of cholesterol-lowering treatment: prospective meta-analysis of data from 90 056 participants in 14 randomised trials of statins. *Lancet* 366: 1267–1278.

HOPE (Heart Outcomes Prevention Evaluation Study Investigators) (2000) Effect of an angiotensin converting enzyme inhibitor, ramipril, on cardiovascular events in high risk patients. *New England Journal of Medicine* 342: 145–152.

Heart Protection Study Collaborative Group (2002) MRC/BHF Heart Protection Study of cholesterol lowering with simvastatin in 20,536 high-risk individuals: a randomised placebo-controlled trial. *Lancet* 360: 7–22.

MHRA (Medicines and Healthcare Products Regulatory Agency) (2008) Drug Safety Update, Volume 1, Issue 6, January. Available at http://www.mhra.gov.uk/Public ations/ Safetyguidance/DrugSafetyUpdate/CON2033505 [Accessed 10 April 2008].

National Prescribing Centre (2005) Update on statins. MeRec Briefing Issue No. 28. February. Available at http://www.npc.co.uk/MeReC_Briefings/2004/briefing_ no_28.pdf [Accessed 3 July 2008].

NICE (National Institute for Health and Clinical Excellence) (2007) Secondary prevention in primary and secondary care for patients following a myocardial infarction. Available at http://www.nice.org.uk/nicemedia/pdf/CG48NICEGuidance.pdf [Accessed 10 April 2008].

General references

Baxter K (ed.) (2008) *Stockley's Drug Interactions*, 8th edn. London: Pharmaceutical Press.
Braunwald E, Antman EM, Beasley JW *et al.* for the American College of Cardiology; American Heart Association. Committee on the Management of Patients With Unstable Angina (2002) ACC/AHA 2002 guideline update for the management of patients with unstable angina and non-ST-segment elevation myocardial infarction – summary article: a report of the American College of Cardiology/American Heart Association task force on practice guidelines (Committee on the Management of Patients With Unstable Angina). *Journal of the American College of Cardiology* 40: 1366–1374.
Haffner SM, Lehto S, Ronnemaa T et al. (1998) Mortality from coronary heart disease subjects with type 2 diabetes and in non-diabetic subjects with and without prior myocardial infarction. *New England Journal of Medicine* 339: 229–234.
Joint Formulary Committee (2008) British National Formulary 55. London: British Medical Association and Royal Pharmaceutical Society of Great Britain, March.
Kumar P and Clark M (eds) (2005) *Kumar and Clark's Clinical Medicine*, 6th edn. London: Saunders Ltd.
Rapilysin, Summary of Product Characteristics. Available at http://emc.medicines.org.uk/ [Accessed 3 July 2008).
Taskforce on the Management of Acute Coronary Syndromes of the European Society of Cardiology (2002) Management of acute coronary syndromes in patients presenting without persistent ST segment elevation. *European Heart Journal* 23: 1809–1840.

Answers

Case study level 1 – Angina – see page 20

1a   What is angina?

Angina pectoris describes the classic symptoms of chest pain, and is caused by transient myocardial ischaemia. In stable angina, the blood flow through the coronary arteries may be limited due to the development of atherosclerotic plaques that restrict blood and therefore oxygen to the cardiac muscle myocardium. Episodes of angina are typically caused by exertion or emotion and are relieved by rest.

1b   What typical symptoms could a patient with angina present with?

Central chest tightness or heaviness, which may be brought on by exertion or relieved by rest. It may radiate to one or both arms, the neck, jaw or teeth. Other associated symptoms include: dyspnoea (shortness of breath), nausea, sweatiness and faintness.

2a   What are the risk factors for developing angina?

Modifiable risk factors (those that we can do something about) for angina and ischaemic heart disease include:

- hyperlipidaemia
- smoking
- hypertension
- lack of exercise
- poor diet
- personality
- obesity
- heavy alcohol consumption
- contraceptive pill
- stress.

Non-modifiable risk factors (those we cannot change) include:

- age
- gender
- positive family history
- diabetes mellitus
- ethnicity.

2b   What, if any, risk factors does Mr AG have for developing stable angina?

- Age
- Indian origin
- Sedentary job/possible lack of exercise
- Smoking
- Gender – men are at increased risk.

3a   What group of drugs does GTN spray belong to?

GTN is a nitrate. This class of drugs are potent vasodilators. At therapeutic doses the main effect of nitrates is to act on vascular smooth muscle to dilate the veins, thus reducing central venous pressure (preload) and ventricular end-diastolic volume. The overall effect is to lower myocardial contraction, wall stress and oxygen demand, thereby relieving the angina. Nitrates also promote vasodilation of the coronary blood vessels.

3b   What are the side-effects of GTN spray?

- Postural hypotension
- Tachycardia
- Throbbing headache
- Dizziness
- Less commonly – nausea, vomiting, heartburn, flushing.

3c   How would you counsel Mr AG on the use of his spray?

The patient should be instructed to:

- remove the cap and to hold the spray upright (vertically),
- prime the spray before using for the first time,
- spray one or two sprays under the tongue and close the mouth immediately afterwards, and
- sit down and rest until the pain subsides.

3d   What other formulations of GTN are available? List their advantages and disadvantages.

Available formulations of GTN are listed in Table A2.1.

4   Mr AG's headache may be caused by his use of GTN spray. What can you recommend to him to help manage his headache?

Check how Mr AG is using his spray in the first instance. The correct approach is at the onset of an attack or prior to a precipitating event: one or two 400-micrograms metered doses sprayed under the tongue. It is recommended that no more than three metered doses are taken at any one time and that there should be a minimum interval of 15 minutes between consecutive treatments.

For the prevention of exercise-induced angina or in other precipitating conditions one or two 400-micrograms metered doses should be sprayed under the tongue immediately prior to the event.

Mr AG can be advised to take paracetamol up to 4 g daily (i.e. one or two 500 mg tablets, every 4–6 hours; maximum eight tablets per 24 hours) to relieve his headache. If the headache persists or is severe he should arrange to see his GP to discuss his treatment.

5   What advice would you give Mr AG in relation to his smoking?

Anyone with angina who smokes should be advised to stop. Smokers have a higher incidence of ischaemic heart disease, and a greater risk of dying from it. The greater the number of cigarettes smoked, the greater the risk. Nicotine-replacement therapy can be recommended as part of a smoking cessation pro-gramme in people with angina.

Table A2.1 Formulations of glyceryl nitrate

Formulation	Advantages	Disadvantages
1. GTN sublingual tablets 300 micrograms or 500 micrograms	Rapid onset (<30 seconds) Cheap	Chemical degradation occurs, hence discard 8 weeks after first opening Headache and dizziness common
2. GTN spray 400 micrograms	Rapid onset (<30 seconds) Long expiry date (years) compared to sublingual tablets	More expensive than tablets Headache and dizziness common
3. GTN patches	Useful as longer duration of action	Skin reactions may occur, although uncommon (between 0.1 and 1%) Headache and dizziness common
4. GTN buccal tablets	Rapid onset but slightly slower than sublingual tablets (see 1 above)	Headache and dizziness common
5. GTN injection	Dose by infusion can be carefully controlled and titrated against chest pain in acute situations	Not suitable for day-to-day use as injection – only for acute situations (e.g. unstable angina) Requires careful dilution and use of specific types of syringes and infusion lines

Case study level 2 – Hypertension – see page 21

1   What is hypertension?

Hypertension (in people without diabetes) is defined as a sustained systolic blood pressure of (SBP) of ≥140 mmHg, or sustained diastolic blood pressure (DBP) of ≥90 mmHg (Clinical Knowledge Summaries, 2007). Note: Hypertension is considered to be sustained if an initial raised blood pressure measurement persists at two or more subsequent consultations).

2   What are the appropriate treatment targets for this patient's blood pressure?

The aim of treatment is to reduce blood pressure to 140/90 mmHg or below (NICE, 2006). Note: Patients not achieving this target, or for whom further treatment is inappropriate, declined or not tolerated will still receive some worthwhile benefit from the drug treatments if these lower blood pressure.

3   Besides blood pressure, what other advice and treatment does this patient require to ensure his risk of a cardiovascular event is reduced? Give clear reasons for your advice and explain the risks associated with not taking this advice.

This patient should receive appropriate advice on a range of lifestyle measures that may reduce his overall cardiovascular disease risk. In particular he needs to be encouraged to lose weight, stop smoking and to reduce his alcohol intake to within recommended limits.

The Clinical Knowledge Summary on Hypertension (2007) suggests that people with hypertension should be advised on appropriate lifestyle modifications to reduce cardiovascular disease risk. Advice should be given on:

■   alcohol consumption
■   diet
■   physical activity
■   smoking cessation
■   weight reduction.

There is evidence that a healthy diet, regular exercise and moderation of alcohol intake can reduce, delay or remove the need for long-term antihypertensive drug treatment (North of England Hypertension Guideline Development Group, 2006).

Combining dietary and exercise interventions reduces blood pressure by at least 10 mmHg in about a quarter of people with hypertension (North of England Hypertension Guideline Development Group, 2006). Detailed dietary, exercise and weight-loss advice is given in the Dietary Approaches to Stop Hypertension (DASH) eating plan (available from www.nhlbi.nih.gov/health/public/heart/hbp/dash).

Individual lifestyle modifications that are known to reduce blood pressure include (North of England Hypertension Guideline Development Group, 2006):

■   Regular aerobic exercise for 30–60 minutes, three to five times each week
■   Moderating alcohol intake to recommended levels (less than 21 units per week for men; and less than 14 units per week for women)
■   Restriction of dietary sodium salt to less than 6 g per day by reducing intake or substitution with low-sodium salt alternatives
■   Weight reduction in people who are overweight (body mass index [BMI] over 25 kg/m^2)
■   Restricting coffee consumption (and other caffeine-rich drinks) to fewer than five cups per day
■   Relaxation therapies (e.g. stress management, meditation, cognitive therapies, muscle relaxation, biofeedback) – can reduce the blood pressure, and individuals might wish to pursue these as part of their treatment (though routine provision by primary care teams is neither widely available nor currently recommended).

Weight reduction

Up to 30% of all coronary heart disease deaths have been attributed to unhealthy diets. In 1980, 8% of women were obese and 6% of men. By 1998, however, the prevalence had almost trebled to 21% of women and 17% of men. The four most common problems linked to obesity are heart disease, type 2 diabetes, hypertension and osteoarthritis (National Audit Office, 2001).

Healthy, low-calorie diets had a modest effect on blood pressure in overweight individuals with raised blood pressure, reducing systolic and diastolic blood pressure on average by about 5–6 mmHg in trials. However, there is variation in the reduction in blood pressure achieved in trials and it is unclear why. About 40% of patients were estimated to achieve a reduction in systolic blood pressure of 10 mmHg systolic or more in the short term, up to 1 year (NICE, 2006).

Reducing alcohol consumption

Excessive alcohol consumption (men >21 units/week; women >14 units/ week) is associated with raised blood pressure and poorer cardiovascular and hepatic outcomes.

Structured interventions to reduce alcohol consumption can reduce on average SBP and DBP by 3–4 mmHg in clinical trials.

Smoking cessation

There is no strong link between smoking and blood pressure. But the evidence of the link between smoking and cardiovascular and pulmonary diseases is overwhelming. In addition there is evidence that smoking cessation strategies are cost-effective (NICE, 2006).

4   What are the main classes of drug used to treat hypertension?

Thaizide diuretics, calcium channel blockers, angiotensin-converting enzyme (ACE) inhibitors, beta-blockers and angiotensin II receptor blockers.

5   Which class of drug would be appropriate first-line treatment for Mr HA? How would this treatment choice be affected if the patient had been of Afro-Caribbean origin?

Angiotensin-converting enzyme inhibitors (ACE inhibitors) would be the appropriate initial choice in this patient. If the patient had been of Afro-Caribbean origin then a thiazide diuretic or calcium channel blocker would be an appropriate choice.

6   For one of the classes of drugs mentioned in question 4 indicate the following:

■   a drug from that class
■   a suitable starting dose and frequency
■   the maximum dose for hypertension
■   three contraindications
■   three common side-effects.

Suitable starting doses, frequencies and maximum doses for some appropriate drugs are listed in Table A2.2.

Table A2.2 Suitable starting doses, frequencies and maximum doses for some appropriate drugs for Mr HA (hypertension)

Drug	Dose	Frequency	Maximum dose
Ramipril	1.25 mg	Once daily, increased at intervals of 1–2 weeks	10 mg once daily
Lisinopril	10 mg	Daily	40 mg daily
Enalapril	5 mg	Once daily	40 mg once daily
Perindopril	4 mg	Daily	8 mg daily

Three contraindications are: (a) patients with a hypersensitivity to ACE inhibitors (including angioedema), (b) patients with known or suspected renovascular disease, and (c) pregnancy.

Three common side-effects are: (a) first-dose hypotension, (b) persistent dry cough and (c) hyperkalaemia. Other side-effects include: gastrointestinal effects (nausea, vomiting, dyspepsia, diarrhoea, altered liver function tests, blood disorders, angioedema, rash, loss of sense of smell (more likely if also on potassium-sparing agents or potassium supplements).

7   In view of Mr HA's age he requires cardiovascular risk assessment. How would you assess this patient's cardiovascular risks?

According to the Joint British Societies Guidelines on prevention of cardiovascular disease (CVD) in clinical practice (British Cardiac Society *et al.*, 2005) the following patients should be assessed:

■   Adults >40 years with no history of CVD or diabetes who are not already on treatment for blood pressure or lipids should be opportunistically reviewed.
■   Patients <40 years with a family history of premature atherosclerotic disease should also have their cardiovascular risk assessed.

Cardiovascular risk over 10 years >20% is high risk and patients should be targeted for advice to reduce this risk (i.e. blood pressure reduction, aspirin, dietary modification and drug treatment for modification of lipids, stop smoking, etc.).

In order to calculate cardiovascular risk for a primary prevention patient such as Mr HA, use a validted risk calculator. These are JBS CVD Risk Predictor Charts (*Heart*, 2005, 91: 1–52); BNF Extra (contains JBS CVD risk prediction programme. Available at http://www.bnf.org/bnf/extra/current/450024.htm); QRISK (Available at http://www.qrisk.org/).

Case study level 3 – Atrial fibrillation – see page 23

1   What is atrial fibrillation?

Atrial fibrillation is an arrhythmia in which the electrical activity in the atria is disorganised. The AV node receives more electrical impulses than it can conduct and most are blocked resulting in an irregular ventricular rhythm.

2   What are the most common signs and symptoms exhibited by patients with atrial fibrillation? Indicate which of these signs and symptoms the patient is exhibiting.

■   *Symptoms*: Breathlessness/dyspnoea, palpitations, syncope or dizziness, chest discomfort or stroke/transient ischaemic attack.
■   *Signs*: Irregular pulse, ventricular rate usually 120–180 bpm. ECG shows fine oscillations of the baseline with no clear P-waves. Rapid and irregular QRS rhythm.
■   *Causative factors*: This patient's hypertension is a potential causative factor.

3   What are the two options in terms of treatment strategy that may be employed to manage atrial fibrillation? Indicate what would be the most appropriate strategy that you could recommend to the doctor managing this patient and why you think this is the case.

The two options are rate control or rhythm control. Rate control is the most appropriate in this patient as he is over 65 years. Atrial fibrillation appears to be of long standing and may have been present two months ago when the patient experienced a similar episode. His lisinopril should be stopped as he will get blood pressure control with the beta-blocker.

4   Assuming a rate control strategy is to be used what class of drug should be the first-line treatment for this patient? If the first-line drug was contraindicated what class of drug could be used as alternative treatment?

A beta-blocker is suitable first line treatment for rate control. A rate-limiting calcium channel blocker could be used in those in whom a beta-blocker is not suitable, such as asthmatics.

5   What patient parameters should be monitored to assess therapy with the usual first-line treatment and what is an appropriate treatment target for such parameters?

Titrate dose against heart rate. The target is for a resting heart rate of <90 bpm (or 110 for those with recent onset atrial fibrillation) and an exercise heart rate of <110 bpm (inactive) or 200 minus age (active).

6   What are the two options in terms of antithrombotic prophylaxis in this patient and what are the potential side-effects of each? State which of these is the most appropriate for this patient and why.

The two options are warfarin or aspirin. The side-effects are listed in Table A2.3.

Table A2.3 Side-effects of warfarin and aspirin

Drug	Side-effects
Warfarin	Haemorrhage
	Hypersensitivity
	Rash
	Alopecia
	Diarrhoea
	Nausea and vomiting
	Skin necrosis
	Hepatic dysfunction (e.g. jaundice)
	Pancreatitis
Aspirin	Mild stomach upset/irritation (e.g. heartburn). Occasionally severe gastrointestinal side-effects may occur which may lead to stomach ulcers (evidence severe GI pain, black tarry stools, vomiting blood)
	Occasionally ringing or buzzing in the ears
	In very rare cases and only with larger doses, salicylism may occur. Effects include dizziness, ringing or buzzing in the ears, nausea, headache and confusion

The overall risk of stroke should be assessed for each individual with atrial fibrillation. It should also be reassessed regularly, as a person's risk of stroke will change over time. The individual's attitude to anticoagulation will strongly influence the cost/benefit of treatment, and should always be taken into account.

The decision to use warfarin or aspirin should ultimately be based on the balance of an individual's overall risk of stroke compared with the risk of adverse effects and their personal preference.

In this case the patient is 61-years-old with additional risk factors for stroke (hypertension and smoking). He is at moderate risk and could be offered either aspirin or warfarin.

7   Assuming the patient is to be discharged on a beta-blocker and aspirin, what counselling does he require?

Mr Jones needs to be advised to take his medication regularly. If he experiences any problems he should talk to his GP or a pharmacist. As he is poorly compliant it is worthwhile exploring with him why he did not take his previous therapy (lisinopril) regularly.

He should be advised to take his aspirin in the morning after food. The tablet may be dispersed in water or taken whole with some water. The beta-blocker should be taken regularly at the time(s) prescribed, at the same time each day, swallowed whole with a drink of water. Mr Jones should be told that if he experiences side-effects with this medication, such as dizziness, he should not stop taking it suddenly but should speak with his GP or pharmacist.

Case study level Ma – Heart failure – see page 25

1   What signs and symptoms experienced by this patient indicate that he has heart failure? Does he have right- or left-sided heart failure or both? Explain your answer.

Symptoms are:

- shortness of breath (indicates lung congestion and therefore left-sided heart failure)
- tiredness/lethergy (+ only able to walk limited distance)
- swelling of ankles and pitting to the knees (indicates right-sided heart failure).

Signs are:

- increasing weight due to increased fluid retention
- cardiomegaly on CXR
- basal crackles in both lungs (indicate fluid retention in the lungs due to left-sided heart failure)
- increased JVP
- increased urea and creatinine (indicates renal impairment).

The patient has both left- and right-sided heart failure as he is displaying signs and symptoms such as swelling of the ankles and increased jugular venous pressure (right-sided heart failure) and lung congestion (left-sided heart failure).

2   What system is used to classify heart failure according to severity of symptoms?

The New York Heart Association (NYHA) classification is a well-accepted classification of heart failure based on the severity of symptoms:

- Class I – No symptoms with normal physical activity.

- Class II – Slight limitation and shortness of breath on moderate to severe exertion.
- Class III – Marked limitation of activity, less than ordinary activity causes shortness of breath.
- Class IV – Severe disability, dyspnoea at rest, no physical activity possible without discomfort.

3a   What drug treatment should be initiated for the immediate management of the oedema associated with the acute heart failure?

Diuretic therapy should be initiated for the acute heart failure. An agent such as furosemide would be appropriate. The aim of the furosemide treatment is to relieve symptoms such as shortness of breath and to make the patient more comfortable. A dose of furosemide 40 mg twice daily (8am and 2pm) would be appropriate as initial therapy.

3b   What parameters should be monitored to ensure the effectiveness of the drug treatment for oedema and to minimise toxicity?

- *Blood pressure*: The aim is to ensure blood pressure is as near normal as possible and to avoid a precipitous drop in blood pressure. The healthcare staff managing the patient's care should try and ensure that blood pressure is kept above 100/60 mmHg. Blood pressure should be monitored regularly throughout the day, including before furosemide dosing and a few hours after. A pragmatic frequency would be approx 4–5 times a day during this acute phase. In some cases continued monitoring via electronic means may be considered, depending upon the patient's condition.
- *Heart rate*: The aim is to keep as near normal as possible. Normal rate is around 70–80 bpm. If over-diuresis occurs then rate may increase due to compensatory mechanisms.
- *Weight*: The patient's weight should be monitored on a daily basis to ensure that excess fluid is removed. This will improve symptoms and make the patient more comfortable. The aim is for a weight loss of no more than 1 kg per day. Any more is likely to indicate over-diuresis.
- *Fluid balance*: The total amount of fluid the patient takes in (including any from drug therapy) and excretes (urine) must be monitored. In the acute phase the aim is to remove more than is taken in and to limit the patient's fluid intake.
- *Urea and electrolytes*: Sodium, potassium, urea and creatinine require close daily monitoring. The aim is to normalise and to avoid, in particular, drops in electrolytes such as sodium and potassium due to diuretic therapy. Other electrolytes such as magnesium and calcium may need to be checked regularly.

4   What are the overall aims of drug treatment in acute heart failure?

- Ensure that appropriate diuretic therapy is prescribed at a suitable dose and frequency.
- Relieve congestion and to monitor the patient for improvement in signs and

symptoms of heart fluid retention such as shortness of breath, swelling of the ankles and reduce jugular venous pressure.

- Monitor weight loss as a measure of fluid loss.
- Maintain blood pressure and heart rate within normal limits.
- Monitor urea and electrolytes and to ensure they remain within normal ranges.

5a   The patient's symptoms stabilise over the initial 24 hours. What other class of drug treatment should now be initiated at this stage for management of chronic heart failure? Indicate a drug, starting dose and any parameters that need monitoring.

All patients with heart failure due to left ventricular systolic dysfunction must be initiated on an ACE inhibitor. This should be initiated as soon as the patient's acute symptoms have been controlled at the appropriate dose and then titrated up at short intervals to the target dose or maximum tolerated dose. A suitable agent would be ramipril 2.5 mg once daily, which then could be slowly titrated (e.g. approximately every two weeks) to the target of 10 mg once daily or 5 mg twice daily. Parameters that require regular monitoring are blood pressure, urea and electrolytes (particularly serum potassium) at drug initiation then every week and after each dose increase until stable.

5b   What side-effect can occur when first initiating the treatment above and how can this side-effect be minimised?

Profound first-dose hypotension can occur when ACE inhibitors are introduced to patients with heart failure. This effect may be particularly pronounced if the patient is taking a high dose of a loop diuretic. Temporary withdrawal of the loop diuretic could be considered but is not appropriate in this case as it may cause rebound pulmonary oedema. Therefore in this case the steps are to initiate the ACE inhibitor at low dose (e.g. ramipril 1.25 mg daily at night time while the patient is lying down) and then to monitor blood pressure hourly for the first 4 hours.

6   What is the role of beta-blockers in heart failure? Summarise the clinical trial evidence to date.

NICE guidelines state that beta-blockers should be used in patients with heart failure due to left ventricular systolic dysfunction after a diuretic and ACE inhibitor regardless of whether symptoms persist or not.

Beta-blockers have been shown to reduce total mortality, hospitalisation and improve left ventricular ejection fraction in patients with mild, moderate and severe heart failure.

Only two beta-blockers are licensed for the treatment of heart failure, bisoprolol (Cardicor) and carvedilol (Eucardic). Their starting and target doses are listed in Table A2.5.

Table A2.5 Starting and target doses for two beta-blockers licensed for severe heart failure

Drug	Starting dose	Target dose
Bisoprolol	1.25 mg once daily	10 mg once daily
Carvedilol	3.125 mg twice daily	25–50 mg twice daily

Note – see *BNF*; Summary of Product Characteristics for Cardicor and Eucardic for further details on dose titration schedules. The NICE clinical guideline on heart failure provides further detailed guidance on dose titration and monitoring.

7   What advice should be given to the patient at discharge with regard to lifestyle issues?

The patient should be advised to follow standard advice with regard to following a healthy, low-fat diet, stopping smoking, reducing his alcohol intake to within normal limits (<28 units per week). In addition he needs to be advised regarding his fluid and salt intake but the exact restrictions on these will depend on the extent of his heart failure and symptoms.

Case study level Mb – Myocardial infarction – see page 29

1   What further diagnostic and biochemical tests should be ordered to help confirm the diagnosis?

Troponin

Troponin enzymes consist of troponin T, C and I which are located within cardiac and skeletal muscle. Cardiac isoforms of troponin T and I are exclusively expressed in cardiac myocytes. They act as sensitive and specific markers of cardiac damage. An initial rise in troponin may be seen as early as 3–4 hours after a cardiac event, and is usually measured on admission to hospital. However a rise in troponin may be delayed therefore the initial measurement taken on admission is repeated by a further blood sample 12 hours after the onset of chest pain.

The troponin assay has prognostic information that can determine mortality risk in acute coronary syndrome and define which patients may benefit from aggressive medical therapy and early coronary revascularisation.

Creatine kinase

Creatine kinase (CK) occurs in high concentrations in the brain, cardiac and skeletal muscle and is elevated in the blood with muscle damage. A rise in CK is seen in acute myocardial infarction but also in other conditions. A more specific marker is creatine kinase MB (CK-MB), which is an isoenzyme of creatine kinase that is more specific for cardiac muscle damage. CK or CK-MB will rise approximately 4 hours after an acute cardiac event and will reach a peak after approximately 24 hours and will remain raised for 3–4 days.

CK-MB was until recently the standard marker for myocyte damage used in acute coronary syndrome, but the presence of low levels of CK-MB in the serum of normal individuals and in patients with significant skeletal muscle damage has limited its accuracy.

2   What is myocardial infarction and what are the classic symptoms?

Myocardial infarction (also known as a heart attack) occurs when the blood supply to a part of the heart is interrupted. This is most commonly due to occlusion (blockage) of a coronary artery following the rupture of an atherosclerotic plaque in the wall of the artery. The resulting ischaemia and oxygen shortage if left untreated can cause damage and/or death (infarction) of the heart muscle (myocardium).

Severe cardiac pain, chest tightness, sweating, breathlessness and nausea. Some patients may present with atypical features including indigestion, pleuritic chest pain or dyspnoea.

3   Explain the mechanism of action of thrombolytics such as reteplase in acute myocardial infarction.

Fibrinolytic agents such as reteplase enhance the breakdown of occlusive thromboses by the activation of plasminogen to form plasmin.

4   Following the initial dose of heparin (5000 units stat), what dose of heparin should be administered by i.v. infusion and for how long?

Intravenous infusion of heparin 1000 units per hour starting after the second reteplase bolus. Heparin should be administered for at least 24 hours, preferably for 48–72 hours, aiming to keep activated partial thromboplastin time (aPTT) values 1.5–2 times normal.

5   What classes of drugs should be initiated as standard secondary prevention treatment following acute myocardial infarction in this patient?

■   Beta-blockers
■   Statins
■   ACE inhibitors
■   Antiplatelet therapy with aspirin.

6   For each of the classes of drug to be initiated as secondary prevention state (a) a suitable drug choice and (b) a starting dose. Indicate what clinical trial evidence and national guidelines support the use of the drugs that you have mentioned.

Statins – drug choice: simvastatin

Simvastatin 20–40 mg daily (given at night) would be a suitable starting dose. This has been shown in large, well-conducted clinical trials to reduce clinically relevant events such as heart attacks and strokes. The NICE technology appraisal on statins states that there is no evidence that any one statin is superior to another in reducing cardiovascular events. However, only atorvastatin, fluvastatin, pravastatin and simvastatin (and not rosuvastatin) have trials reporting clinical events as outcomes. There are substantial differences in prices between the different statins. Therefore, therapy should usually be initiated with a drug with a low acquisition cost (taking into account required daily dose and product price per dose).

Based on clinical trial evidence and cost, generic simvastatin 20 mg or 40 mg daily would seem a reasonable first-line choice. In the largest statin trial to date, the Heart Protection Study (2002), which included people with and without existing coronary heart disease (CHD), simvastatin 40 mg was associated with a significant 27% reduction in major coronary events (CHD death plus non-fatal myocardial infarction), equating to an NNT (number needed to treat) of 32 over 5 years.

Based on clinical trial evidence, atorvastatin 10 mg daily would be a reasonable alternative to simvastatin. However, branded atorvastatin 10 mg is over four times more expensive than generic simvastatin 40 mg.

See MeReC Briefing No. 28 (National Prescribing Centre, 2005) for further details of the evidence base relating to statins and also the Cholesterol Treatment Trialists' (CTT) Collaborators (2005) meta-analysis.

Beta-blockers – drug choice: atenolol, bisoprolol or metoprolol

There is strong evidence that beta-blockers can reduce mortality by up to 23% post myocardial infarction. Beta-blockers should be used to reduce the risk of further cardiovascular disease events irrespective of whether the blood pressure is raised or not. There is no evidence that any beta-blocker is more effective than another in secondary prevention, hence a beta-blocker which is well tolerated and that can be taken once or twice daily should be used. Atenolol, bisoprolol or metoprolol are suitable agents. These agents are not specifically licensed post myocardial infarction but all are licensed for angina and the doses for this indication should be used i.e.

- atenolol – up to 100 mg daily in one or two divided doses

- bisoprolol – usually 10 mg daily up to a maximum of 20 mg daily (note it is usual to start at lower doses e.g. 2.5–5 mg and increase time)
- metoprolol – 50–100 mg two to three times daily.

ACE inhibitors: drug choice:

ACE inhibitors reduce morbidity and mortality post myocardial infarction in patients with left ventricular systolic dysfunction (LVSD). This is thought to be mediated via their action on the renin–angiotensin system. More recent evidence from the HOPE study (2000) has established that ACE inhibitors given to high risk CVD patients who had not got low ejection fraction or heart failure resulted in benefits in terms of reduced morbidity and mortality.

The NICE clinical guidelines on secondary prevention of myocardial infarction (2007) now recommend that ACE inhibitors should be used in all patients post myocardial infarction with or without LVSD (i.e. ejection fraction <40%).

Within the HOPE study ramipril was the agent of choice and this would be an appropriate ACE inhibitor to use post-myocardial infarction. Ramipril is licensed for use post myocardial infarction at a dose of 2.5 mg twice daily initially (started in hospital 3–10 days after infarction), increased after 2 days to 5 mg twice daily. Maintenance doses are 2.5 mg–5 mg twice daily.

Antiplatelet therapy – drug choice: aspirin

Aspirin 75 mg daily for life is recommended for people with existing cardiovascular disease (secondary prevention). Doses of aspirin from 75 mg to 325 mg daily have been proven to be effective, therefore the lowest effective dose that minimises side-effects (i.e. 75 mg daily) should be used.

7 As this patient has type 2 diabetes mellitus: (a) Which drug/drug class mentioned above as standard secondary prevention may cause problems in this patient? (b) What problems may be experienced in the use of this drug/drug class in a patient with type 2 diabetes mellitus? (c) What alternative drug could you recommend?

Beta-blockers may be a problem in this patient because they can mask the usual signs of hypoglycaemia. But the benefit is considered to outweigh the risks in the majority of patients who should be counselled regarding this effect. An alternative would be a rate-limiting calcium channel blocker such as diltiazem although clinical trial evidence as regards its benefit post myocardial infarction is lacking.

8a If this patient is initiated on a statin as cholesterol-lowering treatment when should the total cholesterol next be checked following drug initiation?

After 6–12 weeks. Minimum interval of at least 4 weeks.

8b   What counselling should the patient receive regarding the side-effects of statins?

Simvastatin, like other inhibitors of HMG-CoA reductase, occasionally causes myopathy manifested as muscle pain, tenderness or weakness with creatine kinase (CK) 10 times above the upper limit of normal (ULN). Myopathy sometimes takes the form of rhabdomyolysis with or without acute renal failure secondary to myoglobinuria, and very rare fatalities have occurred.

The Committee on Safety of Medicines (CSM) has advised that rhabdomyolysis with lipid-regulating drugs is rare (1 case in every 100 000 treatment years) but may be increased in those with renal impairment and/or hypothyroidism.

Concomitant prescribing of drugs that increase the plasma statin concentration (e.g. fibrates) will increase the risk of muscle toxicity.

All patients starting therapy with a statin, or whose dose of statin is being increased, should be advised of the risk of myopathy and told to report promptly any unexplained muscle pain, tenderness or weakness.

9   Mr FG experiences a chest infection 4 days post admission and is prescribed amoxicillin 500 mg three times daily and erythromycin 500 mg four times daily. What problems may this cause with this patient's statin therapy and what advice would you give in order to avoid this problem occurring?

Erythromycin may cause increases in the serum levels of simvastatin. The CSM has advised that this should not be co-prescribed with simvastatin. In the first instance the pharmacist should check local policies for management of hospital acquired chest infections/pneumonia to ascertain first and second line choices. If erythromycin or any macrolide cannot be avoided then a practical way forward may be to avoid taking any dose of simvastatin for the duration of the course of macrolide. In addition a recent Drug Safety Update from the Medicines and Healthcare Products Regulatory Agency (MHRA, 2008) on statins has highlighted statin drug interactions and the appropriate actions to take.

3

Respiratory system case studies

Soraya Dhillon and Andrzej Kostrzewski

Case study level 1 – Asthma – community

Learning outcomes

Level 1 case study: You will be able to:

- describe the risk factors
- describe the disease
- describe the pharmacology of the drug
- outline the formulation, including drug molecule, excipients, etc. for the medicines
- summarise basic social pharmacy issues (e.g. opening containers, large labels).

Scenario

An 18-year-old man, VB, presents with a history of recurrent episodes of wheeze after walking 200 metres. VB has recently started to go to a gym and his episodes of wheeze have worsened. He goes to see his GP. He can talk in sentences but his respiratory rate is increased. His peak flow is 420 L/min which is 80% of predicted result. A diagnosis of mild asthma is made.

He is started on salbutamol metered dose inhaler (MDI) two puffs when required and beclometasone (Qvar) 50 micrograms twice daily.

Questions

1 What is asthma?
2 What are the risk factors for developing asthma? What risk factors does the patient have?

3a   What is the pharmacology of beta$_2$-agonists and inhaled corticosteroids?
3b   What are the side-effects of beta$_2$-agonists?
4   What formulations of salbutamol and inhaled corticosteroids are available and
         what are the advantages and disadvantages?
5   Describe how to use an MDI.
6   What are the social implications of this man's asthma?

General reference

Joint Formulary Committee (2008) *British National Formulary 55*. London: British Medical
    Association and Royal Pharmaceutical Society of Great Britain, March.

Case study level 2 – Asthma – acute on chronic

Learning outcomes

Level 2 case study: You will be able to:

- interpret relevant lab and clinical data
- identify monitoring and referral criteria
- explain treatment choices
- describe goals of therapy including monitoring and the role of the
  pharmacist/clinician
- describe issues – counselling points, adverse drug reactions, drug
  interactions, complementary/alternative therapies and lifestyle advice.

Scenario

HT, a 32-year-old woman, 155 cm, 81 kg, presents to hospital casualty with a
history of increased breathlessness and wheeze, over the last 5 days. She is
known to have had asthma for 20 years and has smoked 10 cigarettes per day
since the age of 15. Her last hospital admission was one month ago. She works
in a small 'do-it-yourself' shop, as a counter assistant. HT lives in a tenth-floor
council flat; she is single.

On medical examination the following is found:

- audible wheeze throughout the chest, using accessory muscles
- not able to speak in sentences – stops for breath after two words
- tachycardia – pulse 130 beats per minute
- tachypnoeic – respiratory rate 25 breaths per minute
- peak expiratory flow rate 150 L/min.

1a Explain why this patient is tachycardic and tachypnoeic.

1b Describe what peak expiratory flow measures and how this value is interpreted in this woman.

1c Describe what other tests would be of importance in this patient at the time of admission.

1d Explain how the severity of acute asthma is estimated and how often investigations should be done.

2 List the medicines available for the acute treatment of asthma and describe the method of administration.

3a Describe the role of the pharmacist in the care of this patient.

3b What are the aims of asthma treatment for the patient and the professional?

4a Explain the social issues this patient will face on discharge.

4b Critically review the non-pharmacological therapies that are available for people with asthma. Would these be of benefit for this patient?

4c Discuss the role of an asthma management plan for this patient.

References

BTS/SIGN (British Thoracic Society and Scottish Intercollegiate Guidelines Network) (2008) British guideline on the management of asthma. Available at http://www.sign.ac.uk/guidelines/fulltext/101/ index.html [Accessed 4 July 2008].

Virchow J, Crompton G, Dal Negro R *et al.* (2007) Importance of inhaler devices in the management of airway disease. *Respiratory Medicine* 102: 10–19.

General reference

Joint Formulary Committee (2008) *British National Formulary* 55. London: British Medical Association and Royal Pharmaceutical Society of Great Britain, March.

Case study level 3 – Chronic obstructive pulmonary disease (COPD) – with co-morbidity

Learning outcomes

Level 3 case study: You will be able to:

- interpret clinical signs and symptoms
- evaluate laboratory data
- evaluate treatment options
- state goals of therapy
- describe a pharmaceutical care plan to include advice to a clinician
- describe the prognosis and long-term complications
- describe the social pharmacy issues which could include supply (e.g. complex treatments at home, concordance and compliance) and lifestyle issues.

Scenario

A 63-year-old woman, 67 kg, is admitted to hospital with chest pain, shortness of breath and sweating. She is seen in casualty and treated using a salbutamol nebuliser. She looks obese. She has been a life-long smoker who stopped one day ago.

Her previous medical history includes chronic obstructive pulmonary disease (COPD) for 10 years, last admission to hospital was two weeks ago; ischaemic heart disease since 1995, myocardial infarction 4 years ago; osteo-porosis diagnosed 3 years ago; hypertension diagnosed 9 years ago; and pulmonary embolism two months ago.

On examination:

- blood pressure 105/90 mmHg
- heart rate 90 bpm
- respiratory rate 20 breaths per minute.

Arterial blood gases on admission

- pH 7.388 on 35% O_2
- PCO_2 9.67 kPa
- PO_2 6.5 kPa.

Oxygen saturation: SpO_2 89%. Lungs hyperinflated, no wheeze, few right base crepitations.

Laboratory tests at admission

WCC	16.5×10^9/L	$(4-11 \times 10^9$/L)
Na⁺	140 mmol/L	(135–145 mmol/L)
K⁺	4.4 mmol/L	(3.5–5 mmol/L)
Creatinine	75 micromol/L	(59–104 micromol/L)
Urea	7.8 mmol/L	(1.7–8.3 mmol/L)
Hb	11.6 g/dL	(13–17 g/dL)

Medication on admission

- prednisolone 10 mg o.d.
- fluticasone inhaler 500 micrograms b.d.
- aspirin 75 mg o.d.
- bumetanide 1 mg o.d.
- Combivent nebs 2 q.d.s.
- enalapril 5 mg o.d.
- Uniphyllin Continus 200 mg bd
- senna 2 tablets nocte
- warfarin 5 mg o.d.
- zopiclone 7.5 mg nocte
- diclofenac 50 mg p.r.n.
- O₂ 2 L nasal specs.

Questions

1a Describe the clinical signs and symptoms of COPD, explain the pathophysiology and how these relate to the patient.

1b What is the interpretation of this patient's pulse oximetry and arterial gases?

1c Describe the clinical difference between asthma and COPD.

2 Comment on the current drug therapy and describe the role of O₂ in this patient.

3 Describe the care plan for this patient, including smoking cessation.

4 What are the key aims for this patient and the professional?

5 Explain how spirometry can be used to monitor this patient.

6 What are the social issues in treating this patient at home?

Reference

NICE (National Institute for Health and Clinical Excellence) (2004) Chronic obstructive pulmonary disease – Management of chronic obstructive disease in adults in primary and secondary care. Available at http://www.nice.org.uk/nicemedia/pdf/CG012_niceguideline.pdf [Accessed 4 June 2008].

Case study level Ma – COPD

Learning outcomes

Level M case study: You will be able to:

- interpret clinical signs and symptoms
- evaluate laboratory data
- critically appraise treatment options
- state goals of therapy
- describe a pharmaceutical care plan to include advice to a clinician
- describe the prognosis and long-term complications
- describe the social pharmacy issues which could include supply (e.g. complex treatments at home, concordance and compliance) and lifestyle issues
- describe the monitoring of therapy.

Scenario

Mr CD, a 75-year-old man, 1.7 m tall, is admitted to hospital very short of breath. He used to work in the docks as a clerk and has smoked 40 cigarettes daily for 30 years and stopped 2 years ago. His previous medical history includes COPD, recurrent infective exacerbations since 1991, no LTOT; type 2 diabetes mellitus on insulin 14 IU b.d. for 20 years, retinopathy; ischaemic heart disease – coronary artery bypass graft (twice), hypertension; myocardial infarction 1986; atrial fibrillation; high cholesterol.

The patient was discharged from hospital three weeks ago with antibiotics. There was some improvement, but he is still very short of breath at rest. Five days ago, with worsening shortness of breath over the previous week, the patient took clarithromycin 500 mg b.d. Four days ago he took prednisolone 30 mg daily but has now stopped, with no improvement. He is using nebulisers 7 times daily (salbutamol + ipratropium). Because he was no better today, his daughter called an ambulance.

On arrival he had shortness of breath on exertion after 2 yards (best 30 yards), cough – chronic, no worse, non-productive, chronic wheeze, no chest pain, no palpitations, ankle swelling no worse then usual, both legs swollen to upper calf, orthopnoea. The patient sleeps upright and gets paroxysmal nocturnal dyspnoea if lying flat.

Systems review

- Bowels – ok
- Genitourinary – poor stream, no haematuria, no dysuria, nocturia × 4–5
- No allergies.

Medicines

The patient's medications comprise:

- aspirin 300 mg o.d.
- diltiazem MR (Tildiem LA) 300 mg o.d.
- bendroflumethazide 2.5 mg o.d.
- losartan 50 mg o.d.
- furosemide 80 mg o.d.
- atorvastatin 10 mg o.d.
- carbocisteine 500 mg q.d.s.
- Insulatard 14 IU b.d.
- ferrous sulphate 300 mg t.d.s.
- omeprazole 20 mg o.d.
- alendronate 70 mg weekly
- salbutamol 2.5 mg nebulised prn
- ipratropium 500 micrograms t.d.s. nebulised.

He is an ex-smoker who stopped 2 years ago, alcohol very occasionally, retired clerk.

On examination: °J °A °C °C °L.

Mr CD's pulse rate is 115 irregular and his respiratory rate is 40 breaths per minute. He has bilateral crepitations and FEV_1 1.2 L.

Laboratory tests

WBC	15.8×10^9/L (4–11×10^9/L)
Hb	11 g/d/L (13–17 g/d/L)
Neutrophils	14.4×10^9/L (1.5–7×10^9/L)
Lymphocytes	0.5×10^9/L (1.2–3.5×10^9/L)
Troponin T	0.02 micrograms (<0.03 micrograms)
Na^+	135 mmol/L (135–145 mmol/L)
K^+	4.0 mmol/L (3.5–5 mmol/L)
Urea	6.9 mmol/L (1.7–8.3 mmol/L)
Creatinine	81 micromol (59–104 micromol)
Mg^{2+}	0.67 mmol/L (0.65–1.05 mmol/L)
GGT	169 IU/L (4–72 IU/L)
ALT	35 IU/L (4–59 IU/L)
Bilirubin	11 mmol/L (<16 mmol/L)
Albumin	47 g/L (40–52 g/L)
CRP	16 mg/L (<4 mg/L)
Glucose	18.2 mmol/L (3.8–5.5 mmol/L)

Diagnosis

Infective exacerbation of COPD with heart failure.

Questions

1   Discuss the clinical signs and symptoms for Mr CD.
2a   Discuss the role of smoking history and calculate the total pack years this patient has been subjected to.
2b   What spirometry should be used to assess Mr CD's lung function and what main factors affect the predicted values?
3   Discuss the role of oxygen and delivery systems during the acute exacerbation.
4a   Critically review Mr CD's list of medicines.
4b   Discuss the place and route of corticosteroids in Mr CD's management.
5   Describe a pharmaceutical care plan for the continued treatment of this patient.

Reference

NICE (National Institute for Health and Clinical Excellence) (2004) Chronic obstructive pulmonary disease – Management of chronic obstructive disease in adults in primary and secondary care. Available at http://www.nice.org.uk/nicemedia/pdf/ CG012_niceguideline.pdf [Accessed 4 June 2008].

Case study level Mb – Brittle asthma

Learning outcomes

Level M case study: You will be able to:

- interpret clinical signs and symptoms
- evaluate laboratory data
- critically appraise treatment options
- state goals of therapy
- describe a pharmaceutical care plan to include advice to a clinician
- describe the prognosis and long-term complications
- describe the social pharmacy issues which could include supply (e.g. complex treatments at home, concordance and compliance) and lifestyle issues
- Describe the monitoring of therapy.

A 22-year-old woman, Ms RJ, is admitted via casualty with sudden breathlessness and wheeze. She has had asthma for 10 years and her last hospital admission was a month ago. She is usually on salbutamol nebs, and at home uses them once or twice weekly, budesonide turbo 800 micrograms q.d.s., ipratropium nebs. Ms RJ was on 40 mg prednisolone daily since last hospital discharge but this was increased by GP a week ago for an upper respiratory tract infection. Recently Ms RJ has bought some painkillers from her local pharmacy.

The patient is allergic to penicillin and house dust. She is single, a money dealer and non-smoker.

On examination:

- audible wheeze (using accessory muscles)
- not able to speak in sentences
- pulse 130 beats/min, respiratory rate 25 per minute, blood pressure 110/80 mmHg
- peak expiratory flow rate 200 L/min (best 450 L/min)
- apyrexial, has a dry cough.

Laboratory tests

WBC	6.7×10^9/L ($4 - 11 \times 10^9$/L)
Hb	11.2 g/dL (13 – 17 g/dL)

Arterial blood gases

- pH 7.388 on 60% O_2 (7.3 – 7.5)
- PCO_2 4.67 kPa (4.0 – 6.7 kPa)
- PO_2 24.7 kPa (11 – 13 kPa)
- Oxygen saturation: 99.6% on oxygen.

After 48 hours she has some spirometry tests which show FEV_1 (L) >20% increase after salbutamol. After 72 hours in hospital Ms RJ is ready for discharge.

Medication on discharge is suggested to be:

- salbutamol nebuliser 5 mg p.r.n.
- salmeterol inhaler 100 micrograms b.d.
- budesonide inhaler 800 micrograms b.d.
- theophylline SR 200 mg bd
- prednisolone 50 mg daily
- omeprazole 20 mg o.d.

Questions

1   Using the data provided, assess the severity of the asthma.
2   Explain the blood gases on admission.
3a   Describe the role of Ms RJ's discharge therapy.
3b   Critically review the role of magnesium in acute asthma.
3c   Discuss the issue of non-steroidal anti-inflammatory drugs in asthma.
4a   Describe the role of theophylline in asthma.
4b   Critically review the role of anti-IgE monoclonal antibody for Ms RJ.
5a   Discuss the issues in variability of peak expiratory flow.
5b   What other therapy could be considered? Devise a care plan.
6   Discuss the factors that predict poor compliance with asthma treatment.

References

Ayres JG, Mikes JF and Barnes PJ (1998) Brittle asthma. *Thorax* 53: 315–321.
BTS/SIGN (British Thoracic Society and Scottish Intercollegiate Guidelines Network) (2008) British guideline on the management of asthma. Available at http://www.sign.ac.uk/guidelines/fulltext/101/index.html [Accessed 4 June 2008].

General references

Aldington S and Beasley R (2007) Asthma exacerbations 5: assessment and management of severe asthma in adults in hospital. *Thorax* 62: 447–458.
Anon (2006) Omalizumab for severe asthma? *Drug and Therapeutics Bulletin* 44: 86–88.
Anon (2007) Adherence to prophylactic asthma medications is affected by many factors. *Drugs and Therapy Perspectives* 23: 25–26.
Hamad AM, Sutcliffe AM and Knox AJ (2004) Aspirin-induced asthma: clinical aspects, pathogenesis and management. *Drugs* 64: 2417– 2432.
Holgate ST and Frew A (2004) Respiratory disease. In: Kumar P and Clark M (eds) *Kumar and Clark's Clinical Medicine*, 5th edn. Philadelphia: WB Saunders, Elsevier Limited, pp. 833–919.
Jenkins C, Costello J and Hodge L (2004) Systematic review of prevalence of aspirin induced asthma and its implications for clinical practice. *British Medical Journal* 328: 434.
Joint Formulary Committee (2008) *British National Formulary* 55. London: British Medical Association and Royal Pharmaceutical Society of Great Britain, March.
Rees J (2006) Asthma control in adults. *British Medical Journal* 332: 770.
Strunk RC and Bloomberg GR (2006) Omalizumab for asthma. *New England Journal of Medicine* 354: 2689–2695.
Weinberger M and Hendeles L (1996) Theophylline in asthma. *New England Journal of Medicine* 334: 1380–1388.

Case study level 1 – Asthma – community – see page 49

1   What is asthma?

Asthma is a chronic inflammatory disease affecting the airways. Symptoms are cough, wheeze, a feeling of tightness in the chest and shortness of breath. Asthma is characterised by:

- airway obstruction (bronchoconstriction), which is usually reversible either spontaneously or with therapeutic intervention,
- airway hyperresponsiveness to a range of stimuli,
- inflammation of the respiratory bronchioles due to eosinophils.

T lymphocytes and mast cells are involved in the production of mucus, oedema, smooth muscle hypertrophy and this can lead to mucus production and epithelial damage. If asthma is chronic it can lead to inflammation associated with irreversible bronchoconstriction.

Asthma can be classified as either extrinsic or intrinsic.

- Extrinsic – there is a known external stimulus. This is usually in patients that are atopic and show reactions to allergens. This is common in childhood asthma
- Intrinsic – there is a causative agent identified. This usually starts in middle life, but there may be some evidence of allergy in younger life.

Patient VB may have had mild asthma as a child and this has now been exacerbated by the increased incidence of wheeze.

2   What are the risk factors for developing asthma? What risk factors does the patient have?

The risk factors for developing asthma are as follows:

- Atopy in a patient, which refers to a group of disorders which include asthma, eczema and hay fever.
- Positive family history.
- Circulating antibodies and developing IgE class against common environmental factors.
- Genetic and environmental factors influencing levels of IgE.
- Occupational hazards (e.g. exposure to reactive chemicals such as isocyanates or IgE-related, such as allergens from animals, flour and grain).
- Non-steroidal anti-inflammatory drugs (NSAIDs) (e.g. aspirin), which can precipitate an attack in 5% of people with asthma.
- Beta-blockers. There is some evidence that beta-adrenergic blocking drugs such as propranolol can cause bronchoconstriction in some patients. Some selectivity with beta$_2$-adrenergic drugs can minimise this effect but caution should be exercised.

- Atmospheric pollutants (e.g. cigarette smoke, car pollutants, dust).
- Cold air and exercise. People with asthma should ensure they are using effective medication since the latter can precipitate hyperresponsiveness of the airway.

This patient has limited risk factors, however recurrent episodes of wheeze and exposure to cold and exercise may have precipitated the attack.

3a   What is the pharmacology of beta$_2$-agonists and inhaled corticosteroids?

Beta$_2$-adrenergic agonists are available as short- and long-acting agents. These drugs have limited gastric absorption and are only effective when inhaled, following which they exert a local effect in the lungs. Beta$_2$-adrenergic agents cause bronchodilation by increasing the levels of cyclic adenosine monophosphate (cAMP) following stimulation of the beta$_2$-receptors in smooth muscle. They act throughout the respiratory tract. Short-acting beta$_2$-adrenergic agents are the drugs of choice for the acute management of asthma. Longer acting beta$_2$-adrenergic agonists are used in patients with moderate to severe asthma in combination with corticosteroids.

Corticosteroids are anti-inflammatory drugs and are available in a range of formulations. These drugs are used in the management of short- and long-term control of asthma. A wide range of formulations and types of corticosteroids varying in potency are available.

Inhaled corticosteroids are minimally absorbed and have a local effect. However, depending on the dose and potency of the inhaled corticosteroid, inhaled forms can produce systemic side-effects. Oral prednisolone is rapidly absorbed and is metabolised by the liver. Some corticosteroids may be administered intravenously.

Corticosteroids have a complex mechanism of action. They can affect the production of cytokines, leukotrienes and prostaglandins. This affects the production of eosinophils and release of other markers of the inflammatory response. Corticosteroids can affect other areas of the body and hence have a range of side-effects.

3b   What are the side-effects of beta$_2$-agonists?

Adverse effects include:

- paradoxical bronchospasm
- tachycardia
- palpitations
- tremor
- restlessness
- headache
- blushing
- dry mouth

- hypertension
- arrhythmia
- low potassium levels.

4   What formulations of salbutamol and inhaled corticosteroids are available and what are the advantages and disadvantages?

Salbutamol

Salbutamol is available as tablets, inhalers, nebuliser solution and intravenous injection. In the management of asthma at step 1 and 2 the inhaled formulation is the best option since it targets the drug and minimises side-effects. Oral tablets of salbutamol are rarely used and there is limited evidence of their effectiveness.

Patients who have difficulty in coordination with inhalers can use a spacer device. These remove the need for coordination between actuation of a pressurised metered dose inhaler and inhalation. The spacer device reduces the velocity of the aerosol and subsequent impaction on the oropharynx. In addition, the device allows more time for evaporation of the propellant so that a larger proportion of the particles can be inhaled and deposited in the lungs. The size of the spacer is important, the larger spacers with a one-way valve (Nebuhaler, Volumatic) being most effective. Spacer devices are particularly useful for patients with poor inhalation technique, for children, for patients requiring higher doses, for nocturnal asthma, and for patients who have poor coordination.

Nebulised and intravenous salbutamol is required for more severe and acute status asthmaticus.

Corticosteroids

Corticosteroids are available in tablet, inhaled and intravenous dosage forms. Inhaled corticosteroids allow the control of asthma with minimal systemic absorption and thus reduce the risks associated with corticosteroids such as osteoporosis and adrenal suppression. These risks are greatly increased when taking systemic corticosteroids.

Oral tablets and intravenous steroids are used in more severe and acute status asthmaticus.

5   Describe how to use an MDI.

Patient education is vital for the management of asthma. Patients should be guided in their use of the asthma inhaler. It is important that you then observe the patient's use. Instructions given to the patient are as follows:

- Sit in a comfortable, upright position.
- Remove the cap of the inhaler.
- Shake the inhaler.
- Breathe out and then put the mouthpiece into your mouth and take a deep inhalation, simultaneously pressing the inhaler.
- Hold your breath, then exhale slowly.
- Wipe the mouthpiece and replace the lid.
- The inhaler should be stored in a cool dry place.

The essential counselling points should be taken from the inhaler package insert

- If you are to take two puffs, wait half a minute before repeating the steps above.

6   What are the social implications of this man's asthma?

VP is entering adult life and will need to be aware of the importance of effective asthma management. He has to be mature enough to take responsibility for his asthma management and must not feel inhibited by having to carry inhalers with him. He needs to ensure prophylactic cover with beta$_2$-agonists when undergoing strenuous exercise. He needs to be counselled on issues of sex education and the regular use of his inhalers. There is limited evidence of genetic malformation from his medicines, but the patient needs to be aware that when he considers a family, his child may be prone to asthma due to the genetic predisposition.

Case study level 2 – Asthma – acute on chronic – see page 50

1a   Explain why this patient is tachycardic and tachypnoeic.

Tachycardia is an increase in the heart rate over 100 per minute. This can be due to excessive use or side-effects of a beta-agonist. It can be induced by anxiety and panic, which a patient may experience during an asthma attack. Tachypnoea is an increase in the respiratory rate due to airway narrowing and constriction, hence the body will increase its respiratory rate to try to increase the intake of oxygen.

1b   Describe what peak expiratory flow measures and how this value is interpreted in this woman.

This is a test to assess the degree of airway limitation. It is easy to perform and relatively inexpensive. The patient takes a full inspiration to total lung capacity and then blows out forcefully into the peak flow meter. The best of three recordings are normally taken. The peak flow measures the expiratory flow rate in the first 2 ms of expiration and can overestimate the extent of lung function in patients with moderate to severe airway limitation. Other tests such as spirometry, forced expiratory volume (FEV_1), forced vital capacity (FVC) and the ratio of FEV_1/FVC are used.

Peak expiratory flow rate

Peak flow measurement of peak expiratory flow rate (PEFR) on waking, before bed, before and after bronchodilator medication is useful to assess the extent of airflow limitation and the characteristic of the disease in terms of reversibility. There is some evidence of diurnal variability. PEFR is also useful in assessing the disease progression longer term and the response to therapy. Patients are advised to keep an asthma diary and record regularly the peak flows to ascertain their diurnal pattern.

The extent of reversibility can be assessed using PEFR: 15% improvement in the PEFR determines the extent of reversibility following bronchodilator therapy.

This patient's PEFR (150 L/min) is very limited. In a patient of her age and weight her normal value would be 300–350 L/min hence she is showing 50% or <50% of her best value which indicates substantial airflow limitation.

1c   Describe what other tests would be of importance in this patient at the time of admission.

Other tests which would be helpful in this woman would be FEV_1, FVC and blood gases. The spirometry values provide data not only on the expiration of air but also on the time taken for forced expiration. Patients with significant airway limitation will show a prolonged forced expiratory time. The FEV_1 expressed as a percentage of the FVC provides a measure of the extent of airway limitation. In normal subjects it would be in the region of 75%. In patients with obstruction, the ratio FEV_1/FVC will be reduced.

Blood gases would need to be checked. The normal for this patient would be:

- oxygen saturation above 95%
- pH 7.3–7.5
- PCO_2 4.0 – 6.7 kPa
- PO_2 11–13 kPa.

1d   Explain how the severity of acute asthma is estimated and how often investigations should be done.

Patients should be routinely assessed by the GP or pharmacists at least every three months. Once a patient is stable, most assessments will be carried out annually by the GP or clinical nurse specialist. Pharmacists should routinely review the patient if medication alters and at least every three months.

The following symptoms should be assessed:

- episodic wheeze
- cough
- shortness of breath
- number of attacks.

Investigations include:

- peak expiratory flow rates
- lung function tests
- histamine or methacholine bronchial provocation tests for severe cases (rare)
- skin prick tests to identify allergens.

The severity is also assessed according to which step of treatment the patient is on (BTS/SIGN, 2008).

Clinical features of acute severe asthma include:

- inability to complete sentences
- respiratory rate >25 breaths per minute
- tachycardia 110 beats/min
- PEFR 33–50% of patient's best or predicted.

Life-threatening characteristics include:

- silent chest and cyanosis
- exhaustion confusion and coma
- bradycardia or hypotension
- PEFR <33% of patient's best or predicted
- blood gases: $PaCO_2$ 4.6–6.0 kPa, PaO_2 < 8 kPa.

2   List the medicines available for the acute treatment of asthma and describe the method of administration.

Patients will be prescribed inhalers and tablets and, at a later stage, nebulisers may be used.

Asthma is managed in a stepwise approach using the British Thoracic Society and Scottish Intercollegiate Guidelines Network (2008). Details are available in the *British National Formulary* (*BNF*).

Summary

- **Step 1 Occasional bronchodilator relief** (inhaled short acting beta$_2$-agonist as required).
- **Step 2 Regular inhaled preventer therapy** (inhaled short acting beta$_2$-agonist as required and regular standard dose inhaled corticosteroid).
- **Step 3 Inhaled corticosteroid and long-acting inhaled beta$_2$-agonists** (inhaled short-acting beta$_2$-agonist as required and regular standard-dose

inhaled corticosteroid and regular inhaled long-acting beta$_2$-agonist PLUS at this step either leukotriene receptor antagonist or modified-release oral theophylline or modified-release oral beta$_2$-agonist therapy may be considered).

■ **Step 4 High-dose inhaled corticosteroid and regular bronchodilators** (inhaled short-acting beta$_2$-agonist as required and regular high-dose inhaled corticosteroid and inhaled long-acting beta$_2$-agonist PLUS six-week sequential trial of one or more of leukotriene receptor antagonist or modified-release oral theophylline or modified-release oral beta$_2$-agonist).

■ **Step 5** Patient would be on step 4 then add in regular corticosteroid tablets.

The most important issues in the management of asthma are effective therapeutic management. Virchow *et al.* (2007) have clearly identified that the use of inhaler devices is crucial to effective clinical management. The study suggests several issues that influence treatment including:

■ poor understanding of treatment guidelines in terms of content, implementation and relevance to everyday clinical life,
■ insufficient patient education,
■ lack of access to healthcare and cost of medication, and
■ poor inhaler technique.

Pharmacists have a key role to play in education since inhalation therapy is a vital component of effective asthma management.

3a Describe the role of the pharmacist in the care of this patient.

Pharmacists are responsible for:

■ ensuring that the patient understands their condition and can recognise the signs of acute deterioration and risk of status asthmaticus,
■ counselling the patient on the medication and ensuring they know why, when and how to take the medicines,
■ ensuring that patients know how to monitor the effectiveness of the therapy,
■ ensuring that patients know how often they should visit their GP and ensure appropriate clinical test are completed, and
■ effective medicines management.

3b What are the aims of asthma treatment for the patient and the professional?

The aims of asthma treatment are:

■ effective control of asthma symptoms,
■ positive quality of life, and
■ minimal acute hospital admissions.

4a Explain the social issues this patient will face on discharge.

HT will need to deal with medicines management including supply, impact on her lifestyle and importance of concordance, and lifestyle issues, such as exercise and sports.

4b Critically review the non-pharmacological therapies that are available for people with asthma. Would these be of benefit for this patient?

Non-pharmalogical recommendations could include:

- lifestyle advice (e.g. exercise management and stop smoking),
- the avoidance of precipitating factors (i.e. pollutants, house dust mite, grass pollen and/or fungal spores) by the use of special vacuum cleaners for the house and regular change of bedding,
- flu vaccinations,
- the avoidance of certain medicines (e.g. NSAIDs, aspirin and beta-blockers),
- occupational hazards (e.g. veterinary medicine, bakery and laundry work).

The above parameters are known to be associated with exacerbation of asthma and hence patients need to have an understanding of how to manage their treatment.

4c Discuss the role of an asthma management plan for this patient.

The object of an asthma management plan is to ensure the patient:

- understands the disease,
- can describe the medicine, why it is prescribed and how it should be used,
- is monitored effectively,
- has appropriate health outcomes,
- has effective chronic disease management and prevents exacerbations and hospital admissions.

The pharmacist is responsible for preparing a pharmaceutical care plan for this patient and must include the issues listed in Table A3.1.

Table A3.1

Care issues	Care plan
Patient understanding of medicines	Discuss with the patient the need for each medicine. Side effects and monitoring. Advise on how to administer the medicine.
Use of medicine devices	Educate, monitor and assess the use of the inhalers.
Advise and monitor the patient if she suffers from colds or chest infection	Educate the patient to watch for signs of deterioration and advise when to refer.
Action plans	Routine asthma diary to record peak flows. Advise on management of acute exacerbations. Lifestyle advice.
Patient organisations	Discuss with the patient the availability of patient support, including the Asthma Association.

Case study level 3 – COPD – with co-morbidity – see page 52

1a Describe the clinical signs and symptoms of COPD, explain the pathophysiology and how these relate to the patient.

The clinical signs and symptoms of COPD, the pathophysiology and how this relates to the patient are explained in Table A3.2.

Table A3.2 Clinical signs and symptoms of COPD, the pathophysiology and how this relates to the patient in Case study level 3

Signs and symptoms	Pathophysiology	Patient
Breathlessness	Airflow obstruction, due to airway and parenchymal damage as a result of chronic inflammation that is progressive, not fully reversible.	Shortness of breath
	Due to increased hydrogen ion concentrations and possible increased metabolic rate stimulating the respiratory centre.	RR 20 per min
	Airway narrowing, mucosal damage, oedema of airway and increased sputum production increases the ventilation/perfusion mismatch.	PCO_2 9.67_2 kPa
	The duration of expiration is insufficient to allow the lungs to deflate (due to airway resistance or increased breathing rate).	Lungs hyperinflated

1b What is the interpretation of this patient's pulse oximetry and arterial gases?

Interpretation of this patient's pulse oximetry and arterial gases is shown in Table A3.3.

This is considered to be type II respiratory failure.

Table A3.3 Interpretation of this patient's pulse oximetry and arterial gases

Oxygen saturation: SpO_2 89% on 35% O_2	Normal range	Low, hypoxic (less than 92%)
pH 7.388	7.3–7.5	Acidotic, due to CO_2 retention
PCO_2 9.67 kPa	4.0–6.7 kPa	Raised, hypoventilation
PO_2 6.5 kPa	11–13 kPa	Low

1c　Describe the clinical difference between asthma and COPD.

Asthma and COPD are compared in Table A3.4.

Table A3.4 Asthma and COPD compared

	Asthma	*COPD*
Smoker or ex-smoker	Possibly	Nearly all
Symptoms under age 35	Common	Rare
Chronic productive cough	Uncommon	Common
Breathlessness	Variable	Persistent and progressive
Night time waking with breathlessness and/or wheeze	Common	Uncommon
Significant diurnal or day to day variability of symptoms	Common	Uncommon

NICE COPD Guidelines 2004

2　Comment on the current drug therapy and describe the role of O_2 in this patient.

This patient's current drug therapy is discussed in Table A3.5.

Table A3.5 Current drug therapy for the patient in Case study level 3

Current therapy		*Comments*
Prednisolone	10 mg od	Need to review the duration and need. Will need bisphosphonate for bone protection as osteoporotic
Fluticasone inhaler	500 micrograms BD	Check which device? Accuhaler or Diskhaler. Patient not taking a long acting beta agonist, so why is she on an inhaled corticosteroid?
Aspirin	75 mg od	NICE guidelines post MI
Bumetanide	1 mg od	Loop diuretic, why? BP is low, what evidence of heart failure is there?
Combivent nebs	2 qds	Salbutamol 2.5 mg, ipratropium 500 micrograms in 2.5 mls. Is there a need for regular short acting beta$_2$-agonist? Change to long acting. Why use nebulisers?

continued

Table A3.5 *continued*

Current therapy		Comments
Enalapril	5 mg od	Low dose for heart failure, or is it for high BP, but patient has a low BP!!! On admission.
Uniphyllin Continus	200 mg bd	Theophylline normally used after a trial of short and long-acting bronchodilators. Needs plasma levels monitored. Increased risk of low potassium when given with prednisolone and bumetanide.
Senna	2 tablets nocte	Review the patient's intake and need for laxatives.
Warfarin	5 mg od	INR will need to be checked, 3–6 months duration. Care with drug interactions, anticoagulant effect may be affected by prednisolone, and aspirin. Patients Hb is already at the lower end of normal.
Zopicolone	7.5 mg nocte	Normally only used for 4 weeks, as a hypnotic.
Diclofenac	50 mg prn	Need to change to different pain control as high risk of bleeding when on warfarin and aspirin. Must not be taken as required.
O_2	2 L nasal specs	Nasal specs: difficult to predict the amount of oxygen inspired Need to investigate LTOT for home use.

Role of oxygen

As this patient has a PaO_2 of less than 7.3 kPa and oxygen saturation of arterial blood of less than 90%, she is eligible for Long-Term Oxygen Therapy (LTOT). She will need to use oxygen at least 15 hours a day and needs to be counselled on the importance of smoking cessation. Ambulatory and short-burst oxygen therapy should also be considered, as per NICE guidelines (NICE, 2004).

3   Describe the care plan for this patient, including smoking cessation.

■   Check patient understanding of therapy:

- – discuss with the patient the role of each medicine.
- – check inhaler technique
- – discuss the need to have regular blood pressure checks.

- Offer smoking cessation:

  - – all patients should be encouraged to stop smoking (NICE guidance available)
  - – initial supply to last two weeks after target stop date
  - – nicotine replacement – bupropion or varenicline can be considered.

- Review the use of nebulisers:

  - – review the need for nebulisation, check inspiratory flow rate
  - – consider use of tiotropium.

- Review of changes in treatment: discuss with GP the changes in medicines, especially the warfarin and pain control.
- Check the plan for acute exacerbations: discuss with patient and GP what plan is in place.
- Review the need for bone protection: osteoporosis is present, need to check why no bone protection medication has been given, therefore start if no contraindications.
- Check understanding of anticoagulation: careful monitoring of INR.

4   What are the key aims for this patient and the professional?

The key aims for the patient and the professional are listed in Table A3.6.

Table A3.6 Key aims for the patient and the professional

Patient	Professional
Keep well and not get worse	Reduce exacerbation rate
To carry out normal daily tasks	Maximise symptom relief
Maintain independence if wanted	Co-operate with the patient
Get treatment quickly when needed	Have a plan for exacerbations

5   Explain how spirometry can be used to monitor this patient.

The degree of airflow obstruction should be assessed using:

- FEV_1 (<80% predicted is airway obstruction)
- FEV_1/FVC ratio (<0.7 is airway obstruction)
- vital capacity (VC)
- peak expiratory flow (less informative than spirometry).

Normal FEV_1 excludes COPD as a diagnosis, a normal peak flow does not. The patient inhales maximally and then exhales as forcefully as possible. The volumes recorded are compared with predicted values based on age, sex and height. The ratio of FEV_1/FVC airflow obstruction is diagnosed, as well as the severity.

The VC in COPD may be greater than the FVC, because of floppy airways. Spirometry does not distinguish between airflow obstruction due to asthma and COPD, but in conjunction with reversibility testing it can do so. FEV_1 can therefore be diagnostic, assess severity and prognosis and monitor progression of disease.

6 What are the social issues in treating this patient at home?

Patients may be anxious and refuse such support. The cultural and social setting of the patient needs to be taken into account. As patients lose their mobility and increase dependence on others for help with day-to-day living, anxiety increases. Patients can become hesitant to seek help because of the perception that their condition was self-inflicted. Poor populations tend to have a higher risk of developing COPD, other factors include poor nutrition, crowding, exposure to pollutants, poor access to healthcare and early respiratory infections. Some evidence suggests women are more susceptible to COPD development than men. A multidisciplinary team should be involved in the support of the patient at home. Additional use can be made of nebulisers, compressors, oxygen, visiting respiratory nurses and increased social service input. The patient remains under care of the hospital but the GP is made aware of the extra support. Health status is better in home-treated patients.

COPD is linked with other co-morbid conditions. Patients are more likely to have ischaemic heart disease, pneumonia and diabetes, making treatment more complicated and requiring a holistic approach to care. This patient demonstrates five co-morbidities. These in turn impact on the medication load she has to cope with, so concordance is important.

Case study level Ma – COPD – see page 54

1 Discuss the clinical signs and symptoms for Mr CD.

The clinical signs and symptoms for Mr CD are outlined in Table A3.7.

2a Discuss the role of smoking history and calculate the total pack-years this patient has been subjected to.

Cigarette smoking is the single most important risk factor for the development of COPD. Stopping smoking as COPD becomes more severe has limited impact on its progression. Smokers with impaired lung function are likely to die from complications of atherosclerotic vascular disease. Far more than 15% of smokers get COPD; with enough smoking, all will have reduced lung function. Some

Table A3.7

Clinical signs & symptoms	Notes
Very short of breath at rest	MRC dyspnoea scale (graded 1–5), based on the level of exertion to get breathless, this patient scores 5 (too breathless to leave the house)
Five days ago worsening SOB over previous week, 2 yards (best 30 yards)	
Cough—chronic, no worse, non-productive, chronic wheeze	Due to lung disease may be contributed by the ACE II blocker.
Orthopnoea, sleeps upright, gets PND if flat	Symptom of congestive heart failure, use of diuretics will need to be reviewed.
Poor urinary stream	May be aggravated by the use of ipratopium, this should be reviewed.
Pulse Rate = 115 irregular	Has AF and is taking frequent doses of salbutamol
Respiratory rate, 40 per minute	Tachypnoea, due to possible hypoxia
Bilateral crepitations	Also called crackles, re-opening of small airways (occluded during expiration) could be due to pulmonary oedema from heart failure
FEV_1 1.2L	low
WBC 15.8×10^9/L	Raised—infection
Hb 11g/dL	Low—adverse effect of aspirin?
Neutrophils 14.4×10^9/L	Raised—infection
GGT 169 u/L	Raised—liver congestion from heart failure
C Reactive protein 16 mg/L	Raised—infection
Glucose 18.2 mmol/L	Raised—uncontrolled diabetes

smokers are very susceptible to impaired lung function. Smoking (including occupational exposure) is not the only cause of COPD.

Total pack-years is calculated by multiplying the number of cigarettes per day by the number of years smoked and dividing by 20. In Mr CD's case this is $(40 \times 30)/20 = 60$ pack-years.

2b   What spirometry should be used to assess Mr CD's lung function and what main factors affect the predicted values?

There is no single diagnostic test for COPD. Airflow obstruction = FEV_1 and FEV_1/FVC less than 0.7. Mr CD's FEV_1 = 1.2 L, and that predicted for 80 kg = 4.7 L (25%); therefore <30% predicted = severe airflow obstruction.

Daily monitoring of PEF should not be performed routinely as changes are very small, but it should be measured before discharge.

Reference values may lead to underdiagnosis in the elderly, this is not applicable in black and Asian populations. The values for the black population are 10–15% lower than for white people of similar build. Chinese have been found to have an FVC about 20% lower and Indians about 10% lower than matched white populations.

3   Discuss the role of oxygen and delivery systems during the acute exacerbation.

Oxygen saturation should be measured if there are no facilities to measure arterial blood gases. Do not exceed oxygen saturation of 93%. Start oxygen at 40% and monitor for drowsiness or saturations rising to 93–94%. Blood gases must be repeated according to response. Oxygen is given to keep saturation greater than 90%.

Driving gas for nebulised therapy must be specified in the prescription. If oxygen is needed during nebuliser therapy, nasal cannulae should be used. Care must be taken with the nasal route, as it is difficult to predict the amount of oxygen inspired.

4a   Critically review Mr CD's list of medicines.

Mr CD's medications are reviewed in Table A3.8.

This patient will need a course of antibiotics.

Table A3.8 Review of Mr CD's medicines

Current therapy		Comment
Aspirin	300 mg OD	*AF and IHD
Diltiazem MR (Tildiem LA)	300 mg OD	AF
Bendroflumethazide	2.5 mg OD	*Hypertension
Losartan	50 mg OD	*CCF
Furosemide	80 mg OD	CCF
Atorvastatin	10 mg OD	High cholesterol
Carbocisteine	500 mg qds	*COPD
Insulatard	14 iu BD	Blood glucose
Ferrous sulphate	300 mg TDS	Iron deficient anaemia
Omeprazole	20 mg OD	Cover for aspirin
Alendronate	70 mg weekly	*Long term steroids
Salbutamol	2.5 mg nebulised PRN	COPD
Ipratropium	500 micrograms TDS nebulised	COPD

(*NICE Guidelines)

4b   Discuss the place and route of corticosteroids in Mr CD's management.

Inhaled corticosteroids do have a role in COPD. They should be prescribed for patients with an FEV_1 ≤50% predicted, with two or more exacerbations in 12 months that require antibiotics or oral corticosteroids. These patients are still breathless despite monotherapy with a long-acting beta$_2$-agonist. Maintenance use of oral corticosteroids is not recommended, but some patients with advanced COPD may require them. Oral corticosteroids should be used in all patients admitted to hospital with an exacerbation of COPD. There is insufficient evidence to establish the minimum dose of inhaled corticosteroids to obtain benefit (NICE, 2004).

5   Describe a pharmaceutical care plan for the continued treatment of this patient.

A pharmaceutical care plan is outlined in Table A3.9.

Table A3.9 Pharmaceutical care plan for Mr CD

Care issues	Care plan
Patient understanding of medicines	Discuss with the patient the need for each medicine. Access the need for mucolytic therapy.
Use of medicine devices	Monitor and assess the use of the nebuliser.
Transfer from nebulisers to inhalers	Change to inhaled long acting beta$_2$-agonist and corticosteroid, at least 24 hours before discharge. Could benefit from the use of tiotropium inhaler in place of ipratropium.
Blood glucose	Check the haemoglobin (HbA_{1c}), should be ≤ 7% and review the dose of insulin.
Monitor for chest infection	Raised WCC, with raised neurophils and CRP, will require a course of antibiotics.
Monitor patients nutrition	Check the patients BMI and record the MRC dyspnoea score.
Verify the use of vaccines	Pneumococcal and flu vaccinations are recommended.
Review the need for long term oxygen (LTOT)	LTOT should be assessed in this patient as FEV1 ≤ 30%, and has peripheral oedema.

continued

Table A3.9 *continued*

Care issues	Care plan
Action plans	Evidence for the use of action plans is lacking. Patients should be encouraged to take prompt action if they experience worsening of symptoms; this may involve the use of a course of antibiotics and oral steroids, in which case the GP should be informed as soon as possible.
Patient organisations	Discuss with the patient the availability of patient support, including the British Lung Foundation.

Case study level Mb – Brittle asthma – see page 56

1   Using the data provided, assess the severity of the asthma.

The severity of Ms RJ's asthma is assessed in Table A3.10.

Table A3.10 Assessment of severity of asthma

Parameter	BTS/SIGN May 2008	Severity
Pulse 130 beats per minute	≥ 110/min	Acute severe
Respiratory rate 25 per minute	≥ 25/min	Acute severe
Not able to speak in sentences	Inability to complete sentences in one breath	Acute severe
PEFR 200 L/min (best 450 L/min) 44% of best	33–50% best or predicted	Acute severe
Sudden severe attack	Sudden severe attacks on a background of well controlled asthma	Brittle asthma Type 2

2   Explain the blood gases on admission.

Ms RJ's blood gases are explained in Table A3.11.

Table A3.11 Explanation of Ms RJ's blood gases

Arterial blood gases:		Range	
pH	7.388 on 60% O_2	7.3–7.5	In normal range
PCO_2	4.67 kPa	4.0–6.7 kPa	In normal range
PO_2	24.7 kPa	11–13 kPa	High due to 60% O_2

Tissue hypoxia occurs within 4 minutes of failure to deliver adequate supply. Hyperventilation due to carotid chemoreceptor stimulation becomes noticeable when PO_2 falls to 5.3. Arterial oxygen saturation should be between 95–100%. This patient has a good saturation figure of 99.6%.

3a   Describe the role of Ms RJ's discharge therapy.

Ms RJ's discharge therapy is outlined in Table A3.12.

3b   Critically review the role of magnesium in acute asthma.

Magnesium has been established in clinical practice in acute emergency therapy as an adjunct to standard treatment with bronchodilators and corticosteroids. Magnesium has bronchodilatory effects, the exact mechanism of action of which is unclear, as it affects a number of pathways. A single dose of i.v. magnesium sulphate 1.2–2 g over 20 minutes is recommended (BTS/SIGN, 2008); repeated doses have not been assessed. Repeated doses can cause hypermagnesaemia, causing respiratory depression.

3c   Discuss the issue of non-steroidal anti-inflammatory drugs in asthma.

Aspirin-induced asthma has an onset of 30 minutes to 3 hours after ingestion. Affected individuals are cross-sensitive to all non-steroidal anti-inflammatory drugs (NSAIDs). Paracetamol is seldom associated with cross-sensitivity in patients with aspirin-induced asthma. Aspirin-induced asthma is believed to involve inhibition of COX-1. Patients should be provided with information on which drugs these are.

4a   Describe the role of theophylline in asthma.

Theophylline has several effects which have been described, especially in asthma:

- bronchial smooth muscle relaxation
- increase in mucociliary clearance
- inhibition of release of mediators
- decrease of pulmonary hypertension and increase in right ventricular ejection fraction

Table A3.12 Ms RJ's discharge therapy

Salbutamol nebuliser 5 mg prn	Short-acting β_2 agonist	At least 24 hours before discharge the patient should have been changed to aerosol or dry powder inhalers.
Salmeterol inhaler 100 micrograms bd	As Accuhaler, Evohaler or Diskhaler. Long-acting β_2 agonist	No evidence to decide which device should be used in patients who cannot use pMDI. Inhaler technique must be reassessed and device found that is suitable for the patient.
Budesonide inhaler 800 micrograms BD	Corticosteroid	The role of high-dose corticosteroids as an adjunct to, or in place of, systemic ones has not been resolved. Using both in life-threatening asthma in those who respond poorly to normal treatment is worthwhile.
Theophylline SR 200 mg bd	Bronchodilator	As Uniphyllin Continus. Brand name should be specified.
Prednisolone 50 mg daily	Corticosteroid, 40–50 mg for at least five days or until recovery.	Can be stopped abruptly provided patient receives inhaled steroids. Patients requiring prednisolone for over three months should be prescribed a long-acting bisphosphonate.
Omeprazole 20 mg OD	Proton pump inhibitor	Gastro-oesophageal reflux should be treated, but this does not have a direct effect on asthma control.

- improved contractility of fatigued diaphragmatic muscle
- central stimulation of ventilation.

Possible mechanisms include:

- inhibition of cyclic nucleotide phosphodiesterases,
- interaction with guanine nucleotide regulatory proteins (G proteins),
- adenosine antagonism,
- effects via increased catecholamine release, and
- inhibition of the formation of intracellular second messengers such as inositol triphosphate.

Intravenous aminophylline is used in patients with a poor response to initial therapy; levels must be measured.

4b   Critically review the role of anti-IgE monoclonal antibody for Ms RJ.

Anti-IgE monoclonal antibody (omalizumab) is of benefit in highly selected patients. It is given fortnightly or monthly as a subcutaneous injection. It is licensed for use by doctors experienced in severe persistent asthma. Published evidence in severe allergic asthma is poor. Trials so far have been relatively short term.

There is a large variation in annual cost. This is partly because the dose is determined by a patient's IgE level and body weight.

There is a lack of data on suppressing serum IgE systems long term.

Omalizumab is licensed as add-on therapy, in patients with the following:

- positive skin test to an aeroallergen
- FEV_1 below 80%
- multiple daytime or night-time symptoms
- frequent documented exacerbations, and
- have been having standard therapy i.e. high dose inhaled corticosteroids (more than 800 micrograms of beclometasone) and long-acting inhaled beta$_2$-agonists.

Omalizumab should only be used if the asthma is IgE-mediated. It has been reported that patients requiring daily prednisolone to control their asthma are unlikely to respond. This lady is already on high dose oral corticosteroids, and long-acting inhaled beta$_2$-agonists, but with no details of her IgE level, and this needs to be checked before a decision is made.

5a   Discuss the issues in variability of peak expiratory flow.

The term 'brittle' asthma was first used in 1977 to describe patients who maintained a wide variation in PEFR despite high-dose inhaled steroids. This has been reviewed and described by Ayres *et al.* (1998) based on the magnitude of diurnal PEFR variability, rather than the pattern of variability. They also describe two subclasses: maintained wide PEF variability (type 1, >40% diurnal variation for >50% of the time over at least 150 days) or sudden onset of acute airway obstruction (type 2, occurring in less than 3 hours without obvious trigger).

PEF is effort dependent and thought to measure large-calibre airway function. FEV_1 has both effort-dependent and effort-independent characteristics. It is thought to measure intermediate and smaller airways.

PEF should be recorded as the best of three forced expiratory blows with a pause of 2 seconds before each. The patient can be either standing or sitting.

PEF variability is calculated as the difference between the highest and lowest PEF, expressed as a percentage of either the mean or highest PEF.

5b   What other therapy could be considered? Devise a care plan.

Other treatments to be considered:

- increase budesonide to 2000 micrograms daily
- leukotriene receptor antagonists
- methotrexate
- ciclosporin
- oral gold
- subcutaneous terbutaline infusion.

Care plan

Before discharge:

- check use of inhalers,
- advise patient to make an early follow-up appointment with GP,
- check patient can use a peak flow meter and that they know at what stage to seek medical help, and
- check patient has an asthma self-mangement plan.

6   Discuss the factors that predict poor compliance with asthma treatment.

Adherence to prophylactic asthma medications is affected by many factors:

- age – younger adults have less adherence than older working-age adults; problems may arise in the elderly due to poor coordination, vision and cognitive impairment,
- cost of treatment,
- educational level,
- lower socioeconomic status,
- fear of dependency and lack of control,
- lack of insight into illness,
- complexity of treatment,
- effect of peer pressure to appear normal,
- duration of disease,
- concern over side-effects of treatment, and
- poor concordance.

Simple written instructions increase compliance.

4

Central nervous system case studies

Fabrizio Schifano

Case study level 1 – A case of insomnia

Learning outcomes

Level 1 case study: You will be able to:

- describe the risk factors
- describe the disease
- describe the pharmacology of the drug
- outline the formulation, including drug molecule, excipients, etc. for the medicines
- summarise basic social pharmacy issues (e.g. opening containers, large labels).

Scenario

Mr AB, a 21-year-old, white European, pharmacy student came to the local pharmacy last week with a 7-day prescription for diazepam 10 mg tablets, one to be taken at night. The drug was prescribed to him by his GP because some five weeks ago Mr AB started suffering from insomnia. In fact, although he is typically supposed to wake up at 7.00am to attend his lectures, at 4.00am he is already fully awake. He does not find it difficult to fall asleep, nor does he wake up too frequently during the night. During the day, he feels very tired, anxious and tearful. It is now 3 days since you dispensed his prescription and the patient has returned to you because he claims he is still not able to sleep properly.

1   How is insomnia defined?
2a What are the risk factors for its development?
2b Does Mr AB have any of the risk factors for developing insomnia?
3a What group of drugs does diazepam belong to? What are the main pharmacokinetic differences between the components of this class of drugs?
3b What is the mechanism of action of diazepam in the treatment of insomnia?
3c What are the side-effects of diazepam?
4a What formulations are available for diazepam?
4b What alternative preparation(s) could you recommend for Mr AB?
5   What counselling could you give Mr AB to help try and resolve the issue?

General references

Breimer DD, Jochemsen R and von Albert HH (1980) Pharmacokinetics of benzodiazepines. Short-acting versus long-acting. *Arzneimittelforschung* 30: 875–881.

Curran HV, Schifano F and Lader MH (1991) Models of memory dysfunctions? A comparison of the effects of lorazepam and scopolamine on memory, psychomotor performance and mood. *Psychopharmacology (Berlin)* 10: 83–90.

Hindmarch I (2005) Medicines in the workplace: the effects of prescribed and OTC drugs on performance. In: Ghodse AH (ed.) *Addiction at Work: Tackling Drug Use and Misuse in the Workplace*. London: Gower Publishing Ltd.

Joint Formulary Committee (2008) *British National Formulary 55*. London: British Medical Association and Royal Pharmaceutical Society of Great Britain, March.

Leger D, Guilleminault C, Dreyfus JP *et al.* (2000) Prevalence of insomnia in a survey of 12,778 adults in France. *Journal of Sleep Research* 9: 35–42.

Schifano F (1991) Ansiolitici benzodiazepinici (alprazolam, bromazepam, camazepam, clobazam, clorazepato dipotassico, clordiazepossido, clotiazepam, delorazepam, diazepam, estazolam, flunitrazepam, fluoresone, flurazepam, glaziovina, lorazepam, lormetazepam, mebutamato, medazepam, meprobamato, nitrazepam, nordiazepam, oxazepam, pinazepam, prazepam, temazepam, triazolam, valnottamide). In: Casiglia E and Gava R (eds) *L'Annuario dei Farmaci. Farmacologia Clinica e Terapia*. Padova: Piccin Nuova Libraria, (I), pp. 111–129.

Schifano F (2005) Substance misuse in the workplace. In: Ghodse AH (ed.) *Addiction at Work: Tackling Drug Use and Misuse in the Workplace*. London: Gower Publishing Ltd.

Schifano F and Magni G (1989) Panic attacks and major depression after discontinuation of long-term diazepam abuse. *Drug Intelligence and Clinical Pharmacy; the Annals of Pharmacotherapy* 23: 989–990.

Case study level 2 – A case of eating disorder (bulimia nervosa)

Learning outcomes

Level 2 case study: You will be able to:

- interpret relevant lab and clinical data
- identify monitoring and referral criteria
- explain treatment choices
- describe goals of therapy including monitoring and the role of the pharmacist/clinician
- describe issues – counselling points, adverse drug reactions, drug interactions, complementary/alternative therapies and lifestyle advice.

Scenario

Ms CD, a 24-year-old white British woman, presents to your pharmacy asking for some information around use of laxatives and diuretics. On further questioning, it appears that she seems to be obsessed with her body weight. Her height is 1.64 m and her weight is 56 kg. Her food intake is quite irregular, being characterised by periodical binges followed by fasting periods. She reports that some recent blood tests have shown a few electrolyte imbalances, including sodium 130 mmol/L, but she doesn't understand what this means.

Questions

1a Calculate Ms CD's body mass index (BMI).
1b What would be causing Ms CD's electrolyte imbalances?
2 Monitoring and referral criteria; what signs and symptoms should you look out for which could indicate a patient may have an eating disorder?
3 What are the treatment choices for the management of bulimia?
4 Ms CD was eventually prescribed fluoxetine 60 mg daily by her GP. What are the goals of therapy, including monitoring and the role of the pharmacist/clinician?
5 What are the social pharmacy issues of this case, including alternative therapies and lifestyle advice?

General references

Newcastle University School of Neurology, Neurobiology & Psychiatry, Faculty of Medical

Sciences (2005) Antidepressants. Available at http://www.ncl.ac.uk/nnp/teaching/management/drugrx/antdep.html [Accessed on 2 April 2007].

NICE (National Institute for Health and Clinical Excellence) (2004a) Eating disorders full guideline. Available at www.nice.org.uk/CG009fullguideline [Accessed 1 July 2008].

NICE (2004b) Anorexia nervosa, bulimia nervosa and related eating disorders. Understanding NICE guidance: a guide for people with eating disorders, their advocates and carers, and the public. Available at www.nice.org.uk/CG009NICE guideline [Accessed 1 July 2008].

NICE (2004c) Depression. Available at www.nice.org.uk/CG023NICEguideline [Accessed 1 July 2008].

Winstead NS and Willard SG (2006) Gastrointestinal complaints in patients with eating disorders. *Journal of Clinical Gastroenterology* 40: 678–682.

Case study level 3 – A case of dementia, Alzheimer's type

Learning outcomes

Level 3 case study: You will be able to:

- interpret clinical signs and symptoms
- evaluate laboratory data
- evaluate treatment options
- state goals of therapy
- describe a pharmaceutical care plan to include advice to a clinician
- describe the prognosis and long-term complications
- describe the social pharmacy issues which could include supply (e.g. complex treatments at home, concordance and compliance) and lifestyle issues.

Scenario

The wife of Mr EF, a 68-year-old black Caribbean male, is asking for some advice from the village pharmacist because she is concerned about the changes in behaviour her husband has been showing over the last few months. In contrast with Mr EF's previous personality, his mood is now very volatile and somewhat unpredictable, his memory and concentration seem to be very poor and, at times, he may be very impulsive indeed. For the first time in his life he is now using words and language expressions that are both rude and vulgar. The assessment carried out by the local old age psychiatrist showed that Mr EF was mildly confused, with both a decrease in blood pressure (100/65 mmHg) and a sodium level of 155 mmol/L. He was finally diagnosed with Alzheimer's type dementia.

Questions

1   What are the Alzheimer's type dementia clinical signs and symptoms?
2   Expand briefly on the neuropathological changes observed in Alzheimer's dementia; comment on Mr EF's clinical and laboratory data.
3   What are the suitable treatment options for Mr EF?
4   Outline a pharmaceutical care plan for Mr EF. What are the goals of therapy in Alzheimer's dementia?
5   Expand on the monitoring of long-term treatment with antidementia medication.
6   Describe the prognosis and long-term complications of Alzheimer's dementia.
7   What are the social pharmacy issues related to the case of Mr EF?

References

Alzheimer's Society (2006) Anger as NICE says no to Alzheimer's appeal. Available at http://www.alzheimers.org.uk/News_and_Campaigns/News/10102006nice_says_no.htm [Accessed 1 July 2008].
NICE (National Institute for Health and Clinical Excellence) (2006) NICE announces Alzheimer's disease drug appeal outcome and NHS guideline to support patients and carers. Available at http://www.nice.org.uk/page.aspx?o=373237 [Accessed 1 July 2008].

General references

Newcastle University School of Neurology, Neurobiology & Psychiatry, Faculty of Medical Sciences (2005) Atypicals. Available at http://www.ncl.ac.uk/nnp/teaching/management/ drugrx/antpsych.html [Accessed 1 July 2008].
Schifano F (2002) Pharmacokinetic and pharmacodynamic considerations in old age psychopharmacology. In: Copeland JRM, Abou-Saleh M and Blazer DG (eds) *Principles and Practice of Geriatric Psychiatry*. Chichester: John Wiley & Sons Ltd, pp. 61–64.

Case study level Ma – A case of schizophrenia

Learning outcomes

Level M case study: You will be able to:

- interpret clinical signs and symptoms
- evaluate laboratory data
- critically appraise treatment options
- state goals of therapy
- describe a pharmaceutical care plan to include advice to a clinician
- describe the prognosis and long-term complications
- describe the social pharmacy issues which could include supply (e.g. complex treatments at home, concordance and compliance) and lifestyle issues
- describe the monitoring of therapy.

Scenario

Mr GH, a 25-year-old white British PhD student, comes to your pharmacy in quite a distressed state. He is totally unkempt and smells of body odours; his mood is volatile and he reports to you that he has sensations of insects crawling under his skin. Over the last few days he has been feeling sick, and he is absolutely convinced that this is because his neighbour somehow put some toxic gases into his flat. He brings you some of his vomit to be analysed, so that his concerns will now be 'demonstrated' and he will be able to take appropriate action against his neighbour.

Questions

1   What are the most typical signs and symptoms of schizophrenia?
2   Is there any routine role of laboratory data in making a diagnosis of schizophrenia?
3   Please evaluate and critically appraise available treatment options for schizophrenia; expand on their side-effects.
4   Describe a pharmaceutical care plan in the case reported here?
5a What are the goals of therapy of schizophrenia?
5b Expand on the monitoring of therapy in schizophrenia and risk of medication non-compliance.
5c What are the social pharmacy issues relevant to the condition of schizophrenia?

6   Please expand on the prognosis and comorbidity issues relevant to the condition of schizophrenia.

7   Are there alternative, non-pharmacological therapies for the treatment of schizophrenia?

References

Gharabawi GM, Greenspan A, Rupnow MF *et al.* (2006) Reduction in psychotic symptoms as a predictor of patient satisfaction with antipsychotic medication in schizophrenia: Data from a randomized double-blind trial. *BMC Psychiatry* 61: 45.

Newcastle University School of Neurology, Neurobiology & Psychiatry, Faculty of Medical Sciences (2005) Antipsychotics. Available at http://www.ncl.ac.uk/nnp/teaching/management/drugrx/antpsych.html [Accessed on 1 July 2008].

Perrella C, Carrus D, Costa E and Schifano F (2007) Quetiapine for the treatment of borderline personality disorder; an open label study. *Progress in Neuropsychopharmacology and Biological Psychiatry* 31: 158–163.

Schifano F, Zamparutti G and Zambello F (2004) Substance misuse in adolescence: theoretical and clinical issues. *Progress in Neurology and Psychiatry* 8: 25–34.

General references

Carr VJ, Lewin TJ and Neil AL (2006) What is the value of treating schizophrenia? *Australian and New Zealand Journal of Psychiatry* 40: 963–971.

NICE (National Institute for Health and Clinical Excellence) (2002a) Treating and managing schizophrenia (core interventions). Understanding NICE guidance – information for people with schizophrenia, their advocates and carers, and the public. Available at http://www.nice.org.uk/nice media/pdf/CG1publicinfo.pdf [Accessed on 1 July 2008].

NICE (2002b) Schizophrenia: core interventions in the treatment and management of schizophrenia in primary and secondary care. Available at http://www.nice.org.uk/nicemedia/pdf/CG1NICEguideline.pdf [Accessed 4 July 2008].

UK Medicines Information (2004) Aripiprazole. Available at www.ukmi.nhs.uk/NewMaterial/html/docs/AripiprazoleNMP0604.pdf [Accessed on 1 July 2008].

Case study level Mb – A case of buprenorphine high-dose prescribing in heroin addiction

Learning outcomes

Level M case study: You will be able to:

- interpret clinical signs and symptoms
- evaluate laboratory data
- critically appraise treatment options
- state goals of therapy
- describe a pharmaceutical care plan to include advice to a clinician
- describe the prognosis and long-term complications
- describe the social pharmacy issues which could include supply (e.g. complex treatments at home, concordance and compliance) and lifestyle issues
- describe the monitoring of therapy.

Scenario

Mr IJ, a 33-year-old white British male, stopped working as an IT engineer 4 years ago. He recently turned out to be both hepatitis B and C positive, whilst his HIV test was negative. He started using heroin at the age of 18, but this became a major problem some 6 years ago. At that time, Mr IJ started to be prescribed with methadone. He came to your pharmacy today because he would like to be switched to buprenorphine high-dose. In fact, some of his acquaintances told him that while buprenorphine is not as addictive as methadone, it is just as successful in controlling drug cravings.

Questions

1 What are the diagnostic criteria for substance dependence?
2 Which biological fluids are usually taken to monitor drug dependence?
3 What are the prominent pharmacological characteristics of methadone and buprenorphine? How is the dosage titration process carried out when a treatment with either methadone or buprenorphine is started?
4 What are the key differences between buprenorphine and methadone?
5 Please expand on the pharmaceutical care plan for Mr IJ and on issues relevant to monitoring of his therapy.
6 What are the buprenorphine-containing formulations licensed for treatment of opiate addiction in the UK? What are the goals of opiate dependence treatment?

7   Please expand on the social pharmacy issues appropriate for this case, including supply, concordance, compliance and lifestyle issues.
8   Describe the prognosis and long-term complications of drug addiction?
9   Is there a role for herbal medicine in the treatment of addiction?

Reference

Ghodse AH, Szendrey K, Schifano F and Carver S (2006) Report to the Home Office by the International Expert Group on Herbal Medicine in the Treatment of Addictions. The International Centre for Drug Policy (ICDP), St George's, University of London.

General references

Corkery J, Schifano F, Ghodse AH and Oyefeso A (2004) Methadone effects and its role in fatalities. *Human Psychopharmacology: Clinical and Experimental* 19: 565–576.
Gilvarry E and Schifano F (2002) Medical use of buprenorphine in the UK. Special report prepared for the WHO, February, pp. 1–93.
Schifano F, Corkery J, Gilvarry E *et al.* (2005) Buprenorphine mortality, seizures and prescription data in the UK (1980–2002). *Human Psychopharmacology: Clinical and Experimental* 20: 343–348.
Schifano F, Zamparutti G, Zambello F *et al.* (2006) Review of deaths related to analgesic- and cough suppressant-opioids, England and Wales, 1996–2002. *Pharmaco-psychiatry* 39: 185–191.

Answers

Case study level 1 – A case of insomnia – see page 80

1   How is insomnia defined?

Insomnia is characterised by the incapacity to sleep and/or to remain asleep for a reasonable period, which may vary from individual to individual. The sleep disturbance is observed at least three times per week and for at least one month.

2a   What are the risk factors for its development?
2b   Does Mr AB have any of the risk factors for developing insomnia?

Some of the most common risk factors for development of insomnia are as follows:

■   Depression; typically, depressed individuals wake up earlier than usual, e.g. at least 2 hours before the scheduled time. For this reason, in the case presented one might suspect the existence of an underlying depression.

■   Excessive use of alcohol; excessive use of caffeine: Mr AB might have recently increased his alcohol intake. A possible recent increase in caffeine intake might be associated with the need to cope with his pending academic commitments.

■   Stress, pain: Mr AB may be suffering from a short-term, exam-related, stressful situation.

■   Hypomanic/manic episodes: in people with bipolar disorder.

■   Circadian rhythm sleep disorders: jet lag; insomnia experienced by shift workers; and delayed sleep phase syndrome (sometimes seen in students who are enjoying their first experiences outside the family environment and who go to bed too late). This is something that should be discussed with the present client.

■   Nocturnal polyuria, sometimes observed in conditions such as: diabetes, kidney diseases, prostate enlargement, hormonal imbalances, use of diuretics.

■   Sleep apnoea: interrupts the normal breathing stimulus of the central nervous system and the person must actually wake up to resume breathing.

3a   What group of drugs does diazepam belong to? What are the main pharmacokinetic differences between the components of this class of drugs?

Diazepam is a benzodiazepine. Diazepam is more reliably absorbed following oral rather than intramuscular admininstration. This may be due to precipitation in the muscle. Diazepam appears to undergo enterohepatic recirculation with a second plasma peak occurring 4–6 hours after initial administration. This may be associated with re-sedation. Diazepam is oxidised in the liver to active metabolites including desmethyldiazepam (nordiazepam), which has a half-life of over 100 hours. Benzodiazepine oxidation may be impaired in patients with liver disease and in some elderly patients. Metabolism of benzodiazepines such as oxazepam and lorazepam is not impaired in the elderly and in those with liver dysfunction.

Benzodiazepines have five major clinical indications:

■   as anti-anxiety agents
■   as sedative hypnotics
■   as anticonvulsants
■   as muscle relaxants
■   as amnestic agents.

This fivefold clinical activity is possessed, to a greater or lesser extent, by all benzodiazepines in current clinical use. The properties of benzodiazepines make them ideally useful for managing anxiety (e.g. diazepam, chlordiazepoxide, lorazepam); insomnia (e.g. diazepam, temazepam, nitrazepam, loprazolam, flurazepam, lormetazepam); epilepsy (e.g. clobazam, diazepam, lorazepam); sports injuries where muscle relaxation is required (e.g. diazepam) and as pre-medications prior to surgery (e.g. midazolam, lorazepam). The benzodiazepines have a number of other uses, including management of alcohol withdrawal syndrome (chlordiazepoxide, diazepam) and restless legs (clonazepam). Short duration of action may be useful (e.g. for falling asleep), although longer duration of action may be desired (e.g. in treatment of sleep-maintenance disturbances or for seizure control).

Among the different benzodiazepines large variation exists in respect to their pharmacokinetic properties. Those benzodiazepines that have the long-acting metabolite N-desmethyldiazepam in common (diazepam, prazepam, clorazepate) are eliminated relatively slowly, others are metabolised rather rapidly (e. g. oxazepam, temazepam, triazolam). Pharmacokinetic parameters constitute the basis for a rational dosage regimen. In anticonvulsant and anti-anxiety treatment stable blood levels of the drug are pursued, so that compounds with long elimination half-lives of parent drug or active metabolites are of advantage. Conversely, if a benzodiazepine is taken as an hypnotic, the duration of action should be restricted to the night, hence a compound with a short elimination half-life is to be preferred.

3b   What is the mechanism of action of diazepam in the treatment of insomnia?

Benzodiazepine agonists and other agonist ligands at the benzodiazepine site achieve their therapeutic effects by enhancing the actions of the inhibitory neurotransmitter gamma-aminobutyric acid (GABA) at its receptor. Benzodiazepines have a binding site on the GABA-A receptor, which forms a channel through the membrane and opens and closes to control chloride flow into the cell. When benzodiazepine agonists act on their receptor site, GABA produces a more frequent opening of the channel, so that the flow of chloride is increased. As a result, the neuron will be less likely to go through depolarisation, which ultimately results in neuronal inhibition. For this reason, all GABAergic drugs produce sedation. Type I and type II GABA receptors have been identified; benzodiazepines bind with relative non-selectivity to both types. There are several other drugs which are also ligands of the GABA–chloride ion receptor complex, notably barbiturates, chloral hydrate and the newer non-benzodiazepine hypnotics, zopiclone, zolpidem and zaleplon ('Z'-drugs). The Z-drugs are likely to possess smaller residual next day sequelae than clinically equivalent doses of most benzodiazepines.

3c   What are the side-effects of diazepam?

Any prescription for benzodiazepines must be preceded by a careful risk–benefit analysis considering the issues of an individual's particular life situation, personality style and psychiatric diagnosis. Risks of both abuse and cognitive/psychomotor impairments have to be balanced against therapeutic benefits.

The most common side-effects of benzodiazepines in routine clinical use are drowsiness, muscle weakness, lightheadedness, dizziness, ataxia, dysarthria, blurring of vision, confusion and apathy. Because of pharmacokinetic changes of pro-nordiazepam molecules (e.g. diazepam) associated with ageing, the elderly may be at increased risk. There may be an association between benzodiazepine use and the risk of falls and/or hip fractures in the elderly. For those benzodiazepines given at bedtime for sleep induction and/or sleep maintenance in patients with insomnia, the problem arises when the clinically desired effect of nocturnal sedation carries over into the early part of the next day. Patients who work in any high accident risk environment (e.g. with heavy machinery) as well as those where cognitive failure could cause accident to themselves or others should be warned about possible interactions of benzodiazepines with alcohol. Finally, increased hostility and aggression ('paradoxical effects') can sometimes be observed following ingestion of these drugs, especially in borderline personality disorders and in the elderly. Both benzodiazepines and newer non-benzodiazepine molecules possess a significant addiction liability; typical rebound and withdrawal symptoms may be observed if the drug is not carefully titrated down.

4a   What formulations are available for diazepam?

Diazepam formulations include: tablets: 2 mg; 5 mg; 10 mg. Oral solution: 2 mg/5 mL. Strong oral solution: 5 mg/5 mL. Injection (solution): diazepam 5 mg/mL. Formulation for intravenous injection or infusion (emulsion): 5 mg/mL. Rectal solution: 2 mg/mL; 1.25 mL (2.5 mg); 2.5 mL (5 mg) tube; 4 mg/mL, 2.5 mL (10 mg). Suppositories: 10 mg. Dental prescribing on NHS: tablets or oral solution 2 mg/5 mL.

4b   What alternative preparation(s) could you recommend for Mr AB?

Diazepam is better indicated if insomnia is associated with daytime anxiety. Other benzodiazepines prescribed for insomnia include: nitrazepam, flurazepam, loprazolam, lormetazepam and temazepam. The non-benzodiazepine hypnotics zaleplon, zolpidem and zopiclone are not licensed for long-term use. The sedative antipsychotic promethazine hydrochloride is sometimes used to facilitate sleep, with a 25–50 mg recommended dose. Melatonin has proved effective for some clients, mostly in regulating the sleep/waking cycle. Although evidence of efficacy is limited, some clients use herbs such as valerian and chamomile. If Mr AB will finally be diagnosed with depression, a trial with an antidepressant will be indicated.

5   What counselling could you give Mr AB to help try and resolve the issue?

Relevant sleep hygiene issues may be discussed with the client. Some traditional remedies for insomnia have included drinking warm milk before bedtime, taking a warm bath in the evening; exercising vigorously for half an hour in the afternoon, having only a light evening meal, avoiding mentally stimulating activities in the evening hours, and making sure to get up early in the morning and to go to bed at a reasonable hour. Mr AB should seriously consider the possibility of tapering down gradually his caffeine intake and might want to avoid any excessive intake of alcohol. Distractions in the bedroom, including excessive light and noise (e.g. from television) should be avoided. Finally, Mr AB should be informed that with a continuous, long-term (e.g. more than 3–12 weeks), prescription of benzodiazepines both tolerance and dependence have been described.

Case study level 2 – A case of eating disorder (bulimia nervosa) – see page 82

1a   Calculate Ms CD's body mass index (BMI).

The calculation of the BMI is given by the following formula: weight (kg)/ height (m)^2 (calculations are not to be carried out using the Imperial system). In this case: $56/1.64^2 = 20.8$. The BMI normal value is in the range of 20–25.

1b   What would be causing Ms CD's electrolyte imbalances?

Due to frequent laxative intake and vomiting induction, a related electrolyte imbalance may be observed in people with bulimia. Sodium normal reference values are in the range of 133–147 mmol/L.

2   Monitoring and referral criteria; what signs and symptoms should you look out for which could indicate a patient may have an eating disorder?

Bulimia nervosa is an illness in which people feel that they have lost control over their eating. People with bulimia nervosa show a cycle of eating large quantities of food (e.g. 'binge eating'), and then either vomiting, taking laxatives and diuretics, or excessive exercising and fasting, in order to prevent weight increase. Most bulimic clients' weight is normal. Low weight or recent significant loss of weight; excessive concern about weight; vomiting are the most obvious warning signs. Referral issues: the first step will often be given by an assessment and possible treatment by a psychiatrist with special training in eating disorders. Most bulimic clients can be treated as outpatients; an inpatient treatment may be considered when either the client's suicide risk or severe self-harm need to be managed.

3   What are the treatment choices for the management of bulimia?

Adults with bulimia nervosa may be offered a trial with an antidepressant drug. Patients should be informed that antidepressant drugs can reduce the frequency of binge eating and purging. Selective serotonin reuptake inhibitors (SSRIs), and specifically fluoxetine, are the drugs of first choice for the treatment of bulimia nervosa. For these clients, the typical dose of fluoxetine (e.g. 60 mg daily) is higher than that for the treatment of depression. These drugs selectively block the reuptake of 5-HT, leading to neuronal adaptive processes that produce the therapeutic effect.

4   Ms CD was eventually prescribed fluoxetine 60 mg daily by her GP. What are the goals of therapy including monitoring and the role of the pharmacist/clinician?

People with bulimia can experience a range of physical problems. Those who are vomiting frequently or taking large quantities of laxatives should have their fluid and electrolyte balance assessed. When supplementation is required to restore electrolyte balance, oral rather than intravenous administration is recommended, unless there are problems with gastrointestinal absorption. Fluoxetine, especially when given at high dosages, might be associated with a number of side-effects, including nausea, anorexia, transient increase in anxiety levels and insomnia, headache and sexual dysfunction (delayed ejaculation, anorgasmia). Both the clinician and the pharmacist should proactively explore these issues with their patients at each assessment.

5   What are the social pharmacy issues of this case, including alternative therapies and lifestyle advice?

Fluoxetine has a long half-life, which may be useful in patients who occasionally forget their medication and in helping to prevent any discontinuation syndrome on tapering down the dosage. Prescribers will gradually reduce the SSRI doses of the drug over a four-week period, although some people may require longer periods. Fluoxetine can usually be stopped over a shorter period. For patients at high risk of suicide, a limited quantity of antidepressants should be prescribed. When a patient with depression is assessed to be at high risk of suicide, the use of additional support such as more frequent direct contacts with primary care staff or telephone contacts should be considered. Particularly in the initial stages of SSRI treatment, healthcare professionals should actively seek out signs of akathisia, suicidal ideation, and increased anxiety and agitation. When prescribing an SSRI, consideration should be given to using a product in a generic form.

When communicating with both clients or carers, healthcare professionals should use a non-technical language. Where possible, all services should provide written material in the language of the patient. Since people with bulimia are typically female, sometimes a same-gender clinician might be preferred by the client. Community-based healthcare professionals often play an important part in first identifying eating disorders. Both the client and the family should be informed about self-help and support groups for people with eating disorders and how to contact them.

Case study level 3 – A case of dementia, Alzheimer's type – see page 83

1   What are the Alzheimer's type dementia clinical signs and symptoms?

Alzheimer's disease is a neurodegenerative disease characterised by progressive cognitive deterioration accompanied by neurological, psychiatric and behavioural disorders. It is characterised by loss of short-term memory (amnesia), accompanied by a relative integrity of older memories. As the disorder progresses, cognitive impairment extends to the domains of language (aphasia), skilled movements (apraxia), recognition (agnosia), decision-making and planning. Either disinhibition and outbursts of violence, or excessive passivity, can be frequently observed. The onset of Alzheimer's disease is insidious and slow, often making diagnosis difficult.

2   Expand briefly on the neuropathological changes observed in Alzheimer's dementia; comment on Mr EF's clinical and laboratory data.

Typical Alzheimer's disease pathological processes include neuronal loss or atrophy at the temporoparietal and frontal cortex, together with an inflammatory response and the deposition of amyloid plaques and neurofibrillary tangles. Functional neuroimaging studies can provide a supporting diagnostic role. However, Alzheimer's disease remains a primarily clinical diagnosis based on the presence of characteristic neurological features and the absence of alternative diagnoses; there are no typical biochemical markers.

For measurement of cognitive outcomes in Alzheimer's disease, the MMSE (Mini Mental State Examination) instrument, scored out of 30 (best), is used. Mild Alzheimer's disease is usually associated with an MMSE of 21–26. Moderate Alzheimer's disease is usually associated with an MMSE of 10–20 (NICE, 2006).

Hypotension, increase in sodium levels and confusion found here might suggest a moderate level of dehydration, which must be corrected.

3   What are the suitable treatment options for Mr EF?

Based on cost–benefit reasons, NICE (2006) recommendations state that:

- donepezil, galantamine and rivastigmine should be used as a treatment for moderate stages of Alzheimer's disease only (i.e. those with an MMSE score of between 10 and 20 points) and
- memantine, previously used to treat more severe stages of the disease, has been withdrawn from the NHS.

4   Outline a pharmaceutical care plan for Mr EF. What are the goals of therapy in Alzheimer's dementia?

People with dementia may at some point in their illness develop symptoms such as depression, restlessness, aggressive behaviour and psychosis (delusions and hallucinations). Possible medications to be prescribed include atypical anti-psychotics, although some of these drugs (risperidone and olanzapine) have been determined to be unsuitable for use in people with dementia because of the high risk of stroke. Furthermore, prescription of these drugs might be associated with accelerating rates of decline and disease progression in people with demen-tia. Sodium valproate and carbamazepine are sometimes also used to reduce aggression and agitation. Antidepressants may be helpful not only in improving persistently low mood but also in controlling both the irritability and the rapid mood swings that often occur in dementia. Tricyclic antidepressants, such as amitriptyline, imipramine or dothiepin, are likely to increase confusion in those who suffer from dementia. They might also cause dry mouth, blurred vision, constipation, difficulty in urination and hypotension, which may lead to falls and injuries. Newer antidepressants are preferable as first-line treatments for depression in dementia. SSRIs are likely to be better tolerated by older people. Sleep disturbances can be distressing for the person with dementia and disturb-ing for carers. Hypnotics are often best used intermittently.

5   Expand on the monitoring of long-term treatment with antidementia medication.

Patients who continue to be prescribed on a long-term basis with one of the above antidementia medication should be reviewed by MMSE score and global, functional and behavioural assessment every six months. The drug should normally only be continued while their MMSE score remains above 10 points, and clients' global, functional and behavioural condition remains at a level where the drug is considered to be having a suitable effect. When the MMSE score falls below 10 points, patients should not normally be prescribed any of the above antidementia medication (NICE, 2006). Any review involving MMSE assessment should be undertaken by an appropriate specialist team.

6   Describe the prognosis and long-term complications of Alzheimer's dementia.

People with Alzheimer's disease eventually lose the ability to carry out routine daily activities such as dressing/undressing; toileting; travelling and handling money. As a result, many people with Alzheimer's disease require a high level of care.

7   What are the social pharmacy issues related to the case of Mr EF?

Whenever possible, the client should be helped to lead an active life, with inter-esting and stimulating daily activities. By minimising distress and agitation it is sometimes possible to limit the use of sedative drugs. The NICE guidelines (NICE, 2006) regarding the use of antidementia drugs have proved to be very controversial (Alzheimer's Society, 2006).

Case study level Ma – A case of schizophrenia – see page 85

1   What are the most typical signs and symptoms of schizophrenia?

Onset of schizophrenia typically occurs in late adolescence or early adulthood; the disease is often described in terms of 'positive' and 'negative' symptoms. Positive symptoms include delusions, auditory hallucinations and thought disorder and are typically regarded as manifestations of psychosis. Negative symptoms include flat, blunted or constricted affect and emotion, poverty of speech and lack of motivation. The client may show both disorganised speech (e.g. frequent derailment or incoherence) and behaviour. One or more major areas of functioning, such as work, interpersonal relations or self-care, are markedly below the level achieved prior to the onset of schizophrenia. Typically, continuous signs of the disturbance persist for at least six months. A diagnosis of schizophrenia is excluded if the symptoms are the direct result of a substance abuse or a general medical condition.

2   Is there any routine role of laboratory data in making a diagnosis of schizophrenia?

Diagnosis is based on the self-reported experiences of the patient, in combination with the signs identified. There are no reliable biological markers for schizophrenia, though studies suggest that genetics and neurobiology are important contributory factors.

3   Please evaluate and critically appraise available treatment options for schizophrenia; expand on their side-effects.

Antipsychotics are classified into 'typical' and 'atypical':

- First-generation (typical) antipsychotics include: amisulpride, chlorpromazine, fluphenazine, haloperidol, promethazine, promazine, trifluoperazine
- Second-generation (atypical) antipsychotics include: clozapine, olanzapine, quetiapine, risperidone, aripiprazole.

The therapeutic effects of typical antipsychotics are due to block of dopamine D_2 receptors, while the extrapyramidal effects (EPS) are due to dopamine antagonism in the basal ganglia. Acute dystonias, often of jaw, neck or external ocular muscles may be observed in the first few days of treatment. Eventually, a parkinsonism (typically characterised by akinesia, rigidity and tremor) may manifest. This may respond to the use of antimuscarinic drugs (e.g. procyclidine, orphenadrine). A subjective restlessness of the legs often leading to pacing (akathisia) may appear within weeks of starting treatment, but does not respond to antimuscarinics. The often irreversible tardive dyskinesia condition may appear after several months; it is characterised by involuntary, choreiform movements mainly of mouth and face but sometimes also of limbs and trunk. Since dopamine is the prolactin inhibitory factor, dopamine blockade in the hypothalamus may also lead to hyperprolactinaemia. In turn, this is associated with gynaecomastia, galactorrhoea and amenorrhoea, which are the typical signs and symptoms of an increase in prolactin levels. Neuroleptic malignant syndrome is a rare but potentially fatal syndrome of rigidity, hyperpyrexia and confusion. Other side-effects include: blood dyscrasias, hepatitis, skin rashes and photosensitivity. Contraindications include: cardiovascular and cerebrovascular disease, parkinsonism, epilepsy, pregnancy and breastfeeding, renal and hepatic impairment, prostatism, glaucoma. Interactions: increased effect of other hypotensives or sedatives.

Typical antipsychotics may be usefully grouped according to their adverse effects' profile (Table A4.1).

Table A4.1 Classification of typical antipsychotics according to their adverse effects profile

Sedation	Anticholinergic	Extrapyramidal	Examples
+++	++	++	Chlorpromazine
++	+++	+	Thioridazine[a]
+	+	+++	Haloperidol,
+	+	+++	Flupentixol decanoate[b],
+	+	+++	Fluphenazine decanoate[b]

[a]The intrinsic anticholinergic activity of these drugs may limit their extrapyramidal effects but bears a higher risk of ECG changes.
[b]Decanoate formulations are used in depot preparations.

Recently, several 'atypical' antipsychotics have entered the UK market. All these medications tend to be better tolerated than typical antipsychotics but may be more expensive as well. There is an ongoing debate about whether they should be prescribed 'first line' or reserved for patients who fail to respond or do not tolerate typical antipsychotics (Newcastle University, 2005; Gharabawi et al., 2006).

Since clozapine is associated with potentially fatal agranulocytosis, it is only indicated in schizophrenia which has not responded to other antipsychotics. In addition, patients must have regular (initially weekly) blood counts performed before being prescribed the medication. Other adverse events include marked sedation, hypersalivation and anticholinergic effects, but EPS are less frequently seen than with typical antipsychotics. Risperidone, olanzapine and quetiapine show varying degrees of $5\text{-HT}_2/\text{D}_2$ antagonism and are associated with weight gain but fewer EPS compared with typical antipsychotics.

Risperidone can cause EPS, anticholinergic effects and hyperprolactinaemia at higher doses. Olanzapine is reasonably sedative; apart from its use in psychosis, some data have emerged for the use of quetiapine in borderline personality conditions as well (Perrella *et al.*, 2007). Aripiprazole seems to have little effect on prolactin, glucose and lipid levels and QT interval in short- and long-term trials. Weight gain is similar to risperidone and less than olanzapine.

4   Describe a pharmaceutical care plan in the case reported here?

In a case like the one reported here, the only meaningful approach a pharmacist/health professional could take is to make sure that the client is appropriately referred to the GP for an immediate assessment by the Community Mental Health Team. The client may need to be compulsorily admitted to the local psychiatric ward. On specific occasions, it may be necessary to involve the police to cope with the situation.

5a   What are the goals of therapy of schizophrenia?
5b   Expand on the monitoring of therapy in schizophrenia and risk of medication non-compliance.
5c   What are the social pharmacy issues relevant to the condition of schizophrenia?

The most important action is to ensure that the client receives appropriate pharmacological treatment. One of the main problems in schizophrenia is lack of medication compliance. This is often caused by lack of client collaboration, often explained by the intrinsic pathological characteristics of the disease itself. Both typical and atypical 'depot' antipsychotics' formulations are available. Depot preparations are typically administered by intramuscular injection every 1–4 weeks. This may be of great advantage in patients with poor compliance.

6   Please expand on the prognosis and comorbidity issues relevant to the condition of schizophrenia.

It is generally considered that a third of people will make a full recovery, about a third will show improvement over time, but not a full recovery, and a third will remain ill. Women tend to show higher recovery rates than men. Acute and sudden onset of schizophrenia is associated with higher rates of recovery, while gradual onset is associated with lower rates. Patients diagnosed with schizophrenia are highly likely to be diagnosed with other medical disorders as well. The lifetime prevalence of substance abuse is typically around 40% (Schifano *et al.*, 2004). Comorbidity is also high with both depression and anxiety disorders.

7   Are there alternative, non-pharmacological therapies for the treatment of schizophrenia?

Cognitive behavioural psychotherapeutic approach may be offered. This may focus on direct symptom reduction, self-esteem, social functioning and insight.

Case study level Mb – A case of buprenorphine high-dose prescribing in heroin addiction - see page 87

1   What are the diagnostic criteria for substance dependence?

Typically, criteria for substance dependence include cognitive, behavioural and physiological signs and symptoms indicating ongoing substance use despite significant problems associated with such use. Usually this continuous use will result in tolerance, withdrawal and a pattern of compulsive use.

2   Which biological fluids are usually taken to monitor drug dependence?

To monitor a drug misuse condition, toxicology screening is typically performed on urine or, much less frequently, blood specimens.

3   What are the prominent pharmacological characteristics of methadone and buprenorphine? How is the dosage titration process carried out when a treatment with either methadone or buprenorphine is started?

Methadone is a synthetic opioid which is used mainly for the treatment of opioid dependence. It is widely prescribed in oral liquid formulations and sometimes tablets. Injectable forms are also still fairly common in the UK. Methadone dominates the substitute opiate-prescribing market in the UK. Methadone advantages include: reducing criminal activity, improving social integration and employment prospects, and reducing the morbidity and mortality of opiate users. Complications may arise from the crushing, dilution and injecting of methadone tablets. Methadone should only be administered following a thorough clinical assessment of opiate/opioid dependence and current level of drug consumption. For outpatient stabilisation the initial dose of methadone will be less than 30 mg. Titration of methadone doses is of paramount importance in avoiding the risk of overdose: small increases in dosage of 5–10 mg/day when patients are commencing a course of methadone treatment are advisable. It has been shown that the metabolism of methadone is very slow in individuals who have just started titration with the drug and/or are methadone-naive. Clearance of methadone is significantly lower in opiate addicts at the start of treatment than in those who had reached the steady-state level. This clearly poses a risk of overdose, especially during the initial phase of methadone treatment.

    Buprenorphine is a semi-synthetic, partial mu-agonist, highly lipophilic, opioid drug. Because it is a partial agonist, when buprenorphine competes with morphine or heroin for mu-receptors it can reduce their maximum effect. Buprenorphine binds strongly to mu and kappa opiate receptors; it associates with the mu-receptor slowly (30 minutes), but with high affinity, low intrinsic activity and slow and incomplete dissociation. The slow dissociation from the receptor probably limits the intensity of withdrawal by preventing the rapid recovery of the receptor upon discontinuation of buprenorphine treatment. Buprenorphine might have a ceiling effect on respiratory depression with increasing doses; a ceiling on the respiratory depression is possibly a valuable therapeutic safeguard. After sublingual administration, the peak concentration is reached slowly (90 minutes–4 hours) and the bioavailability is 56%. Because of its properties as a partial agonist, buprenorphine may precipitate withdrawal effects in those who are given high doses of opiate agonists.

Patients on methadone should be reduced to a maximum of 30 mg daily before starting buprenorphine. Buprenorphine should be used with caution in patients who are administered high doses of benzodiazepines, since both buprenorphine and benzodiazepines are CYP3A substrates. Most common side-effects include: drowsiness and sleep disturbance; nausea, vomiting, constipation (less severe than other opiates); sweating, dizziness, fainting; headache; rashes, blurring of vision. Buprenorphine high dose should be administered initially at 0.8–4 mg (sublingual) as a single daily dose; maximum dosage is 32 mg daily. In those who have not undergone opioid withdrawal, buprenorphine should be administered at least 4 hours after last use of opioid or when signs of craving appear.

4   What are the key differences between buprenorphine and methadone?

Buprenorphine differs from methadone in the following ways:

- Because it is a sublingual tablet and so takes time to dissolve, it is more difficult to supervise administration.
- It is relatively easy to misuse, by crushing and injecting.
- It might be safer than methadone in overdose, but more evidence is needed.

Suggestions of selection criteria for use of buprenorphine as opposed to methadone may include:

- younger clients with less established dependence,
- those wanting detoxification from methadone who had difficulty ceasing methadone in the past, and
- those refusing methadone treatment for a variety of reasons.

5   Please expand on the pharmaceutical care plan for Mr IJ and on issues relevant to monitoring of his therapy.

The minimum requirements for any prescribing and dispensing of substitute drugs, including buprenorphine, are as follows:

- Ensure that the patient following assessment and compilation of treatment goals has the correct dose, with particular care on induction and with appropriate measures taken to prevent diversion.
- Supervised consumption in the pharmacy for at least the first three months with relaxation only on clinical stability (i.e. no illicit drug use).

- No more than one to two weeks' drugs should be dispensed at any one time unless in exceptional circumstances and after consultant review.
- Clinical review and monitoring regularly (at least every three months) for those whose drug use is stable.
- Clear liaison between pharmacist and other clinicians involved.
- Careful and adequate recording of prescriptions.

6   What are the buprenorphine-containing formulations licensed for treatment of opiate addiction in the UK? What are the goals of opiate dependence treatment?

The only formulation containing buprenorphine *only* licensed in the UK for management of opiate dependence is Subutex. Recently, the product Suboxone has entered the UK market. This is a combination of buprenorphine and naloxone (a pure opiate antagonist). If the patient tried to inject this formulation, the naloxone would antagonise the buprenorphine pharmacological effects at the central level. Conversely, when the sublingual tablet is appropriately administered, naloxone will not exert its antagonist activities. Temgesic, the other marketed product that contains buprenorphine *only* (albeit at low dose), should not be supplied for substitution treatment.

The main goal of therapy with either buprenorphine or methadone maintenance treatment is to achieve stabilisation (i.e. no illicit drug use; attending appointments on time; no further involvement in criminal activities). Eventually, whenever the above targets are achieved, in collaboration with both the GP and the professionals of the Community Drug and Alcohol Team, a gradual reduction of the dosage will be planned. This may require anything between a few weeks and many months.

7   Please expand on the social pharmacy issues appropriate for this case, including supply, concordance, compliance and lifestyle issues.

When a patient collects his or her first instalment of methadone/buprenorphine an appropriate information leaflet should be supplied, giving advice on how to use the product, special warnings, precautions and drug instructions.

The introduction of supervised methadone consumption appears to have helped to reduce the number of fatalities. There is a substantial 'grey'/black market in all forms of diverted methadone. Some clinicians suggest the need for supervised dispensing for buprenorphine, though there is difficulty with supervision. Sublingual tablets, with an average of 8–12 mg dosage, may take up to 5 minutes to dissolve fully. Anecdotal reports from some services are of crushing the sublingual tablet prior to in-house dispensing (rather than pharmacy supervision) to avoid any possible diversion or injecting the drug. The drug crushed in this manner is not licensed.

8   Describe the prognosis and long-term complications of drug addiction?

Drug addiction should be seen as a chronic condition, subject to relapses. If clients comply with the services offered to them by healthcare professionals, the prognosis may be favourable. However, it must be emphasised that clients will have to maintain a long-life condition of abstention from illicit drugs. Sometimes, this will require long-term attendance of self-help groups (e.g. Narcotics Anonymous).

9   Is there a role for herbal medicine in the treatment of addiction?

Recent reviews of approved pharmacotherapies for the treatment of addictions demonstrate both a striking paucity of novel treatment agents and the modest efficacy of traditionally prescribed medication (Ghodse *et al.*, 2006). Recent population surveys indicate a growing popularity of alternative medicines among drug addicts seeking help or undergoing treatment. A considerable proportion of drug users are seeking help from alternative treatment options, including herbal, complementary and alternative medicines (CAM). A number of reports indicate the extensive use of such medications in Asia (China, Thailand, Burma, Laos), designed to treat opium/heroin addicts. Similar herbal preparations are marketed in various European countries for the symptomatic treatment of alcohol- and nicotine-addicted people. The know-how for such herbal remedies usually comes from local systems of traditional medicine. Published yet insufficient evidence suggests that some of these remedies may have potential value and deserve further investigation and possible development into marketed products (Ghodse *et al.*, 2006).

5

Infections case studies

Kieran Hand

Case study level 1 – Sore throat

Learning outcomes

Level 1 case study: You will be able to:

- describe the risk factors
- describe the disease
- describe the pharmacology of the drug
- outline the formulation including drug molecule, excipients, etc. for the medicines
- summarise basic social pharmacy issues (e.g. opening containers, large labels).

Scenario

A mother and her 6-year-old son present a post-dated prescription for penicillin V syrup 250 mg q.d.s. × 10 days and ask to speak to the pharmacist. The child is irritable, complains of pain when swallowing and appears flushed. The mother is anxious to start antibiotic treatment straight away so that her son can get back to school and she can get back to work, but the prescription is not valid for 3 more days.

Questions

1 What are the causes of sore throat and how are they differentiated?
2a Who is at risk of sore throat and how common is it?
2b How serious is acute throat infection?

2c   Are antibiotics effective for the treatment of sore throat and for how long should you treat?

2d   When are antibiotics indicated for the treatment of sore throat?

3a   What group of drugs does penicillin V belong to and how do they work?

3b   What are the side-effects of penicillin V?

3c   What are the alternatives to penicillin V for treatment of sore throat?

4a   What is the oral bioavailability of penicillin V and what is the impact of administration with food?

4b   What are the storage conditions and shelf-life of penicillin V oral solution?

5a   What are the disadvantages of prescribing antibiotics for sore throat?

5b   How should this patient's mother be counselled regarding the post-dated prescription and symptom relief?

References

Clinical Knowledge Summaries (2008) Sore throat – acute. Available at http://www.prodigy.nhs.uk/sore_throat_acute [Accessed 3 July 2008].

Del Mar CB, Glasziou PP and Spinks AB (2006) Antibiotics for sore throat. *Cochrane Database of Systematic Reviews* no. 4, CD000023.

Joint Formulary Committee (2008) *British National Formulary 55*. London: British Medical Association and Royal Pharmaceutical Society of Great Britain, March.

National Prescribing Centre (UK) (2003) MeReC Briefing. Antibiotic resistance and prescribing practice. Available at http://www.npc.co.uk/MeReC_Briefings/2002/briefing_no_21.pdf [Accessed 3 July 2008].

NICE (National Institute for Health and Clinical Excellence) (2001) Referral advice – a guide to appropriate referral from general to specialist services. Available at http://www.nice.org.uk/page.aspx?o=Referral Advice [Accessed 3 July 2008].

General references

BMJ Clinical Evidence (2006) Sore throat. www.clinicalevidence.com [Accessed 3 July 2008].

Little P, Watson L, Morgan S and Williamson I (2002) Antibiotic prescribing and admissions with major suppurative complications of respiratory tract infections: a data linkage study. *British Journal of General Practice* 52: 187–190, 193.

Case study level 2 – Urinary tract infection (UTI)

Learning outcomes

Level 2 case study: You will be able to:

- interpret relevant lab and clinical data
- identify monitoring and referral criteria
- explain treatment choices
- describe goals of therapy, including monitoring and the role of the pharmacist/clinician
- describe issues – counselling points, adverse drug reactions, drug interactions, complementary/alternative therapies and lifestyle advice.

Scenario

A 27-year-old woman presents a prescription for nitrofurantoin tablets 50 mg q.d.s. for 3 days and asks to speak to the pharmacist. She explains that her GP has checked her urine with a 'coloured strip' and diagnosed a urinary tract infection (UTI). She is suffering considerable discomfort on urination due to a burning/stinging sensation and her GP has suggested she purchase some Effercitrate over the counter. A friend has recommended she also purchase cranberry extract tablets and the patient would like your advice.

Questions

1   What are the symptoms and signs of a UTI and what is the role of dipstick testing?
2a When can a patient with cystitis be safely treated with over-the-counter products and when should they be referred to their GP?
2b When is antibiotic treatment indicated for UTI?
3a What are the typical UTI pathogens and what are the treatment choices for lower UTI in a non-pregnant woman?
3b What are the treatment choices for lower UTI in a pregnant woman?
4a What should be considered by the pharmacist when dispensing nitrofurantoin?
5a What alternative therapies are available for cystitis and how effective are they?
5b What lifestyle advice can be offered to patients with cystitis?

References

Kucers A, Crowe SM, Grayson ML and Hoy JF (1997) *The Use of Antibiotics: A Clinical Review of Antibacterial, Antifungal, and Antiviral drugs*, 5th edn. Boston: Butterworth-Heinemann.

Richards D, Toop L, Chambers S and Fletcher L (2005) Response to antibiotics of women with symptoms of urinary tract infection but negative dipstick urine test results: double blind randomised controlled trial. *British Medical Journal* 331(7509): 143.

SIGN (Scottish Intercollegiate Guidelines Network) (2006) Management of suspected bacterial urinary tract infection in adults. Available at http://www.sign.ac.uk/guidelines/fulltext/88/index.html [Accessed 3 July 2008].

General references

Bint AJ and Berrington AW (2003) Urinary tract infections. In: Walker R and Edwards C (eds) *Clinical Pharmacy and Therapeutics*, 3rd edn. Edinburgh: Churchill Livingstone, pp. 533–542.

Blenkinsopp A, Paxton P and Blenkinsopp J (2005) *Symptoms in the Pharmacy*, 5th edn. Oxford: Blackwells.

Briggs GG, Freeman RK and Yaffe SJ (2005) *Drugs in Pregnancy and Lactation*, 7th edn. London: Lippincott Williams & Wilkins.

Gillespie S and Bamford K (2003) *Medical Microbiology and Infection at a Glance,* 2nd edn. Oxford: Blackwells.

Case study level 3 – Pneumonia

Learning outcomes

Level 3 case study: You will be able to:

- interpret clinical signs and symptoms
- evaluate laboratory data
- evaluate treatment options
- state goals of therapy
- describe a pharmaceutical care plan to include advice to a clinician
- describe the prognosis and long-term complications
- describe the social pharmacy issues which could include supply (e.g. complex treatments at home, concordance and compliance) and lifestyle issues.

Mrs CP, a 74-year-old woman, presents at A&E at 11pm with a 3-day history of productive cough, fever, shortness of breath and pleurisy. A portable chest X-ray taken in A&E shows consolidation in the right lower lobe of her lungs and she is admitted to hospital.

Mrs CP is 162 cm weighs 82 kg, is a smoker and has a medical history of ischaemic heart disease. She had a myocardial infarction 3 years previously and underwent coronary artery bypass grafting.

Her current medication includes:

- aspirin 75 mg o.d.
- simvastatin 40 mg o.n.
- atenolol 25 mg o.d.
- ramipril 5 mg o.d.
- furosemide 20 mg o.d.
- amlodipine 10 mg o.d.
- isosorbide mononitrate slow release 60 mg o.d.
- glyceryl trinitrate sublingual spray p.r.n.

On examination, her vital signs are recorded as follows:

- heart rate 110 bpm
- temperature 38.2°C
- respiratory rate 26 breaths per minute
- blood pressure 140/92 mmHg
- oxygen saturation 89% on 2 L/min oxygen.

Planned investigations include:

- blood cultures
- sputum cultures
- urea and electrolytes and full blood count
- C-reactive protein
- liver function tests
- electrocardiogram (ECG)
- Troponin I
- D-dimer
- urine for bacterial serology.

The patient is diagnosed with community-acquired pneumonia and the treatment plan is as follows:

- continue oxygen
- salbutamol nebulised 2.5 mg q.d.s.
- ceftriaxone i.v. 1 g o.d.
- erythromycin i.v. 500 mg q.d.s.
- paracetamol p.o./p.r. 1 g q.d.s.
- enoxaparin s.c. 40 mg o.d.

Questions

1   How is the diagnosis of pneumonia made and how is the severity of illness assessed?

The patient is assessed on the post-take ward round at 8am the following morning and is noted to have improved slightly with saturations currently at 95% on 2 L/min of oxygen. Her ECG is unremarkable.

The following laboratory investigations (normal ranges) are relevant:

Creatinine	110 micromol/L (estimated creatinine clearance 40 mL/min)
Urea	9.6 mmol/L (2.5–8 mmol/L)
CRP	164 mg/L (<10 mg/L)
WCC	28×10^9/L ($4–11 \times 10^9$/L)
Neutrophils	25×10^9/L ($2–7.5 \times 10^9$/L)

2a   What is the significance of these laboratory findings?

Blood culture results have been phoned to the ward reporting Gram-positive cocci in one culture bottle; further identification and antibiotic sensitivity testing are pending.

2b   What are the possible interpretations of this microbiology result?

3   What are the important pathogens and appropriate treatment options for severe community-acquired pneumonia?

4   Outline a pharmaceutical care plan for this patient with severe community-acquired pneumonia, including advice to the clinician.

5   What are the goals of therapy in community-acquired pneumonia?

6   How should therapy be monitored?

7   What are the prognosis and potential complications of community-acquired pneumonia?

8   What are the relevant social pharmacy issues in this case?

Reference

British Thoracic Society (2001) BTS Guidelines for the management of community acquired pneumonia in adults. *Thorax* 56 (Suppl 4): IV1–IV64. Available at http://thorax.bmj.com/cgi/content/full/56/suppl_4/iv1 (Updated 2004) http://thorax.bmj.com/cgi/content/full/59/5/364 [Accessed 03 July 2008].

General references

Cohen J and Powderly WG (2004) *Infectious Diseases,* 2nd edn. St. Louis: Mosby.
Lewis SA and Macfarlane JT (2003) Defining community acquired pneumonia severity on presentation to hospital: an international derivation and validation study. *Thorax* 58: 377–382.

Lim WS, van der Eerden MM, Laing R *et al.* (2003) Respiratory infections. In: Walker R and Edwards C (eds) *Clinical Pharmacy and Therapeutics*. Edinburgh: Churchill Livingstone, pp. 519–532.

Wallach J (2000) *Interpretation of Diagnostic Tests*, 7th edn. Philadelphia: Lippincott Williams & Wilkins.

Case study level Ma – Meningitis

Learning outcomes

Level M case study: You will be able to:

- interpret clinical signs and symptoms
- evaluate laboratory data
- critically appraise treatment options
- state goals of therapy
- describe a pharmaceutical care plan to include advice to a clinician
- describe the prognosis and long-term complications
- describe the social pharmacy issues which could include supply (e.g. complex treatments at home, concordance and compliance) and lifestyle issues
- describe the monitoring of therapy.

Scenario

Mr JD, a 19-year-old university student, presents to the campus GP in the afternoon with severe headache, vomiting and photophobia since early morning of the same day. On examination, the patient has a fever and he is unable to touch his chin to his knees. He does not have a rash and is alert and oriented. The GP administered benzylpenicillin i.v. 1.2 g and the patient was transferred urgently by ambulance to A&E.

Mr JD weighs 70 kg, is a smoker and has an unremarkable medical history. He takes occasional caffeine tablets prior to examinations but otherwise takes no regular medication. He remembers receiving a meningitis vaccine at school.

On arrival at A&E, his vital signs are recorded as follows:

- heart rate 124 bpm
- temperature 39.0°C
- respiratory rate 26 breaths per minute
- blood pressure 95/65 mmHg
- oxygen saturation 97%.

Planned investigations include:

- lumbar puncture and cerebrospinal fluid (CSF) analysis
- CSF PCR for herpes simplex virus (HSV)
- blood cultures
- coagulation screen
- urea and electrolytes and full blood count
- C-reactive protein
- liver function tests.

The patient is diagnosed with suspected meningitis and the treatment plan is as follows:

- cefotaxime i.v. 2 g q.d.s.
- dexamethasone p.o. 10 mg q.d.s.
- aciclovir i.v. 700 mg t.d.s.
- paracetamol p.o./p.r. 1 g q.d.s.
- cyclizine i.v. 50 mg t.d.s. p.r.n.
- enoxaparin s.c. 40 mg o.d. (post lumbar puncture).

Questions

1   What are the signs and symptoms of meningitis and meningococcal septicaemia (bloodstream infection)?

The following lumbar puncture cerebrospinal fluid (CSF) results (normal ranges) are reported from the biochemistry and pathology laboratories within 4 hours of admission.

White blood cells	1350 cells/mm^3 (<5 cells/mm^3), 90% polymorphs
CSF protein	1.31 g/L (<0.4 g/L)
CSF glucose	1.4 mmol/L (2.2–4.4 mmol/L)
CSF:blood glucose ratio	0.22 (>0.6)
Gram-negative diplococci identified in the CSF	

2   What is the significance of these laboratory findings?

3a What are the important pathogens and appropriate treatment options for bacterial meningitis, including alternatives in penicillin allergy?

3b Which antibiotic regimens achieve therapeutic concentrations in the cerebrospinal fluid and which should be avoided?

3c What is the rationale for prescribing aciclovir in cases of suspected meningitis?

4   Outline a pharmaceutical care plan for this patient with meningitis, including advice to the clinician.

5   What are the goals of therapy in community-acquired bacterial meningitis?

6   How should therapy be monitored?

7   What are the prognosis and potential long-term complications of meningitis?

8   What are the relevant social pharmacy issues in this case, including lifestyle issues?

References

Davison KL, Crowcroft NS, Ramsay ME *et al.* (2003) Viral encephalitis in England, 1989–1998: what did we miss? *Emerging Infectious Disease* 9: 234–240.

Health Protection Agency (UK) (2005a) Meningococcal Reference Unit, laboratory confirmed *Neisseria meningitidis*: England and Wales, by age group, 1989/1990 to 2004/2005. Available at http://www.hpa.org.uk/infections/topics_az/meningo/data_meni_t02.htm [Accessed 3 July 2008].

Health Protection Agency (UK) (2005b). Numbers of laboratory confirmed pneumococcal meningitis cases in England and Wales, 1996–2005. Available at http://www.hpa.org.uk/webw/HPAweb&HPAwebStandard/HPAweb_C/1195733815884?p=1203409671918cases.htm [Accessed 3 July 2008].

Hoen B, Viel JF, Paquot C *et al.* (1995) Multivariate approach to differential diagnosis of acute meningitis. *European Journal of Clinical Microbiology and Infectious Diseases* 14: 267–274.

Spanos A, Harrell FE Jr and Durack DT (1989) Differential diagnosis of acute meningitis. An analysis of the predictive value of initial observations. *Journal of the American Medical Association* 262: 2700–2707.

van de Beek D, de Gans J, McIntyre P and Prasad K (2004) Steroids in adults with acute bacterial meningitis: a systematic review. *The Lancet Infectious Diseases* 4(3): 139–143.

van de Beek D, de Gans J, Tunkel AR and Wijdicks EF (2006) Community-acquired bacterial meningitis in adults. *New England Journal of Medicine* 354: 44–53.

General references

Attia J, Hatala R, Cook DJ and Wong JG (1999) The rational clinical examination. Does this adult patient have acute meningitis? *Journal of the American Medical Association* 282: 175–181.

Beers MH, Porter RS, Jones TV *et al.* (2005) Encephalitis. In: *The Merck Manual of Diagnosis and Therapy*. Available at http://www.merck.com/ mmpe/sec16/ch217/ch217c.html [Accessed 3 July 2008].

Gray JW (2003) Infective meningitis. In: Walker R and Edwards C (eds) *Clinical Pharmacy and Therapeutics*, 3rd edn. Edinburgh: Churchill Livingstone, pp. 555–568.

Case study level Mb – Diabetic foot infection

Learning outcomes

Level M case study: You will be able to:

- interpret clinical signs and symptoms
- evaluate laboratory data
- critically appraise treatment options
- state goals of therapy
- describe a pharmaceutical care plan to include advice to a clinician
- describe the prognosis and long-term complications
- describe the social pharmacy issues which could include supply (e.g. complex treatments at home, concordance and compliance) and lifestyle issues
- describe the monitoring of therapy.

Scenario

Mr SA, a 59-year-old author is taken to A&E by his daughter due to increasing fatigue, weakness, confusion and drowsiness.

Mr SA is 185 cm tall, weighs 83 kg and has a 15-year history of type 2 diabetes mellitus and hypercholesterolaemia. He is under the care of the diabetes clinic at the hospital for management of Charcot's arthropathy of the foot and diabetic foot ulcer. He also has a 5-year history of ischaemic heart disease and underwent coronary artery bypass grafting one year ago. He drinks half-a-bottle of red wine per day and smokes a pipe. He is allergic to penicillin. His current medications are:

- metformin tablets 850 mg t.d.s.
- rosiglitazone tablets 4 mg b.d.
- atorvastatin tablets 40 mg o.d.
- ezetimibe tablets 10 mg o.d.
- amlodipine tablets 10 mg o.d.
- furosemide 40 mg o.d.
- aspirin 75 mg tablets o.d.
- perindopril 4 mg tablets o.d.
- gabapentin 600 mg tablets t.d.s.
- isosorbide mononitrate slow release tablets 60 mg o.d.
- glyceryl trinitrate spray sublingually 400–800 micrograms p.r.n.

On examination, he appears confused and disoriented and clinically dehydrated. He has an inflamed, malodorous foot ulcer with obvious purulent slough. Dorsalis pedis and posterior tibial pulses were palpable, suggesting adequate arterial supply to the foot. On close inspection, the wound is deep – penetrating to the ligaments and muscle – but a probe-to-bone test for osteomyelitis with a steel probe is negative. The area surrounding the ulcer appears cellulitic.

His vital signs are recorded as follows:

- heart rate 117 bpm
- temperature 38.8°C
- respiratory rate 23 breaths per minute
- blood pressure 92/59 mmHg
- oxygen saturation 96%.

A urine dipstick indicates a urinary glucose of >25 mmol/L but is negative for nitrites and leucocyte esterase.

The patient's most recent microbiology results from one month previously are as follows:

- wound swab from foot ulcer
- *Enterococcus faecalis* +++
- lactose fermenting coliforms +++.

Planned investigations include:

- blood cultures
- wound cultures
- blood glucose
- creatinine
- urea and electrolytes and full blood count
- C-reactive protein
- liver function tests
- arterial blood gases
- X-ray
- magnetic resonance imaging if X-ray inconclusive.

The patient is diagnosed with hyperosmolar non-ketotic (HONK) syndrome secondary to infection of a diabetic foot ulcer and the treatment plan is as follows:

- sodium chloride 0.9% i.v. 1 L per hour initially
- insulin (Actrapid) i.v. 12 unit bolus then 8 units per hour after first litre of saline
- piperacillin-tazobactam i.v. 4.5 g t.d.s.
- co-codamol 30/500 mg two tablets q.d.s. prn
- cyclizine i.v. 50 mg t.d.s. p.r.n.
- enoxaparin s.c. 40 mg o.d.

Questions

1a   What are the signs and symptoms of foot infection in diabetic patients and when are antibiotics indicated?

1b   What are the likely pathogens?

2a What are the primary issues to be considered when choosing empirical anti-infective therapy in this case?

2b Comment on the choice of anti-infective regimen in this case and discuss alternative regimens.

Laboratory findings (normal ranges) reported within 12 hours of admission

Blood glucose   34 mmol/L (3–7.8 mmol/L)
Creatinine   186 micromol/L (estimated creatinine clearance 44 mL/min)
WCC 11.2×10^9/L ($4–11 \times 10^9$/L)
Neutrophils 7.6×10^9/L ($2–7.5 \times 10^9$/L)
C-reactive protein 110 mg/L (<10 mg/L)
Blood culture positive for Gram-positive cocci in both bottles
Magnetic resonance imaging does not indicate osteomyelitis

3 What is the significance of these laboratory findings?

4 Critically appraise the management options in this case.

5 Outline a pharmaceutical care plan for this patient with infected diabetic foot ulcer including advice to the clinician.

6 What are the goals of therapy in diabetic foot infection?

7 How should therapy be monitored?

8 What are the prognosis and potential long-term complications of diabetic foot ulcers?

9 What are the relevant social pharmacy issues in this case, including lifestyle issues?

References

Cavanagh PR, Lipsky BA, Bradbury AW and Botek G (2005) Treatment for diabetic foot ulcers. *Lancet* 366(9498): 1725–1735.

Jeffcoate WJ and Harding KG (2003) Diabetic foot ulcers. *Lancet* 361(9368): 1545–1551.

Lipsky BA, Berendt AR, Deery HG *et al.* (2004) Diagnosis and treatment of diabetic foot infections. *Clinical Infectious Diseases* 39: 885–910.

NICE (National Institute for Health and Clinical Excellence) (2004) Type 2 diabetes: prevention and management of foot problems. Available at http://www.nice.org.uk/guidance/index.jsp?action=byID&o=10934 [Accessed 03 July 2008].

General references

Cohen J and Powderly WG (2004) *Infectious Diseases*, 2nd edn. St. Louis: Mosby.

Gemmell CG, Edwards DI, Fraise AP *et al.*(2006) Guidelines for the prophylaxis and treatment of methicillin-resistant *Staphylococcus aureus* (MRSA) infections in the UK. *Journal of Antimicrobial Chemotherapy* 57: 589–608.

Stevens DL, Bisno AL, Chambers HF *et al.* (2005) Practice guidelines for the diagnosis and management of skin and soft-tissue infections. *Clinical Infectious Diseases* 41: 1373–1406.

Case study level 1 – Sore throat – see page 103

1   What are the causes of sore throat and how are they differentiated?

Sore throat is most often caused by viral infection, often associated with cough and cold symptoms or flu-like illness. Bacterial throat infections are commonly caused by streptococci ('strep throat'), usually *Streptococcus pyogenes* also known as group A beta-haemolytic *Streptococcus*. Clinical examination is not reliable for differentiating between bacterial and viral throat infection except in the case of a scarlet fever rash (red eruption with sandpaper texture which usually begins on the chest and spreads to the abdomen and extremities; flushed face with pale area around the mouth; and a 'strawberry tongue'), which is usually indicative of *Streptococcus*. Although group A strep can be isolated from throat swabs of up to 30% of patients with a sore throat, asymptomatic carriage of the organism in the population is estimated at between 6% and 40%. Throat swabs cannot differentiate between infection and carriage.

2a   Who is at risk of sore throat and how common is it?

Children aged 5–10 years and young adults aged 15–25 years are most frequently affected by acute throat infection. GPs can expect to see around 60 cases of sore throat per year for every thousand patients on their list but the majority of patients with sore throat do not consult their GP (Clinical Knowledge Summaries, 2008).

2b   How serious is acute throat infection?

Sore throat is a self-limiting condition and symptoms will resolve within 3 days in 40% of patients and within one week in 85% of patients, regardless of whether the infection is caused by *Streptococcus*. Patients with group A strep throat infection are at risk of complications (<5% of cases) including: otitis media, sinusitis, peritonsillar abscess (quinsy), cervical adenitis (lymph node inflammation), and scarlet fever. In rare cases, patients may develop a streptococcal toxic shock syndrome. In developing countries, other complications of group A strep infection such as rheumatic fever and glomerulonephritis remain problematic (Clinical Knowledge Summaries, 2008).

2c   Are antibiotics effective for the treatment of sore throat and for how long should you treat?

A systematic review found that antibiotics reduced the proportion of people with symptoms of sore throat at 3 days (47%) compared with placebo (66%) (Del Mar *et al.*, 2006). This represents a shortening in duration of illness by an average of 1 day. Antibiotics were found to be more effective in patients with throat swabs positive for *Streptococcus*. Antibiotics also reduce the risk of developing complications but because the absolute risk of complications is low, a considerable number of patients need to be treated with antibiotics to prevent one complication (200 patients in the case of otitis media for example). A 10-day treatment course is recommended for reliable eradication of group A strep (Joint Formulary Committee, 2008).

2d When are antibiotics indicated for the treatment of sore throat?

The Centor criteria are specific clinical signs predictive of group A strep and may be useful for targeting antibiotics to at-risk patients. Three of the following four criteria are required in an unwell patient: history of fever, tonsillar exudate, absence of cough, or tender cervical lymph nodes. However, the Centor criteria are merely predictive of positive throat swab and so cannot distinguish carriage from infection. The National Institute for Health and Clinical Excellence (NICE) recommends antibiotics for the following situations: features of marked systemic upset secondary to the acute sore throat, unilateral peritonsillitis, a history of rheumatic fever, or an increased risk from acute infection (such as a child with diabetes mellitus or immunodeficiency) (NICE, 2001).

3a What group of drugs does penicillin V belong to and how do they work?

Penicillin V or phenoxymethylpenicillin is a beta-lactam antibiotic. The beta-lactam ring at the centre of the penicillin molecule mimics a pair of amino acids in the pentapeptide cross-links that form between linear peptidoglycan polymer chains in the bacterial cell wall. Beta-lactam antibiotics disrupt formation of the cross-links resulting in bactericidal activity. Both Gram-positive and Gram-negative bacteria possess a peptidoglycan cell wall but Gram-negative bacteria possess an outer phospholipid membrane that may confer penicillin resistance by hindering access of the drugs to the cell wall. Streptococci are Gram-positive bacteria.

3b What are the side-effects of penicillin V?

Hypersensitivity is the most important side-effect of penicillins and is manifest usually by rashes and rarely anaphylactic reactions. Allergic reactions to penicillins occur in 1–10% of exposed individuals; anaphylactic reactions occur in fewer than 0.05% treated patients (Joint Formulary Committee, 2008). General side-effects of antibiotics include: nausea, vomiting, abdominal pain, diarrhoea, headache and vaginitis.

3c What are the alternatives to penicillin V for treatment of sore throat?

Ampicillin and amoxicillin are not recommended for blind treatment of sore throat because of their propensity to cause maculopapular rashes in patients with glandular fever. Development of a rash can consequently cause a patient to be wrongly labelled as penicillin-allergic.

Erythromycin is a suitable alternative to penicillins for the treatment of sore throat and a 5–10 day course is recommended.

4a   What is the oral bioavailability of penicillin V and what is the impact of administration with food?

Estimates of bioavailability of penicillin V following oral administration range from 25% to 60%. Penicillin V should be administered an hour before food or on an empty stomach. Administration with food decreases the peak serum concentration but does not affect overall absorption of the drug.

4b   What are the storage conditions and shelf-life of penicillin V oral solution?

Once reconstituted with water, penicillin V oral solution becomes susceptible to degradation by hydrolysis and should be stored in a refrigerator and used within 7 days. If not refrigerated, as much as 10% of the active ingredient will degrade within 24 hours. Preservatives such as sodium benzoate may be included in the formulation. A second bottle should be supplied as dry powder with reconstitution instructions to allow completion of a 10-day course. Penicillin V is also available in a tablet formulation which may be suitable for older children.

5a   What are the disadvantages of prescribing antibiotics for sore throat?

Approximately a third of patients who attend their GP with a sore throat want or expect a prescription for antibiotics. There is evidence to suggest that prescribing antibiotics increases re-attendance rates for further episodes of sore throat and exposes patients to side-effects. Indiscriminate use of antibiotics also increases antibiotic resistance selection pressure (National Prescribing Centre, 2003).

5b   How should this patient's mother be counselled regarding the post-dated prescription and symptom relief?

The patient's mother should be reassured that the majority of sore throats are caused by viral infection and that symptoms often resolve within 3–7 days without antibiotics. Post-dated prescriptions are a means of providing access to antibiotic therapy following a short period of time during which symptoms may resolve and the patient may choose not to 'cash in' the prescription. Evidence suggests that deploying post-dated prescriptions is associated with comparable cure rates to immediate prescriptions but reduces patients' intentions to consult the GP in the future to obtain antibiotics for sore throat. The patient's mother should be reassured that should symptoms persist, the prescription will be honoured on the prescribed date and her child will not suffer any untoward consequences from the delay to starting antibiotics. The risks of adverse effects with antibiotics should also be explained. Paracetamol and ibuprofen are appropriate and effective for symptomatic relief of sore throat. Aspirin is contraindicated in children under 16 due to the risk of Reye's syndrome and aspirin gargle is of unproven efficacy in adults. Salt water gargle is reported to relieve pain in some patients. A number of over-the-counter products are available for the relief of sore throat, including lozenges such as Strepsils, Merocets, Tyrocets and Bradosol Sugar-Free and local anaesthetic sprays such as AAA Sore Throat Spray containing benzocaine. Not all of these products are suitable for young children.

Case study level 2 – Urinary tract infection (UTI) – see page 105

1   What are the symptoms and signs of a UTI and what is the role of dipstick testing?

Typical symptoms of a lower UTI are dysuria (pain on urination), urgency, frequency of urination and polyuria (passing an excessive amount of urine). Patients complaining of flank or back pain may have an upper UTI, often associated with fever and suprapubic tenderness on examination.

The urinary tract is normally sterile and dipsticks or reagent test strips are used to detect bacteriuria (presence of bacteria in the urine) by testing for nitrites (all common UTI bacteria convert nitrate to nitrite) or leucocyte esterase (enzyme indicating the presence of white blood cells).

Where only one symptom or sign of UTI is present, a dipstick test positive for leucocyte esterase or nitrites is associated with a high probability of bacteriuria (80%). If both leucocyte esterase and nitrites are negative, this is associated with a much lower probability of bacteriuria (approximately 20%) (SIGN, 2006).

However, a small study of younger women (16–59 years of age) presenting with a history of two symptoms – dysuria and frequency – but dipstick negative for both leucocyte esterase and nitrites, demonstrated that treatment with short-course trimethoprim significantly decreased the median time to resolution of dysuria (76% of women in trimethoprim group were free of dysuria by day 3 compared with 26% of placebo group). The authors concluded that their results supported the use of symptoms alone to diagnose and treat UTI without urinalysis (Richards *et al.*, 2005).

2a   When can a patient with cystitis be safely treated with over-the-counter products and when should they be referred to their GP?

Treatment with over-the-counter preparations is reasonable for non-pregnant women with mild cystitis of short duration (less than 2 days). The majority of over-the-counter products for cystitis contain potassium or sodium salts to alkalinise the urine, reducing stinging or burning pain and rendering conditions less favourable for bacterial growth. Examples include Canesten Oasis (sodium citrate), Cymelon (sodium salts) and Effercitrate (potassium citrate).

Warning signs that should prompt referral include the following:

- Fever, nausea and/or vomiting, loin pain or tenderness – suggesting upper UTI.
- Haematuria – may be caused by inflammation of the bladder or urethra due to cystitis but requires further investigation to exclude a kidney stone or a tumour in the bladder or kidney.
- Vaginal discharge – indicative of a local fungal or bacterial infection and pelvic examination may be required.

Patient groups requiring medical referral for investigation and treatment of cystitis include children, pregnant women and men. Children with UTI are at risk of damage to the kidneys or bladder and should always be referred to the doctor. Symptomatic bacteriuria is common in pregnancy (17–20% of pregnancies) and 10–30% of women with bacteriuria in the first trimester develop upper UTI in the second or third trimesters. Cystitis in men is an indication for referral to exclude more serious problems including kidney stones or prostate problems. Cystitis is less common in men than women due to their longer urethra and the antibacterial properties of prostatic fluid.

In addition, patients with recurrent cystitis or who have failed medication should be referred to the GP due to the risk of kidney damage.

2b   When is antibiotic treatment indicated for UTI?

Bacteriuria is present in over 70% of younger women (<50 years of age) presenting with acute symptoms suggestive of UTI (dysuria, frequency, urgency, loin/flank pain or back pain). The likelihood of bacteriuria in women presenting with dysuria and frequency but no vaginal irritation or discharge is even higher (77%). The Scottish Intercollegiate Guidelines Network (SIGN) recommends that if dysuria and frequency are both present, the probability of a UTI is greater than 90% and antibiotic treatment is indicated (SIGN, 2006).

In patients with symptoms or signs of UTI who also have a history of fever or back pain, the possibility of an upper UTI should be considered; a urine culture should be obtained and empirical antibiotic treatment started.

In contrast, asymptomatic bacteriuria does not require treatment in non-pregnant women and there is no evidence that treatment of asymptomatic bacteriuria reduces the risk of symptomatic episodes. Antibiotic treatment of bacteriuria in pregnant women, however, has been shown to reduce the risk of upper UTI, pre-term delivery and low birth weight babies and therefore asymptomatic bacteriuria detected during pregnancy should be treated with a 3- to 7-day course of antibiotics.

3a   What are the typical UTI pathogens and what are the treatment choices for lower UTI in a non-pregnant woman?

The most common pathogen associated with UTI in patients in the community is *Escherichia coli*, accounting for up to 90% of infections. Other pathogens include *Proteus mirabilis*, enterococci and staphylococci, along with yeasts from the candida species. The source of these organisms is usually the gastrointestinal tract.

First-line treatment for an uncomplicated lower UTI may vary according to local pathogen epidemiology and antibiotic sensitivity data but SIGN recommends a 3-day course of trimethoprim or nitrofurantoin. The SIGN guideline recommends that ciprofloxacin should not be used for empirical treatment of a lower UTI in women due to concerns over increasing resistance with overuse and its value in treating upper UTI. Suitable alternatives may include cefalexin and pivmecillinam.

3b   What are the treatment choices for lower UTI in a pregnant woman?

Pregnant women with symptomatic UTI should have a urine sample taken for culture before starting empirical antibiotics and treatment should be guided by local sensitivity patterns. Clinical Knowledge Summaries recommends nitrofurantoin, trimethoprim and cefalexin as first-line treatment options for pregnant women with lower UTI. Nitrofurantoin should be avoided close to delivery due to the risk of neonatal haemolysis. The *BNF* cautions against using trimethoprim during the first trimester due to its anti-folate activity and resulting teratogenic risk but short-term use of trimethoprim is unlikely to be harmful in women of normal folate status. Beta lactam antibiotics such as cefalexin and co-amoxiclav are considered safe in pregnancy but quinolones are contra-indicated due to arthropathy in animal studies.

4a   What should be considered by the pharmacist when dispensing nitrofurantoin?

Nitrofurantoin works by inactivating bacterial ribosomal proteins and other large molecules and has a bactericidal effect. The drug is concentrated in the urine and relies on adequate renal function (glomerular filtration rate (GFR) >30 mL/min) to guarantee activity. Nitrofurantoin is ineffective for upper UTI because it does not achieve adequate concentrations in the blood. The use of nitrofurantoin in patients with moderate-to-severe renal failure (GFR <50 mL/min) is not recommended due to increased risk of peripheral neuropathy (Kucers *et al.*, 1997).

Urinary pH significantly affects the activity of nitrofurantoin, with loss of potency as the urine becomes more alkaline. For this reason, women with lower UTI who are prescribed nitrofurantoin should be advised not to take alkalinising agents such as potassium citrate (Effercitrate).

The incidence of gastrointestinal side-effects including nausea, vomiting and diarrhoea with nitrofurantoin is as high as 30% with standard microcrystalline formulations and patients should be advised to take the doses with food. Other important but less common adverse reactions include pulmonary fibrosis, peripheral neuropathy and hypersensitivity. Patients should also be warned that nitrofurantoin can colour the urine yellow or brown.

Patients who do not respond to initial therapy should be referred to their family doctor to have urine taken for culture to guide change of antibiotic.

5a   What alternative therapies are available for cystitis and how effective are they?

There is good evidence to support the effectiveness of cranberry products in the prevention of symptomatic UTI in adult women with a history of recurrent infection and these patients should be advised to take cranberry products to reduce the frequency of recurrence. However, there are currently no randomised trials to evaluate the use of cranberry products in the treatment of symptomatic UTI (SIGN, 2006).

Alkalinising the urine may provide symptomatic relief but has no antibacterial effect.

5b   What lifestyle advice can be offered to patients with cystitis?

A common practice is to encourage patients to drink large quantities of fluids to facilitate physical removal of bacteria from the bladder, but this is not evidence-based.

Sexual intercourse may precipitate an episode of cystitis due to minor trauma or infection arising from bacteria being pushed along the urethra (so-called 'honeymoon cystitis'). Post-coital voiding of urine has been suggested as a means of reducing the risk of cystitis but again this is not evidence-based.

SIGN recommends that routine advice about lifestyle factors should not be offered to patients with bacterial UTI (SIGN, 2006).

Case study level 3 – Pneumonia – see page 106

1   How is the diagnosis of pneumonia made and how is the severity of illness assessed?

Community-acquired pneumonia in hospital is defined as:

■   Symptoms and signs consistent with an acute lower respiratory tract infection associated with new X-ray shadowing for which there is no other explanation (e.g. pulmonary oedema or pulmonary embolism).

The British Thoracic Society (BTS) guidelines state that a diagnosis of community-acquired pneumonia on the basis of history and clinical findings is inaccurate without a chest X-ray (British Thoracic Society, 2001).

The BTS endorses a severity assessment model for community-acquired pneumonia which allows patients to be stratified into groups at specific risk of mortality and therefore suitable for different clinical management pathways. A validated six-point scoring system was proposed with one point for each of: confusion; urea >7 mmol/L; respiratory rate ≥30/min; blood pressure low (systolic <90 mmHg or diastolic ≤60 mmHg); and age >65 years. This is known as the CURB-65 score. In the community, where serum urea is not routinely available a modified version – the CRB-65 score – is used. Patients who have a CRB-65 score of 3 or more are at high risk of death (33%) and require urgent hospital admission. Mrs CC has a CRB-65 score of 2 on admission.

Patients with a CURB-65 score of 3 or more should be managed as severe community-acquired pneumonia with appropriate antibiotics, whereas those with a CURB-65 score of 2 or less should be managed as non-severe community-acquired pneumonia.

2a   What is the significance of these laboratory findings?

Mrs CP has mild renal impairment which may be related to her infection or may be a chronic condition. Historical measurements are required for comparison.

The serum urea result puts Mrs CP's CURB-65 score at 3, indicating a severe community-acquired pneumonia.

C-reactive protein (CRP) is a protein produced by the liver during episodes of acute inflammation. CRP is not a specific test, however, and a positive CRP may indicate a number of things including inflammatory disease, malignancy, muscle necrosis (e.g. myocardial infarction) and trauma, as well as infection. A normal CRP is unlikely in the presence of a bacterial infection and a very high CRP (>100 mg/L) is more likely to occur in bacterial than viral infection. In this case, the patient's high CRP is consistent with a bacterial infection. CRP may be used to monitor a patient's response to therapy.

Elevated white blood cells and a predominance of neutrophils is consistent with a bacterial infection, although other possible causes include steroid administration, myeloproliferative disorders, inflammation (e.g. vasculitis) and acute haemorrhage.

2b   What are the possible interpretations of this microbiology result?

Blood for microorganism culture is typically collected into two bottles – the aerobic and anaerobic bottles. The majority of bacteria are facultative anaerobes which means they will grow in the presence or absence of oxygen, but strict anaerobes will only grow in the absence of oxygen. If the venepuncture site is not sterilised effectively or if poor aseptic technique is used, there is a risk of contamination of the sample with Gram-positive skin bacteria such as *Staphylococcus epidermidis*. With good phlebotomy technique, contamination rates can be as low as 2%. Contamination may be suspected if a single blood culture bottle is positive, as in this case, however, the result should not be dismissed as a contaminant in a patient with obvious signs of sepsis. One of the most common pneumonia pathogens, *Streptococcus pneumoniae*, is a Gram-positive coccus. Bacteraemia (bacteria in the blood) is associated with high mortality and should prompt urgent initiation of appropriate antibiotic therapy.

3   What are the important pathogens and appropriate treatment options for severe community-acquired pneumonia?

Studies of community-acquired pneumonia in the UK indicate that no organism is isolated in over 30% of cases (British Thoracic Society, 2001). Viruses are isolated in approximately 13% of patients. Of the bacterial pathogens associated with community-acquired pneumonia, *Streptococcus pneumoniae* is the most important (isolated in almost 40% of cases), typically sensitive to benzylpenicillin and cephalosporin antibiotics.

So-called atypical bacteria such as *Chlamydia pneumoniae* and *Mycoplasma pneumoniae* are the next most important group of community-acquired pneumonia pathogens, accounting for around one case in every eight in hospitalised patients. Atypical bacteria are not sensitive to beta-lactam antibiotics such as penicillins and cephalosporins and the treatment of choice is a macrolide such as erythromycin.

Other less common pathogens include *Staphylococcus aureus*, *Haemophilus influenzae* and Gram-negative rods from the gastrointestinal tract. In severe community-acquired pneumonia, these pathogens must also be covered due to the high risk of mortality, hence the use of more broad-spectrum cephalosporins or co-amoxiclav.

For a severe hospital-treated community-acquired pneumonia, the BTS guidelines suggest intravenous treatment with a broad-spectrum beta-lactam such as co-amoxiclav or a second- or third-generation cephalosporin. In addition, a macrolide such as erythromycin or clarithromycin should be added to cover atypical bacteria.

For a patient with a history of penicillin/cephalosporin allergy, expert advice should be sought from a clinical microbiologist. Newer quinolone antibiotics such as levofloxacin and moxifloxacin are possible options but the BTS does not recommend monotherapy with these agents at present.

4   Outline a pharmaceutical care plan for this patient with severe community-acquired pneumonia, including advice to the clinician.

For a severe pneumonia, the dose of ceftriaxone may be increased to 2 g once daily and no dose adjustment is required in moderate renal impairment. Intravenous therapy is indicated in severe or life-threatening infection or where there are concerns about absorption of oral therapy.

Erythromycin should be administered slowly and at an appropriate dilution to avoid thrombophlebitis and a risk of prolonged QT interval. Erythromycin is an inhibitor of cytochrome P450 enzymes and concomitant administration with simvastatin is not recommended. Simvastatin treatment may be suspended or azithromycin substituted for erythromycin.

Treatment should continue for 10 days for a severe infection and longer for certain pathogens such as *Staphylococcus aureus* and *Legionella pneumophila*.

Switching from intravenous to oral antibiotics should be considered as soon as clinically appropriate. Prolonged intravenous therapy is associated with risk of intravascular device-related infection and delays discharge. Indicators for switch include resolution of fever, tachycardia, tachypnoea, hypotension and hypoxia and the patient should be clinically hydrated with good oral intake and no gastrointestinal absorption concerns.

5   What are the goals of therapy in community-acquired pneumonia?

The primary goal of therapy in community-acquired pneumonia is to reduce mortality. The secondary goal is to ensure prompt clinical response and symptom resolution with minimum risk of recurrence at an acceptable risk of treatment adverse effects. Other goals include reducing unnecessary disturbance of the patient's normal flora and the associated risk of superinfection with resistant pathogens such as *Clostridium difficile.*

Antibiotic treatment should be appropriate for the likely pathogens and severity of infection, and prescribed at the correct dose, via the optimal route and for the appropriate duration.

Switch from parenteral to oral therapy should be initiated as soon as clinically appropriate.

6   How should therapy be monitored?

The patient's vital signs provide the most sensitive indicator of response to therapy and normalisation of heart rate, respiratory rate, oxygenation, blood pressure and temperature should be confirmed. Laboratory markers of infection such as CRP and WCC should be monitored to ensure normalisation. Failure to improve may indicate an incorrect diagnosis, a resistant pathogen, poor absorption of antibiotic, immunocompromise or local or distant complications of community-acquired pneumonia such as lung abscess.

7   What are the prognosis and potential complications of community-acquired pneumonia?

UK studies report mortality rates for adult patients hospitalised with community-acquired pneumonia ranging from 6% to 12%. Mortality increases to over 50% in patients admitted to the intensive care unit. Parapneumonic effusions develop in up to half of patients hospitalised with community-acquired pneumonia, requiring chest tube drainage; it may be the cause of persisting pyrexia. Lung abscess is a relatively rare complication of community-acquired pneumonia, and metastatic infection such as meningitis, peritonitis, endocarditis and septic arthritis can occasionally develop.

8   What are the relevant social pharmacy issues in this case?

Patients at high risk of mortality from pneumonia should be offered influenza vaccine and pneumococcal vaccine should also be considered. Smoking is an important risk factor and Mrs CP should be offered advice on smoking cessation and referred to an appropriate smoking cessation service.

Case study level Ma – Meningitis – see page 109

1   What are the signs and symptoms of meningitis and meningococcal septicaemia (bloodstream infection)?

The clinical signs of meningitis include the classical triad of fever, stiff neck and impaired consciousness found together in around 44% of cases (van de Beek *et al.*, 2006). Over 90% of patients with community-acquired bacterial meningitis present with at least two of four symptoms:

- fever
- neck stiffness
- altered mental state (drowsy, less responsive, vacant, confused)
- headache.

Three other classical signs of meningitis are:

- a dislike of bright lights (photophobia)
- vomiting
- rash.

Additional signs and symptoms that may indicate septicaemia include:

- severe pains and aches in the limbs and joints
- very cold hands and feet
- shivering
- rapid breathing
- red or purple spots that do not fade under pressure (non-blanching)
- diarrhoea and stomach cramps.

Physical examination should include testing for Kernig's and Brudzinski's signs. Kernig's sign is positive when extension of the knee elicits resistance or pain in the lower back or posterior thigh in a patient lying supine with the hip flexed at 90 degrees. Brudzinski's sign is present when passive neck flexion in a patient lying supine elicits a flexion of the knees and hips.

Lumbar puncture is considered mandatory in patients with suspected bacterial meningitis but the procedure can be hazardous with a risk of brain herniation in patients with raised intracranial pressure, and imaging with computed tomography or MRI is recommended for selected patients to detect brain shift. Patients who are in an immunocompromised state, have new-onset seizures, moderate-to-severe impairment of consciousness or signs that are suspicious of space-occupying lesions (e.g. papilloedema – oedema of the optic disk) should undergo neuroimaging prior to lumbar puncture.

2   What is the significance of these laboratory findings?

CSF white blood cell counts are usually raised above 50 cells/mm^3 in all causes of infective meningitis (up to 600 cells/mm^3 in tuberculous and viral meningitis, up to 1000 cells/mm^3 in cryptococcal meningitis and greater than 1000 cells/mm^3 in bacterial meningitis). Lymphocytes predominate in tuberculous, viral and cryptococcal meningitis, as well as early or partially treated bacterial meningitis. Polymorphonuclear leucocytes (immature and mature neutrophils) usually predominate in bacterial meningitis.

CSF protein is usually raised above 1 g/L in bacterial, tuberculous and cryptococcal meningitis and above 0.5 g/L in viral meningitis.

CSF glucose is usually less than 50% of blood glucose in bacterial, tuberculous and cryptococcal meningitis but normal in viral meningitis. This is due to impaired CNS glucose transport and consumption of glucose by micro-organisms and neutrophils.

Gram's staining of the CSF usually yields the organism in approximately 80% of cases of bacterial meningitis and yields are similar whether or not the patient has received prior antibiotics. The finding of Gram-negative cocci in the CSF is strongly indicative (99%) of bacterial meningitis (Spanos *et al.*, 1989; Hoen *et al.*, 1995).

3a   What are the important pathogens and appropriate treatment options for bacterial meningitis, including alternatives in penicillin allergy?

The main organisms causing bacterial meningitis in adults in the UK are *Neisseria meningitidis,* a Gram-negative diplococcus and *Streptococcus pneumoniae,* a Gram-positive streptococcus, accounting for approximately 1500 and 300 laboratory-confirmed cases per year respectively in England Wales (Health Protection Agency (UK), 2005a, 2005b).

There are a number of serogroups of *Neisseria meningitidis* including A, B, C and the less common W135 and Y. In 1999 a vaccine against *Neisseria meningitidis* group C (MenC) was introduced into the routine immunisation schedule and has now been extended to include everyone under 25 years of age. Hence the incidence of infection with this serogroup has decreased markedly. There is currently no vaccine available for the B serogroup, which is accountable for almost 90% of meningococcal meningitis in England and Wales and is the likely pathogen in this case.

Haemophilus influenzae type B, a Gram-negative cocco-bacillus, accounts for approximately 40 cases per year. The incidence of meningitis caused by *Haemophilus influenzae* type B has fallen considerably following introduction of the Hib vaccine in 1992.

GPs are advised to give benzylpenicillin before urgent transfer to hospital, particularly if meningococcal disease is suspected. Due to increasing resistance to penicillin in pneumococci and *H. influenzae,* the third-generation cephalosporins, cefotaxime and ceftriaxone, are currently recommended as first-line agents for patients hospitalised with suspected bacterial meningitis. Benzylpenicillin remains an option, however, for treatment of confirmed meningococcal infection. The drug of choice in penicillin/cephalosporin-allergic patients is chloramphenicol.

Addition of ampicillin or amoxicillin is recommended in patients over 55 years of age to cover *Listeria*.

Randomised clinical trials have demonstrated a significant beneficial effect of dexamethasone on mortality and morbidity in pneumococcal meningitis, although no benefit was seen for patients with meningococcal meningitis. Steroid treatment is now recommended routinely with or before the first dose of antibiotics, beyond which time dexamethasone begins to lose its effectiveness (van de Beek *et al.*, 2004).

3b Which antibiotic regimens achieve therapeutic concentrations in the cerebrospinal fluid and which should be avoided?

Ampicillin, amoxicillin, cefotaxime and ceftriaxone administered intravenously all achieve peak CSF levels of at least 10 times the typical MIC_{90} (minimum concentration of antibiotic that is inhibitory for 90% of isolates) of *Streptococcus pneumoniae*, *Neisseria meningitidis* and *Haemophilus influenzae*. At dosing intervals of 3–4 half-lives, this ensures that concentration of the drug remains above the MIC_{90} for at lest 50% of the dose interval, thus maximising beta-lactam antibiotic therapeutic effectiveness. Chloramphenicol peak CSF levels following intravenous administration are at least six times the typical MIC_{90} for the three major organisms.

Benzylpenicillin achieves peak CSF levels that are reliable for treating sensitive strains of *Streptococcus pneumoniae* and *Neisseria meningitidis* but not *Haemophilus influenzae* and therefore cefotaxime or ceftriaxone are more reliable for suspected *H. influenzae* meningitis.

Of the other broad-spectrum antibiotics commonly used in hospitals, gentamicin does not penetrate the CNS to achieve therapeutically useful concentrations and ciprofloxacin is not reliable against *S. pneumoniae*. Of the carbapenems, meropenem achieves better CNS penetration than imipenem. Vancomycin has poor CNS penetration but is prescribed routinely in countries with penicillin-resistant *S. pneumoniae*, often with rifampicin which achieves CSF concentrations effective against *S. pneumoniae* but not *Neisseria meningitidis* or *Haemophilus influenzae*.

3c What is the rationale for prescribing aciclovir in cases of suspected meningitis?

Aciclovir is prescribed empirically to cover encephalitis (inflammation of the brain parenchyma) caused by the herpes simplex virus (HSV). Confirmed HSV encephalitis is relatively rare (170 laboratory confirmed cases per annum in

England) but has a high mortality (10%) and survivors may be left with serious neurological sequelae including paralysis and speech loss (Davison *et al.*, 2003). Symptoms of encephalitis include fever, headache and altered mental status (e.g. lethargy, irritability, behavioural and personality changes), often accompanied by seizures and focal neurological deficits. Meningeal signs are typically mild. There is a predominance of lymphocytes in the CSF and glucose is normal with protein mildly elevated. Bacterial pathogens are not typically found on Gram stain.

Aciclovir is an analogue of the nucleic acid guanosine and interrupts viral DNA synthesis by inhibiting viral DNA polymerase.

4   Outline a pharmaceutical care plan for this patient with meningitis, including advice to the clinician.

The clinician should be prompted to review the decision to prescribe aciclovir. If the PCR for HSV is negative and provided the patient has no recent history of cold sores or genital herpes, then aciclovir should be stopped.

If meningococcus is confirmed by the microbiology laboratory and antibiotic sensitivity data suggest the strain is sensitive, the patient's therapy may be streamlined to benzylpenicillin i.v. 2.4 g every 4 hours. However, in practice it may be difficult to persuade the clinician to discontinue the initial therapy if the patient shows signs of improving.

The duration of therapy for meningococcal meningitis is at least 5 days (usually 7 days), 10–14 days for pneumococcal meningitis and at least 10 days for *H. influenzae* meningitis. Steroid therapy should continue for 4 days.

Rifampicin (600 mg orally twice daily for 2 days) should be administered to patients with meningococcal or *H. influenzae* meningitis who have not been treated with ceftriaxone, as soon as they can tolerate oral medication to eliminate nasal carriage of the organisms. Alternatively ciprofloxacin (500 mg orally stat) has proven efficacy for elimination of nasal carriage of meningococcus only.

5   What are the goals of therapy in community-acquired bacterial meningitis?

The goals of therapy are to rapidly control the infection and stabilise the patient to minimise morbidity and mortality. Early recognition of septicaemia and shock is essential to permit timely intervention, including securing the airway, administering high-flow oxygen and providing volume resuscitation. Identification of the pathogen is valuable for diagnostic and treatment purposes but administration of antibiotics should not be delayed until lumbar puncture in an acutely ill patient.

6   How should therapy be monitored?

Patients require close observation and monitoring of vital signs during treatment to ensure response to therapy. Serum C-reactive protein and white cell counts should be monitored and repeated examination of CSF may be required during therapy.

7   What are the prognosis and potential long-term complications of meningitis?

Fatality rates in patients with meningitis due to *Streptococcus pneumoniae* and *Neisseria meningitidis* are 19–37% and 3–13% respectively (van de Beek *et al.*, 2006). Long-term neurologic sequelae including hearing loss and other focal neurological deficits occur in up to 30% of survivors of *Streptococcus pneumoniae* meningitis and 3–7% of survivors of meningococcal meningitis.

8   What are the relevant social pharmacy issues in this case, including lifestyle issues?

Patients with meningococcal meningitis should be isolated until after at least 48 hours of antibiotic therapy to prevent infection spreading to other patients.

Spread of meningococcus between family members and close contacts is well recognised and chemoprophylaxis is recommended for close contacts as soon as possible, preferably within 24 hours. Rifampicin 600 mg every 12 hours for 2 days is licensed for chemoprophylaxis but ciprofloxacin 500 mg orally as a single dose (unlicensed) is also effective and often recommended for convenience.

Close contacts are considered to be individuals who have slept in the same house as the patient at any time in the 7 days before onset of symptoms, and boyfriends or girlfriends of the patient. Only healthcare workers who have administered mouth-to-mouth resuscitation or had prolonged face-to-face contact with the patient require prophylaxis and this should be initiated after consultation with the hospital infection control team. Prophylaxis for other contacts from closed communities such as nurseries, schools or universities should be considered where two or more linked cases have occurred and this should be initiated by a public health doctor.

Smoking is a risk factor for carriage of the meningococcal bacteria and the patient should be referred to a stop smoking service.

Case study level Mb – Diabetic foot infection – see page 112

1a   What are the signs and symptoms of foot infection in diabetic patients and when are antibiotics indicated?

Neuropathy of the sensory, motor and autonomic nerves, along with microvascular and macrovascular disease and impaired neutrophil function all contribute to the development of foot ulcers in diabetic patients. This patient has a neuropathic rather than an ischaemic ulcer.

Features associated with infection include cellulitis, lymphangitis, purulent drainage, sinus tract formation, osteomyelitis, septic arthritis, abscess

formation and sometimes the development of gangrene. Systemic manifestations may include fever, tachycardia, confusion and hypotension. Vesicles and
bullae filled with clear fluid are common.

Clinical diagnosis of infection is generally based on the presence of purulent secretions (pus) or at least two of the four cardinal signs of inflammation –
warmth, erythema (redness), swelling (or induration) and pain/tenderness.
Neuropathy and ischaemia may obscure or mimic these cardinal signs of inflammation in patients with diabetes and experts have suggested that antibiotics are
indicated in patients with evidence of cellulitis, fever, leucocytosis, foul-
smelling wounds or deep tissue infection (Cavanagh *et al.*, 2005).

1b   What are the likely pathogens?

Diabetic foot ulcers are often colonised by multiple organisms that may or may
not be pathogenic, therefore a swab of the ulcer surface is unreliable for identifying causative organisms in infection. The most reliable sample for culture is
a specimen of deep tissue obtained by aspiration or biopsy without contact with
the ulcer surface or draining lesions.

Mild ulcers are frequently infected by *Staphylococcus aureus* and
Streptococcus pyogenes (group A strep). Other pathogens include Gram-negative
rods and anaerobic bacteria (although anaerobes are seldom successfully cultured). Monomicrobial infection is not uncommon in mild ulcers.

Severe ulcers tend to have polymicrobial infection. Gram-positive
pathogens include *Staphylococcus aureus*, *Staphylococcus epidermidis* (coagulase-
negative staphylococcus), streptococci, enterococci, corynebacteria (diph-
theroids) and clostridia. Gram-negative pathogens include Enterobacteriaceae
(coliforms) such as *Escherichia coli*, *Klebsiella*, *Proteus* and *Pseudomonas* species.
Bacteroides bacteria are the predominant anaerobic pathogen.

2a   What are the primary issues to be considered when choosing empirical anti-
infective therapy in this case?

The need to be right

This is an important principle which governs selection of empirical therapy. If
a patient has a severe or life-threatening infection or if they are vulnerable (for
example due to immunocompromise), the empirical therapy regimen must be
broad spectrum enough to encompass the majority of likely pathogens. Bearing
in mind that broad-spectrum anti-infectives are not necessarily the most effective agents against specific pathogens, the regimen can later be streamlined to
narrower spectrum agents once the pathogen(s) and anti-infective sensitivities
are known. Previous microbiology results may influence the choice of empirical
treatment providing they are within a reasonable timeframe and representative
of infection rather than colonisation.

The risk of resistant organisms

Whether an infection is community-acquired or healthcare-acquired is of fundamental importance in choosing empirical therapy. Community-acquired infections tend to be caused by pathogens that are typically sensitive to a wide range of first-line anti-infectives. Healthcare-acquired infections in contrast are often caused by multi-resistant pathogens by virtue of the characteristics of the healthcare environment, including intensive anti-infective use and close cohorting of vulnerable patients. Patients who have failed an anti-infective regimen at adequate dosing are also more likely to have resistant organisms.

Contraindications and cautions

The major groups of patients to whom contraindications may apply are patients with a history of hypersensitivity, pregnant or breastfeeding women, patients with organ dysfunction and the very old and very young. Co-morbidity and current medications may also represent a contraindication (e.g. fluoro-quinolones in patients with epilepsy).

2b   Comment on the choice of anti-infective regimen in this case and discuss alternative regimens.

Piperacillin-tazobactam is a broad-spectrum penicillin-based anti-infective. In this case, the use of piperacillin-tazobactam may be contraindicated depending upon the nature of this patient's penicillin allergy. An assessment of risk–benefit should be made before dispensing.

A broad-spectrum regimen is indicated due to the severity of infection, the risk of losing the patient's foot and the fact that he is immunocompromised due to his diabetes mellitus. Bactericidal agents are preferred in immunocompromised patients. The regimen should ideally cover the organisms identified from his previous microbiology specimens, although these may be unreliable if taken from the surface of the ulcer. Intravenous administration affords greater penetration of the anti-infective to areas of poor perfusion.

The patient is on gabapentin but this is for neuropathic pain rather than epilepsy so fluoroquinolones may be used. He may have renal or hepatic impairment.

Alternatives to piperacillin-tazobactam for a penicillin-allergic patient with infected diabetic foot ulcer include:

- Clindamycin (to cover staphylococci, streptococci and anaerobes) plus gentamicin, ciprofloxacin, ceftazidime or aztreonam (to cover Gram-negative organisms including *Pseudomonas*).
- Ceftriaxone (to cover staphylococci, streptococci and Gram-negative organisms) plus metronidazole (to cover anaerobes) ± ciprofloxacin (to cover *Pseudomonas*).

- Vancomycin, daptomycin or linezolid (to cover staphylococci including methicillin-resistant *Staphylococcus aureus* (MRSA), streptococci and enterococci) plus metronidazole (to cover anaerobes) plus gentamicin, ciprofloxacin, ceftazidime or aztreonam (to cover Gram-negative organisms including *Pseudomonas*).
- Tigecycline (to cover staphylococci including MRSA, streptococci, enterococci and anaerobes) ± ciprofloxacin (to cover *Pseudomonas* and *Proteus*).

3　What is the significance of these laboratory findings?

Hyperglycaemia supports a diagnosis of HONK syndrome and severe hyperglycaemia has been shown to have a deleterious effect on immune function and is a significant predictor of infection rates.

Serum creatinine indicates mild renal impairment which may influence choice and monitoring of antibiotic therapy.

Leucocytosis is an indication of infection but this may be absent in patients with diabetes. Erythrocyte sedimentation rate (ESR) is usually raised. Raised C-reactive protein is consistent with infection.

Gram-positive bacteraemia is a predictor of poor outcome and prompt treatment with Gram-positive antibiotics active against MRSA is critical.

If osteomyelitis is ruled out, then shorter courses of antibiotic therapy are likely to be required for successful clinical outcome.

4　Critically appraise the management options in this case.

Debridement and drainage are critical aspects of management of the infected diabetic foot ulcer and delayed debridement of necrotic or infected tissue and drainage of purulent collections increases the risk of amputation. Wound management is also extremely important and use of vacuum foam dressing may be required to remove exudate and slough and promote granulation. Medicated dressings such as hydrofibre dressings impregnated with silver provide a local antiseptic effect where poor blood supply may limit antibiotic penetration. Strict bed rest is indicated and non-weight-bearing positioning.

An evidence-based guideline for diabetic foot infections from the Infectious Diseases Society of America highlights the lack of published clinical trials of antibiotics for this indication. The use of differing definitions of infection severity and clinical outcome makes comparison of antibiotic efficacy between studies unreliable. The guideline concludes that on the basis of available studies, no single drug or combination of agents appears to be superior to others (Lipsky *et al.*, 2004). Choice of empirical regimen is likely to be dictated by severity of infection, likelihood of resistant organisms such as MRSA and individual patient contraindications and side-effect risks.

The identification of Gram-positive cocci in blood cultures in this case mandates use of reliable Gram-positive cover such as vancomycin or teicoplanin or one of the newer agents: linezolid, daptomycin or tigecycline. These agents are all suitable for patients with penicillin allergy. The patient has mild renal impairment but vancomycin may still be used providing appropriate dose adjustments are made and therapeutic drug monitoring is carried out.

The severity of infection suggests that Gram-negative cover would also be prudent. Gentamicin is associated with increased nephrotoxicity in combination with vancomycin and ciprofloxacin offers an alternative option providing the patient is not at significant risk of seizures.

A malodorous wound is consistent with an anaerobic infection requiring suitable anaerobe cover such as metronidazole or clindamycin.

5   Outline a pharmaceutical care plan for this patient with infected diabetic foot ulcer including advice to the clinician.

Establish the nature of the patient's penicillin allergy and if a history of type 1 hypersensitivity is suspected, suggest an alternative regimen to the clinician to incorporate MRSA cover such as vancomycin plus ciprofloxacin plus metronidazole. Do not delay treatment to allow time for a deep tissue specimen to be taken.

Advise on a suitable starting dose and dose interval for vancomycin to achieve a trough serum concentration in the range 10–15 mg/L, taking into consideration the patient's mild renal impairment.

Monitor the patient's response to therapy and streamline the antibiotic regimen when microbiology results from a reliable clinical specimen become available.

Infections limited to soft tissue will require between 7 and 10 days of intravenous therapy followed by an additional 14 days of oral therapy (total duration 2–4 weeks). If MRSA is isolated, intravenous vancomycin must not be switched to oral vancomycin which has negligible absorption from the gastrointestinal tract. Oral agents may be selected from rifampicin, tetracyclines, fusidic acid or trimethoprim depending on sensitivity data and a combination of two agents is recommended. Oral linezolid monotherapy is an effective alternative.

6   What are the goals of therapy in diabetic foot infection?

The goals of therapy are to rapidly control the infection and stabilise the patient to minimise morbidity and mortality and reduce the risk of amputation.

7   How should therapy be monitored?

Resolution of local and systemic symptoms and signs of infection are the primary indicators of improvement. Blood test results including white blood cell counts, C-reactive protein and ESR are of limited use for monitoring response to treatment although failure of elevated levels to decrease should prompt review of management.

8   What are the prognosis and potential long-term complications of diabetic foot
ulcers?

Foot ulcers cause significant morbidity and impaired quality of life and are the
most important risk factor for lower extremity amputation. The lifetime risk of
a foot ulcer is up to 15% for patients with diabetes and 15–27% of all ulcers
result in surgical removal of bone (Jeffcoate and Harding, 2003). Major amputation incidence is around 0.5% of patients with diabetes per year (NICE, 2004).
Peri-operative mortality for major amputations is 10–15% and 3-year survival
rates can be as low as 50%.

9   What are the relevant social pharmacy issues in this case, including lifestyle
issues?

The National Institute for Clinical Excellence published a guideline on diabetic
footcare in 2004 which recommends regular (at least annual) visual inspection
of patients' feet with assessment of foot sensation and palpation of foot pulses
by trained personnel (NICE, 2004). Pharmacists can play an important role in
patient education around self-care and self-monitoring of the feet.

Patients should be advised to check their feet daily for problems and to
wash in warm (not hot) water and carefully dry their feet daily. They should be
encouraged to wear well-fitted shoes and hosiery and cautioned against skin
removal, including corn removal, without expert help. Over-the-counter preparations for foot problems such as corn removal are not suitable for patients
with diabetes.

Good control of blood glucose is paramount in preventing complications
of diabetes mellitus including diabetic foot ulcers. Pharmacists should support
concordance with oral hypoglycaemic and insulin regimens and regular blood
glucose monitoring.

6

Endocrine case studies

Russell Foulsham

Case study level 1 – Myasthenia gravis

Learning outcomes

Level 1 case study: You will be able to:

- describe the risk factors
- describe the disease
- describe the pharmacology of the drug
- outline the formulation, including drug molecule, excipients, etc. for the medicines
- summarise basic social pharmacy issues (e.g. opening containers, large labels).

Scenario

Mr Jones, a regular customer in your shop, hands you over a prescription. He has some difficulty with signing the back of the prescription as he can't focus properly due to his eyelids drooping, and his hand is a bit shaky. He recently took early retirement from his job as an Office Clerk as he was getting extreme fatigue in all his muscles, especially after a long day at work. The fatigue improved after having a rest.

He had spoken to you a few months ago about the fatigue and thought that it may be due to stress or poor diet, as he had been working very long hours to complete a contract on time. He bought some multivitamins with ginseng, but his tiredness did not improve except when he had a few days holiday.

Mr Jones had been referred to a neurologist at the local hospital who ran some tests and has asked his GP to write him a prescription for pyridostigmine bromide 60 mg tablets with half a tablet to be taken four times daily initially then increased up to six tablets a day if the muscle weakness does not improve.

The GP also prescribed hyoscine butylbromide 10 mg tablets, two of which were to be taken up to four times daily.

1   What is myasthenia gravis?
2   What are the risk factors?
3   What tests would Mr Jones have had at the hospital to diagnose this condition?
4   Why choose pyridostigmine as the anticholinesterase (consider the duration of action, side-effects and the formulations available)?

General references

Joint Formulary Committee (2008) *British National Formulary 55.* London: British Medical Association and Royal Pharmaceutical Society of Great Britain, March.
National Institute of Neurological Disorders and Stroke (2008) Myasthenia gravis fact sheet. Available at http://www.ninds.nih.gov/disorders/myasthenia_gravis/detail_myasthenia_gravis.htm [Accessed 30 June 2008].

Case study level 2 – Thyroid dysfunction

Learning outcomes

Level 2 case study: You will be able to:

■ interpret relevant laboratory and clinical data
■ identify monitoring and referral criteria
■ explain treatment choices
■ describe goals of therapy including monitoring and the role of the pharmacist/clinician
■ describe issues – counselling points, adverse drug reactions, drug interactions, complementary/alternative therapies and lifestyle advice.

Scenario

Mrs Smith, who is 35-years-old, comes into your pharmacy with her 1-year-old daughter and gives you a prescription for levothyroxine 50-microgram tablets take one daily. This is the first time she has taken the drug. She has gained a lot of weight since the birth of her daughter and has not been able to shift it even by sticking to a calorie-controlled diet. She feels cold all the time, even on a hot day, and her hair is thinning. She has no energy at all, whereas before the birth of her daughter she used to go to aerobics at least three times a week.

Questions

1   What do the patient's signs and symptoms indicate?
2   What are the possible causes of the disease?
3   What blood tests would she have for this condition? What should the normal range be for the laboratory test results and what levels would you expect Mrs Smith to have before treatment?
4   What monitoring is required for this condition?
5   Does she have to pay for her prescription?

General references

Joint Formulary Committee (2008) *British National Formulary* 55. London: British Medical Association and Royal Pharmaceutical Society of Great Britain, March.

National Prescribing Centre (2002) Management of common thyroid diseases. *MeReC Bulletin* 12(3) February. Available at http://www.npc.co.uk/MeReC_Bulletins/2001 Volumes/pdfs/v0112n03.pdf [Accessed 3 July 2008].

Clinical Knowledge Summaries (2007) Hyperthyroidism. Available at www.prodigy.nhs. uk/hypothyroidism/view_whole_guidance [Accessed 4 July 2008].

Case study level 3 – Hormone replacement therapy

Learning outcomes

Level 3 case study: You will be able to:

- interpret clinical signs and symptoms
- evaluate laboratory data
- evaluate treatment options
- state goals of therapy
- describe a pharmaceutical care plan to include advice to a clinician
- describe the prognosis and long-term complications
- describe the social pharmacy issues which could include supply (e.g. complex treatments at home, concordance and compliance) and lifestyle issues.

Scenario

Sally Harris has come in to your pharmacy and asks to speak to you privately. You take her into the counselling area and sit down. She tells you that she has been having severe hot flushes at night and thinks that she is 'going through the change of life'. She asks your advice.

Questions

1   What condition does Sally have and what are the usual signs and symptoms?
2   What is the cause of the condition and how is it diagnosed?
3   What hormonal treatments are available? Consider the risks and benefits.
4   What non-hormonal treatments are available on prescription and what symptoms do they act on?
5   What alternative therapies are available? Discuss their efficacy.
6   What other information should Sally be given?

General references

Joint Formulary Committee (2008) *British National Formulary* 55. London: British Medical Association and Royal Pharmaceutical Society of Great Britain, March.

National Prescribing Centre (2001) The benefits and risks of HRT. MeReC Briefing issue 16, October 2001. Available at http://www.npc.co.uk/MeReC_Briefings/2001/briefing_no_16.pdf [Accessed 4 July 2008].

National Prescribing Centre (2004) Hormone replacement therapy: an update. *MeReC Bulletin* 15(4). Available at http://www.npc.co.uk/MeReC_Bulletins/2004Volumes/Vol 14 no 4.pdf [Accessed 4 July 2008].

Case study level Ma – Osteoporosis

Learning outcomes

Level M case study: You will be able to:

- interpret clinical signs and symptoms
- evaluate laboratory data
- critically appraise treatment options
- state goals of therapy
- describe a pharmaceutical care plan to include advice to a clinician
- describe the prognosis and long-term complications
- describe the social pharmacy issues which could include supply (e.g. complex treatments at home, concordance and compliance) and lifestyle issues
- describe the monitoring of therapy.

Scenario

Mrs Patel is a frail (BMI 18) lady of 72 with well-controlled asthma using high-dose steroid inhalers and occasional oral courses during an exacerbation. She came in to show you her wrist, which is in a plaster cast. She wants your opinion as the orthopaedic consultant has said she has got osteoporosis and wants to send her for a special X-ray and start treatment.

Questions

1   How is osteoporosis characterised?
2   What are the risk factors for this condition, and which of these is relevant to Mrs Patel?
3   What is the special X-ray and what do the results indicate?
4   What are the goals of therapy in this case?
5   What drug treatments are available? Comment on their advantages and disadvantages with regards to Mrs Patel, using the latest evidence.
6   What monitoring would be required if Mrs Patel was prescribed alendronate 70 mg weekly?
7   What other measures would patients with this condition need to take, including falls prevention?

General references

Clinical Knowledge Summaries (2006) Osteoporosis-treatment-management (May 2006). Available at www.cks.library.nhs.uk/osteoporosis_treatment [Accessed 4 July 2008].

Joint Formulary Committee (2008) *British National Formulary 55.* London: British Medical Association and Royal Pharmaceutical Society of Great Britain, March.

National Prescribing Centre (2001) Common issues in osteoporosis. *MeReC Bulletin* 12(2), December. Available at http://www.npc.co.uk/MeReC_Bulletins/2001Volumes/pdfs/v0112n02.pdf [Accessed 4 July 2008].

NICE (National Institute for Health and Clinical Excellence) (2005) Bisphosphonates (alendronate, etidronate, risedronate), selective oestrogen receptor modulators (raloxifene) and parathyroid hormone (teriparatide) for the secondary prevention of osteoporotic fragility fractures in postmenopausal women. Available at www.nice.org.uk/nicemedia/pdf/TA087guidance.pdf [Accessed 4 July 2008].

NICE (2004) Falls: the assessment and prevention of falls in older people. Available at www.nice.org.uk/CG21 [Accessed 4 July 2008].

Royal College of Physicians (2002) Glucocorticoid-induced osteoporosis. Available at www.rcplondon.ac.uk/pubs/books/glucocorticoid/ [Accessed 4 July 2008].

SIGN (Scottish Intercollegiate Guidelines Network) (2003) Guideline, management of osteoporosis. Available at www.sign.ac.uk/guidelines/fulltext/71/index.html [Accessed 4 July 2008].

Case study level Mb – Type 2 diabetes

Learning outcomes

Level M case study: You will be able to:

- interpret clinical signs and symptoms
- evaluate laboratory data
- critically appraise treatment options
- state goals of therapy
- describe a pharmaceutical care plan to include advice to a clinician
- describe the prognosis and long-term complications
- describe the social pharmacy issues which could include supply (e.g. complex treatments at home, concordance and compliance) and lifestyle issues
- describe the monitoring of therapy.

You are a supplementary prescriber working in a diabetes clinic when John Stephens comes in to see you. He is still overweight despite being on the maximum dose of metformin and gliclazide. His HbA1c is 9.0% and on examination he has neuropathy developing in his feet. He is also on ramipril 10 mg, simvastatin 40 mg and aspirin 75 mg daily. His blood pressure was 130/80 mmHg and his total cholesterol was 4.0 mmol/L (reading from three months ago). There is no microalbuminuria present.

1   What are the clinical issues for this patient? What leads you to this conclusion?
2   What are the macrovascular and microvascular complications of the condition, and which of them is he exhibiting?
3   What is HbA1c and what does this result mean?
4   Assuming the cardiovascular complications are controlled, critically appraise the treatment options available.
5   How should insulin therapy be introduced and give examples of suitable regimens?
6   What insulin administration devices are there and what different types of insulin are available?
7   Produce a pharmaceutical care plan for this patient and include the goals of therapy.
8   What monitoring does John require?

General references

Clinical Knowledge Summaries (2002) Type 2 diabetes-blood glucose. Available at www. nice.org.uk/page.aspx?o=guidelineg [Accessed 4 July 2008].

Joint Formulary Committee (2008) *British National Formulary 55.* London: British Medical Association and Royal Pharmaceutical Society of Great Britain, March.

National Prescribing Centre (2004) Drug management of type 2 diabetes: summary. *MeRec Bulletin* 15(1), October. Available at www.npc.co.uk/MeReC_bulletins/2004 volumes/v0115n01.pdf [Accessed 4 July 2008].

Case study level 1 – Myasthenia gravis – see page 135

1   What is myasthenia gravis?

This is an autoimmune disease in which there is muscle weakness without any change in the individual's ability to feel things. In myasthenia gravis antibodies block, alter or destroy the receptors for acetylcholine at the neuromuscular junction, which prevents the muscle contraction from occurring. Hence with fewer receptor sites available the muscles receive fewer nerve signals.

The patient has muscle weakness which increases after a period of activity and improves with rest. He has drooping of the eyelids (ptosis) with blurred vision due to weakness of the muscles that control eye movement.

2   What are the risk factors?

Myasthenia gravis most commonly affects young adult women (under 40) and older men (over 60) and is not inherited. Risk factors include fatigue, illness, stress, extreme heat and other medication (including beta-blockers, calcium channel blockers, quinine and quinolones).

3   What tests would Mr Jones have had at the hospital to diagnose this condition?

- The presence of acetylcholine receptor antibodies.
- Edrophonium test. An intravenous injection of edrophonium chloride which is a drug that blocks the degradation of acetylcholine and temporarily increases the levels of acetylcholine at the neuromuscular junction.
- Nerve conduction study. This tests for specific muscle 'fatigue' by repetitive nerve stimulation. It should demonstrate decrements of the muscle action potential due to impaired nerve-to-muscle transmission.

4   Why choose pyridostigmine as the anticholinesterase (consider the duration of action, side-effects and the formulations available)?

It is less powerful and slower in action than neostigmine but it has a longer duration of action. It has relatively mild gastrointestinal effect but an antimuscarinic drug may still be required for the stomach cramps. A total daily dose of 450 mg should not be exceeded in order to avoid acetylcholine receptor downregulation. Immunosuppressant therapy is usually added if the dose of pyridostigmine exceeds 360 mg daily. It is only available as a tablet, unlike neostigmine which comes as a tablet and injection.

Case study level 2 – Thyroid dysfunction – see page 136

1 What do the patient's signs and symptoms indicate?

Hypothyroidism – Low metabolic rate signified by weight gain whilst on a calorie-controlled diet, feeling cold and her hair thinning.

2 What are the possible causes of the disease?

Primary hypothyroidism most commonly presents as an autoimmune disease (Hashimoto's disease) where the body produces antibodies that attack the thyroid gland. Possible causes are:

- congenital – poor development of the thyroid gland
- lack of iodine in the diet
- enzyme defects in the thyroid gland
- overtreatment with antithyroid drug
- lithium and amiodarone
- surgical removal of the thyroid
- radioactive iodine therapy.

Secondary hypothyroidism results from an underproduction of thyroid hormones from the thyroid caused by deficient thyroid-stimulating hormone (TSH) stimulation by the pituitary.

3 What blood tests would she have for this condition? What should the normal range be for the laboratory test results and what levels would you expect Mrs Smith to have before treatment?

- Blood concentrations of levothyroxine (T4), liothyronine (T3) and thyroid stimulating hormone (TSH) need to be taken.
- T4 normal value is 9–25 pmol/L, in hypothyroidism <9 pmol/L.
- T3 normal value is 3–9 pmol/L.
- TSH normal value is <6 mU/L, in hypothyroidism >6 mU/L.

4 What monitoring is required for this condition?

Symptomatic improvement occurs within 2–3 weeks of starting levothyroxine, although it can take about six weeks for TSH to return to normal. TSH levels should be measured every six weeks following a change in dose, then once yearly once the condition is stable. The usual dose range of levothyroxine is 100–200 micrograms daily. Oral contraceptives and hormone replacement therapy can falsely raise total T4 levels, so free T4 should be measured if Mrs Smith takes these drugs.

5 Does she have to pay for her prescription?

No – she will tick for medical exemption as she will require continuous replacement therapy.

Case study level 3 – Hormone replacement therapy – see page 137

1   What condition does Sally have and what are the usual signs and symptoms?

Menopause – hot flushes, night sweats, sleep disturbance, vaginal dryness and discomfort.

2   What is the cause of the condition and how is it diagnosed?

Reduction in circulating oestrogen levels. Levels of serum follicle-stimulating hormone (FSH) will be above 30 IU/L.

3   What hormonal treatments are available? Consider the risks and benefits.

Due to the presence of oestrogens there is increased risk of breast, endometrial and ovarian cancer, venous thromboembolism and stroke, but they alleviate vaginal atrophy and vasomotor instability, and reduce osteoporosis.

Transdermal formulations may be preferred as they require a lower dose (and hence have lower risk) as they do not undergo the first-pass effect in the liver – although patient preference is usually based on convenience.

- Urogenital symptoms only – vaginal preparations carry less risk.
- Without uterus – oral or non-oral oestrogen (does not require progesterone to reduce the risk of endometrial cancer).
- With uterus and perimenopausal – sequential HRT (to allow a bleed).
- With uterus and postmenopausal – continuous combined HRT.
- High-dose progestogen (medroxyprogesterone) – useful to treat vasomotor symptoms with no increased risk of cardiovascular conditions.

4   What non-hormonal treatments are available on prescription and what symptoms do they act on?

Non-hormonal treatments include:

- clonidine – for hot flushes
- selective serotonin reuptake inhibitor (SSRI) drugs – for hot flushes
- gabapentin – for hot flushes, aches, pains and paraesthesia.

5   What alternative therapies are available? Discuss their efficacy.

There are many alternative therapies available, but there is very little clinical trial data so much of the evidence is anecdotal:

- Phytoestrogens (dietary sources such as cereals/seeds, linseed/pulses, particularly soya/vegetables) may help to reduce most symptoms.
- Red clover may reduce hot flushes in some women.
- Agnus castus has a hormone-regulating effect useful in the perimenopausal phase.
- Black cohosh has a serotonin effect which may help with mood swings and depression associated with hormone fluctuation. When used short-term it has been shown to reduce hot flushes in patients with breast cancer.

- Dong quai has no effect.
- Evening primrose oil at therapeutic doses may be useful for mood swings.
- Sage has some evidence of reducing hot flushes.
- St John's wort is an antidepressant.
- Wild yam has no effect as body cannot synthesise sex hormones from it.

6   What other information should Sally be given?

- She will need to consider barrier methods of contraception as she can still conceive for up to 2 years after her periods stop.
- The risk of osteoporosis is reduced while using HRT.
- There is an increased risk of thomboembolism, endometrial cancer and breast cancer while using HRT.

Case study level Ma – Osteoporosis – see page 139

1   How is osteoporosis characterised?

Osteoporosis is characterised by micro-architectural deterioration of bone tissue and low bone mass, leading to increased bone fragility and risk fracture.

2   What are the risk factors for this condition, and which of these is relevant to Mrs Patel?

Mrs Patel has a low body mass index (<21) and a history of long-term steroid use.

Other risk factors include: poor intake of dietary calcium, lack of weight-bearing exercise, previous fracture, premature menopause (before age of 45), family history (maternal side), excessive alcohol intake, long episodes of amenorrhoea before menopause, medical conditions that may affect the absorption of food, hyperparathyroidism.

3   What is the special X-ray and what do the results indicate?

Bone mineral density (BMD) is measured using dual energy X-ray absorptiometry (DEXA) usually at the neck of femur (on the hip). The World Health Organization defines a diagnosis of osteoporosis if the BMD is 2.5 standard deviations or more below the young adult female mean value. This difference is known as the T-score. Patients are considered to have osteopenia if the T-score is between –1 and –2.5.

Other methods of measuring bone density such as ultrasonography of the heel are available.

4   What are the goals of therapy in this case?

The goals are to increase bone mineral density and reduce the likelihood of fracture.

5   What drug treatments are available? Comment on their advantages and disadvantages with regards to Mrs Patel, using the latest evidence.

- Bisphosphonates – must be taken on an empty stomach as they chelate with metal ions in food. Available as daily, weekly or monthly formulations to improve compliance. Increases bone mass by 3% per year when given in conjunction with calcium and vitamin D.
- HRT – will reverse urogenitory symptoms but increased risk of breast cancer.
- Calcitonin – available as a nasal spray, but requires dietary calcium intake.
- Calcitriol – oral, but need to monitor plasma calcium and creatinine.
- Raloxifene – does not reduce menopausal vasomotor symptoms.
- Strontium ranelate – must be taken on an empty stomach as it chelates with metal ions in food.
- Teriparatide – only by injection.

6   What monitoring would be required if Mrs Patel was prescribed alendronate 70 mg weekly?

Monitoring should include:

- U&E – mainly plasma calcium and creatinine
- DEXA scan annually
- possible endoscope to check for oesophageal strictures if complaining of difficulty in swallowing.

7   What other measures would patients with this condition need to take, including falls prevention?

Lifestyle measures, such as smoking cessation and weight-bearing exercise plus calcium and vitamin D supplements would be appropriate.

Patient risk factors for falls include:

- balance, gait or mobility problems (including joint disease, stroke and Parkinson's disease)
- polypharmacy (i.e. taking four or more medicines, particularly centrally sedating or blood pressure-lowering drugs)
- visual impairment
- impaired cognition or depression
- postural hypotension.

Environmental risk factors include:

- poor lighting, particularly on the stairs
- steep stairs
- loose carpets or rugs
- slippery floors
- badly fitting footwear or clothing
- inaccessible lights or windows
- lack of safety equipment (e.g. grab rails).

Older people who fall should be referred to a specialist falls service, particularly those who:

- have had previous fragility fractures,
- have attended accident and emergency following a fall,
- have called an ambulance following a fall,
- have two or more patient risk factors,
- have frequent unexplained falls,
- fall in hospital or in a nursing or residential home,
- live in unsafe housing conditions, or
- are very afraid of falling.

Interventions to reduce the risk of falls and damage from falling include:

- assessment and correction of vision, if possible
- correction of postural hypotension
- medication review and discontinuation of inappropriate medication
- rehabilitation, including physiotherapy, to improve confidence
- occupational therapy to identify and correct hazards in the home
- repairs and improvements to the home
- exercise and balance training
- use of hip protectors (from hospital or community services; not available on FP10)
- treatment of osteoporosis.

Case Study Level Mb – Type 2 diabetes – see page 140

1   What are the clinical issues for this patient? What leads you to this conclusion?

His diabetes is not well controlled as he has neuropathy and high blood sugar levels. His weight must be controlled by diet and exercise otherwise he will develop insulin resistance and require injections.

2   What are the macrovascular and microvascular complications of the condition, and which of them is he exhibiting?

- Macrovascular complications are related to the cardiovascular system. His blood pressure and cholesterol are being controlled.
- Microvascular complications will arise from prolonged high levels of glucose in the blood as signified by the high HbA1c reading. These will include neuropathy, nephropathy and retinopathy. He is starting to demonstrate neuropathy, which could lead to amputation if not controlled.

3   What is HbA1c and what does this result mean?

Red blood cells are composed of haemoglobin. Glucose sticks to the haemoglobin to make a glycosylated haemoglobin molecule (HbA1c). The more glucose present in the blood, the more HbA1c will be present.

Red blood cells live for 8–12 weeks before they are replaced. HbA1c indicates how high a patient's blood glucose has been on average over the previous 8–12 weeks. A normal non-diabetic HbA1c is 3.5–5.5%. In diabetes about 6.5%

is good. Glucose levels averaging 6.5 mmol/L is equivalent to 7% HbA1c. John's reading of 9% is equivalent to average blood glucose of 13 mmol/L which indicates poor control.

4   Assuming the cardiovascular complications are controlled, critically appraise the treatment options available.

The aim of treatment is for the patient to attain the target HbA1c level of 6.5%, but not below this, to reduce the risk of suffering with microvascular complications. All patients should be given structured education (such as diet and exercise) and self-monitor their plasma glucose to ensure that they attain their individually agreed target. All choices are based on patient acceptability and cost-effectiveness. The following steps are recommended if HbA1c is not maintained below 7.5%:

- If metformin alone does not control the HbA1c, then metformin and a sulfonylurea should be given. A thiazolidinedione can be substituted for either agent if unacceptable side effects occur, such as nausea or hypoglycaemia. A rapid-acting insulin secretagogue may be added for people with erratic lifestyles, as it can be given once daily.
- Add insulin or a thiazolidinedione (only if insulin is likely to be unacceptable or ineffective). Exenatide may be considered if the criteria are met, such as a BMI of > 35 kg/m², on a cost effectiveness basis.
- Increase insulin dose and intensify regimen over time. May consider pioglitazone in combination with insulin if thiazolidinedione has been effective previously or high dose insulin is providing inadequate control.

5   How should insulin therapy be introduced and give examples of suitable regimens?

If fasting glucose >6 mmol/L add intermediate-acting insulin 6–10 units at bedtime. Increase dose by 1–2 units every 3 days until blood glucose target is reached.

If fasting glucose is normal but daytime glucose levels are above target level, add intermediate acting insulin, 6–10 units at breakfast time. Increase by 1–2 units every 3 days until target is reached.

6   What insulin administration devices are there and what different types of insulin are available?

Devices include:

- vial + syringe
- penfill cartridge + injection device
- Flexpen (ready filled) – InnoLet device has a large dial on it
- continuous subcutaneous infusion.

Types of insulin:

- short acting – soluble/aspart/glulisine/lispro
- intermediate acting – isophane/biphasic aspart/biphasic lispro/biphasic isophane
- long acting – protamine zinc/detemir/glargine.

Most come in highly purified animal and human sequence versions. Animal versions are used in patients with large titres of antibodies to human insulin.

7   Produce a pharmaceutical care plan for this patient and include the goals of therapy.

Goals include:

- lifestyle – smoking cessation, weight loss and increased exercise levels
- blood glucose control – HbA1c <7.0%
- blood pressure <135/75 mmHg
- lipids – total cholesterol maintain <5.00 mmol/L
- antiplatelet treatment.

8   What monitoring does John require?

Monitoring should include:

- twice daily blood glucose levels at different times of the day
- six monthly HbA1c and blood pressure
- annual lipid, U&Es, microalbuminuria and review with clinician.

7

Obstetrics, gynaecology and UTI case studies

Alka Mistry

Case study level 1 – Primary dysmenorrhoea

Learning outcomes

Level 1 case study: You will be able to:

- describe the risk factors
- describe the disease
- describe the pharmacology of the drug
- outline the formulation including drug molecule, excipients, etc. for the medicines
- summarise basic social pharmacy issues (e.g. opening containers, large labels).

Scenario

Fifteen-year-old Miss SM comes to your pharmacy accompanied by her mother with a prescription for mefenamic acid 500 mg t.d.s. (three times a day) p.r.n. (when necessary). Supply 42 tablets. You recognise the mother as she has recently been in to purchase over-the-counter ibuprofen for her daughter.

Questions

1 What is primary dysmenorrhoea?
2 What are the risk factors for developing primary dysmenorrhoea?
3a What group of drugs does mefenamic acid belong to?

3b   How does mefenamic acid work in the treatment of primary dysmenorrhoea?
3c   What are the side-effects of mefenamic acid tablets (see *BNF*)?
4a   Which non-drug treatments are advocated in primary dysmenorrhoea?
4b   What else could the GP prescribe if mefenamic acid did not adequately control the symptoms of primary dysmenorrhoea?
5   What counselling must be given as you know the mother has previously purchased ibuprofen OTC?
6   What other formulations of mefenamic acid are there?

General references

Clinical Knowledge Summaries (2006) Dysmenorrhoea. Available at http://cks.library. nhs.uk/dysmenorrhoea [Accessed 4 July 2008].
Joint Formulary Committee (2008) *British National Formulary 55.* London: British Medical Association and Royal Pharmaceutical Society of Great Britain, March.
Kennedy S (2005) Dysmenorrhoea: explaining its causes and treatment. *Prescriber* 19 May: 27.

Case study level 2 – Urinary tract infections in pregnancy

Learning outcomes

Level 2 case study: You will be able to:

- interpret relevant laboratory and clinical data
- identify monitoring and referral criteria
- explain treatment choices
- describe goals of therapy, including monitoring and the role of the pharmacist/clinician
- describe issues – counselling points, adverse drug reactions, drug interactions, complementary/alternative therapies and lifestyle advice.

Scenario

A 30-year-old pregnant woman presents to your pharmacy with a new prescription for cefalexin 500 mg three times a day for one week. She is worried about possible effects on the developing baby.

1   What organisms cause urinary tract infections (UTI)?
2a   What is the incidence of UTI in pregnancy?
2b   What are the presenting features, signs and symptoms of UTI?
2c   What are the possible complications of UTI during pregnancy?
3   What are the management recommendations for cystitis in pregnancy?
4a   Which antibiotics used to treat UTI can be safely prescribed in pregnancy?
4b   Which antibiotics used to treat UTI can be used with caution during pregnancy?
4c   Which antibiotics used to treat UTI should be avoided or are contraindicated during pregnancy?
5a   How would you counsel the patient on the medication she has been prescribed?
5b   What nutritional advice could you offer the patient to aid a healthy pregnancy?

General references

Clinical Knowledge Summaries (2006) Urinary tract infection (lower) – women. Available at http://cks.library.nhs.uk/uti_lower_women [Accessed 4 July 2008].
Joint Formulary Committee (2008) *British National Formulary 55*. London: British Medical Association and Royal Pharmaceutical Society of Great Britain, March.
PJ Practice Checklist (2001) Nutrition and pregnancy. Produced by *The Pharmaceutical Journal* (updated January).

Case study level 3 – Pelvic inflammatory disease

Learning outcomes

Level 3 case study: You will be able to:

- interpret clinical signs and symptoms
- evaluate laboratory data
- evaluate treatment options
- state goals of therapy
- describe a pharmaceutical care plan to include advice to a clinician
- describe the prognosis and long-term complications
- describe the social pharmacy issues which could include supply (e.g. complex treatments at home, concordance and compliance) and lifestyle issues.

A 25-year-old woman, Miss AK, presents at a walk-in centre with pelvic pain, specifically lower abdominal and post-coital bleeding. On examination the patient has mild fever and adnexal tenderness. Sexual history reveals a recent change of partner. Endocervical swabs are taken with initiation of immediate antibiotic treatment. Miss AK is told to return to surgery for review within 2 days if she is not getting better.

1a What is pelvic inflammatory disease (PID)?
1b What symptoms may be associated with PID and which apply to Miss AK?
2a Where is the ideal place to manage a case of PID?
2b In which circumstances would a patient be referred to hospital?
2c What are the implications for sexual partners?
3   What are long-term complications if PID is untreated?
4a Which antibiotics can be used to treat PID and which would you suggest?
4b What adverse effects do the antibiotics prescribed to treat PID commonly cause?
4c What is the reason for including metronidazole?
4d Which analgesics would be useful?
5   What counselling is essential in this case?
6   Miss AK is on the combined oral contraceptive (COC) pill. What advice would you give her?

General references

Joint Formulary Committee. *British National Formulary 55*. London: British Medical Association and Royal Pharmaceutical Society of Great Britain, March 2008.

McBride D. Talking to patients about pelvic inflammatory disease. *Prescriber* 5 April 2004: 18–23.

Clinical Knowledge Summaries. Pelvic inflammatory disease (2006). Available from, http://cks.library.nhs.uk/pelvic_inflammatory_disease (Accessed 04 July 2008).

Case study level Ma – Endometriosis management in secondary care

Learning outcomes

Level M case study: You will be able to:

- interpret clinical signs and symptoms
- evaluate laboratory data
- critically appraise treatment options
- state goals of therapy
- describe a pharmaceutical care plan to include advice to a clinician
- describe the prognosis and long-term complications
- describe the social pharmacy issues which could include supply (e.g. complex treatments at home, concordance and compliance) and lifestyle issues
- describe the monitoring of therapy.

Scenario

A 39-year-old patient, Mrs DS, known to urology (as had left ureteric obstruction which was stented), presents with back pain and lower left-sided abdominal pain with rigors and nausea. She has lost 2 stone (12.7 kg) in weight and cannot work.

Her previous medical history includes:

- irregular periods; bleeds for 5–7 days per cycle
- mild dysmenorrhoea
- no dyspareunia
- never pregnant; does not want children.

Investigation results are:

- ultrasound – endometriotic chocolate cysts
- CT scan – cystic mass in pelvis embedding left ureter.

A laparoscopy is performed and the cysts drained. The patient is prescribed GnRh analogue plus add-back therapy. Two months later she is readmitted with left loin pain, hot, cold and dizzy symptoms. The impression is a flare-up of the endometriosis. The pain team prescribed morphine 2 hourly. Patient had radical operation: subtotal abdominal hysterectomy and bilateral salpingo-oophorectomy.

1   What is endometriosis and why does it occur?
2   What are the presenting signs and symptoms? Which does Mrs DS exhibit?
3   How is it diagnosed and how common is it?
4   What are the treatment aims/options?
5   What is the theory behind hormonal treatments?
6   What are the range of hormonal treatments available, their limitation and side-effects?
7   What counselling should be offered for the hormonal treatments?

General references

Clinical Knowledge Summaries (2006) Endometriosis. Available at http://cks.library. nhs.uk/endometriosis [Accessed 4 July 2008].

Dos Reis R (1999) Familial risk among patients with endometriosis. *Journal of Assisted Reproduction and Genetics* 16: 500–503.

Habiba M (2002) Endometriosis – current approaches to treatment. *Prescriber* 19 December: 23–30.

Joint Formulary Committee (2008) *British National Formulary* 55. London: British Medical Association and Royal Pharmaceutical Society of Great Britain, March.

Royal College of Obstetricians and Gynaecologists (2006) The investigation and management of endometriosis. Green-top Guideline No. 24. October. Available at http://www.rcog.org.uk/resources/Public/pdf/endometriosis_gt_24_2006.pdf [Accessed 4 July 2008].

The National Endometriosis Society – Treatment options for endometriosis fact sheet. Available at http://www.endometriosis-uk.org/information/treatment.html [Accessed 4 July 2008].

Case study level Mb – Management of severe pre-eclampsia/eclampsia

Learning outcomes

Level M case study: You will be able to:

- interpret clinical signs and symptoms
- evaluate laboratory data
- critically appraise treatment options
- state goals of therapy
- describe a pharmaceutical care plan to include advice to a clinician
- describe the prognosis and long-term complications
- describe the social pharmacy issues which could include supply (e.g. complex treatments at home, concordance and compliance) and lifestyle issues
- describe the monitoring of therapy.

Scenario

Mrs MB is a daily ward attender with increased blood pressure for last week. Primigravida. Gestation 38 weeks. Scarred left kidney with 11% function. Her notes are given in Table Q7.1.

Questions

1   Define the terms eclampsia/pre-eclampsia and severe pre-eclampsia.
2   List the clinical features of severe pre-eclampsia (in addition to hypertension and proteinuria).
3a Comment on the significance of Mrs MB's test results.
3b What is HELLP syndrome and how is this diagnosis confirmed?
4a What are the treatments used in the management of hypertension during pregnancy? Critically appraise the evidence for options available.
4b What would you recommend for Mrs MB?
4c Mrs MB's condition worsens – now what treatment would you suggest?
5   What signs and symptoms should be monitored if a woman is prescribed magnesium sulphate and what is prescribed if signs of magnesium toxicity are observed?
6   How should fluid balance be managed in a patient with pre-eclampsia?
7   How should Mrs MB be managed post delivery?

Table Q7.1 Notes for patient Mrs MB

Time	Symptoms	Observations	Actions
18:30		bp 160/108 mmHg	15-minute observations
19:45		bp 164/114 mmHg	Nifedipine 10 mg SR prescribed
21:00	Epigastric tenderness		Fluid reduced to 85 mL/h Labetalol 200 mg p.o.stat
22:30	Headache Vomiting	bp 210/150 mmHg ALT 296 IU/L	Transfer to HDU. Labetalol i.v. 50 mg stat + infusion
00:30		bp 146/69 mmHg	Magnesium sulphate i.v. stat + infusion Labetalol 200 mg p.o. t.d.s.
04:15		HELLP syndrome ALT 1132 IU/L Platelets 53×10^9/L Reduced Hb	Emergency LSCS
09:10	Epigastric pain Photophobia	bp 155/115 mmHg	Returned to HDU for CVP monitoring and fluid optimisation post HELLP and PET

General references

Abalos E, Duley L, Steyn DW, Henderson-Smart DJ (2007) Antihypertensive drug therapy for mild to moderate hypertension during pregnancy. *Cochrane Database of Systematic Reviews* Issue 1. Art. No.: CD002252. DOI: 10.1002/14651858.

Duley L, Meher S, Abalos E (2006a) Management of pre-eclampsia. *British Medical Journal* 332: 463–467.

Duley L, Henderson-Smart DJ, Meher S (2006b) Drugs for treatment of very high blood pressure during pregnancy. *Cochrane Database of Systematic Reviews* Issue 3. Art. No.: CD001449. DOI: 10.1002/ 14651858.

Joint Formulary Committee (2008) *British National Formulary 55*. London: British Medical Association and Royal Pharmaceutical Society of Great Britain, March.

Royal College of Obstetricians and Gynaecologists (2006) The management of severe pre-eclampsia/eclampsia. Guideline No. 10 (A) March. Available at http://www.rcog.org.uk/resources/Public/pdf/management_pre_eclampsia_mar06.pdf [Accessed 4 July 2008].

Answers

Case Study Level 1 – Primary dysmenorrhoea – see page 150

1   What is primary dysmenorrhoea?

Dysmenorrhoea is cyclical, lower abdominal or pelvic pain which may also radiate to the back and thighs, occurring before or during menstruation or both. Primary dysmenorrhoea occurs in the absence of any obvious underlying disease that may be cause of pain.

2   What are the risk factors for developing primary dysmenorrhoea?

Risk factors include:

- nulliparity
- obesity
- cigarette smoking
- being sexually inactive
- late child-bearing
- positive family history.

3a   What group of drugs does mefenamic acid belong to?

Mefenamic acid is a non-steroidal anti-inflammatory drug (NSAID). It exhibits anti-inflammatory, analgesic and antipyretic activities. The mechanism of action is not completely understood but may be related to prostaglandin synthetase inhibition.

3b   How does mefenamic acid work in the treatment of primary dysmenorrhoea?

Elevated prostaglandin levels are present in the endometrial fluid of dysmenorrhoeic women and correlate well with the degree of pain. NSAIDs are inhibitors of prostaglandin synthesis and probably work by decreasing uterine prostaglandin levels and uterine contractility.

3c   What are the side-effects of mefenamic acid tablets (see *BNF*)?

Diarrhoea or rashes (withdraw treatment), vomiting, flatulence, constipation, ulcerative stomatitis. Less commonly paraesethesia and fatigue. Rarely, thrombocytopenia, haemolytic anaemia and aplastic anaemia are reported. Convulsions in overdosage.

4a   Which non-drug treatments are advocated in primary dysmenorrhoea?

High-frequency transcutaneous electrical nerve stimulation (TENS) is an option for women who prefer not to take medication. TENS seems to work by altering the body's ability to receive or perceive pain signals, rather than having a direct effect on the uterine contractions.

4b   What else could the GP prescribe if mefenamic acid did not adequately control the symptoms of primary dysmenorrhoea?

Combined oral contraceptives (COCs) are helpful, especially when prostaglandin inhibition fails. COCs are thought to relieve dysmenorrhoea by inducing endometrial thinning and inhibiting ovulation, resulting in low levels of uterine prostaglandins.

5   What counselling must be given as you know the mother has previously purchased ibuprofen OTC?

You have been prescribed with mefenamic acid 500-mg tablets. Take one tablet three times a day while having period pain. Some women find that it helps to start taking these painkillers a day or so before the period is expected to start. Alternatively, start to take them at the onset of pain or bleeding, whichever happens first. Take them regularly while the pain lasts. Mefenamic acid is a drug in the same group of drugs as ibuprofen; it is important that both mefenamic acid and ibuprofen are not taken together as this will increase side-effects in the stomach.

6   What other formulations of mefenamic acid are there?

If mefenamic acid tablets are too big for Miss SM to swallow then a branded capsule formulation (Ponstan) is available. The GP would need to be contacted to agree the change for Drug Tariff reimbursement purposes.

Case study level 2 – Urinary tract infections in pregnancy – see page 151

1   What organisms cause urinary tract infections (UTI)?

Urinary tract infections are usually caused by bacteria from the gastrointestinal tract; *Escherichia coli* accounts for about 90% of UTIs acquired in the community.

Other organisms responsible for UTIs are *Staphylococcus* species, *Proteus mirabilis, Enterococci* and *Candida albicans*.

Candida albicans UTI is rarely found in patients within the community setting but is common in hospital patients with risk factors such as indwelling catheters, immunosuppression, diabetes mellitus and those on antibiotic treatment.

2a   What is the incidence of UTI in pregnancy?

A review of UTI in pregnancy reported that:

- the incidence of asymptomatic bacteriuria (presence of bacteria in urine with no associated symptoms) was 2–10%,
- the incidence of acute cystitis (infection of the bladder) was in the range 1–4%, and
- about 20–40% of women with asymptomatic bacteriuria develop pyelonephritis (kidney infection) later in pregnancy.

2b   What are the presenting features, signs and symptoms of UTI?

Typical symptoms or signs of UTI include:

- dysuria
- frequency of urination
- haematuria
- back pain
- flank/loin tenderness
- no vaginal irritation or discharge.

2c   What are the possible complications of UTI during pregnancy?

Possible complications include:

- development delays in the infant
- cerebral palsy in the infant
- fetal death.

3   What are the management recommendations for cystitis in pregnancy?

Before initiating treatment it is important that a sample of urine be sent for culture and sensitivities. A mid-stream urine sample (MSU) and clean catch urine are the most commonly collected specimens and are recommended for routine use. The first part of the voided urine is discarded and without interrupting the flow approximately 10 mL is collected in a sterile container.

Empirical treatment is then initiated with trimethoprim, nitrofurantoin or cefalexin.

Once the sensitivity of the cultured organism is known treatment can be adjusted accordingly.

A repeat urine culture should be done at approximately 7 days after the completion of treatment to confirm eradication of the bacteria has been achieved.

Symptoms of pain and raised temperature due to infection may be treated with paracetamol.

Urine cultures should be repeated monthly throughout the rest of the pregnancy to screen for asymptomatic infection.

4a   Which antibiotics used to treat UTI can be safely prescribed in pregnancy?

Amoxicillin is recommended only if the organism is known to be sensitive to penicillins. Penicillins are not associated with any increased risk to the fetus.

Cefalexin is a first-generation cephalosporin. It is not associated with any increased risk to the fetus and is effective against most urinary pathogens.

4b   Which antibiotics used to treat UTI can be used with caution during pregnancy?

Trimethoprim can be used during pregnancy except in women with a known folate deficiency or those who are taking folate antagonists, because it may limit availability of folic acid to the fetus and impair normal development. There is equivocal evidence to suggest that folate supplementation reduces the risk of neural tube defects in offspring of pregnant women treated with trimethoprim. Therefore, folate supplementation is recommended in all women treated with trimethoprim during the first trimester as a precautionary measure. Trimethoprim should not be used if the woman has recently had a course (some clinicians recommend avoiding repeating treatment with trimethoprim within three months) or if the woman has a history of recurrent infections resistant to this drug.

Co-amoxiclav can be separated into amoxicillin (see above 4a) and clavulanic acid; no adverse effects in newborn or fetus attributed to the combination of amoxicillin and clavulanic acid during pregnancy. Nitrofurantoin is effective against most UTIs. It should not be prescribed if the mother is glucose-6-phosphate dehydrogenase (G6PD) deficient. Nitrofurantoin can otherwise be used in pregnancy, but may cause haemolysis in a G6PD-deficient infant if used close to term. Nitrofurantoin is thus contraindicated in pregnant women during the third trimester. For most people the standard tablet formulation is suitable. The microcrystalline capsules and the twice-daily modified-release formulation may be better tolerated if nausea is troublesome and are offered as alternatives.

Second-generation cephalosporins are not as well absorbed orally as the first-generation cephalosporins, have a greater incidence of gastrointestinal adverse effects, and are more expensive than first-generation agents – thus they should only be used where specifically indicated.

Third-generation cephalosporins generally require parenteral administration and are reserved for use in secondary care for serious infections.

Pivmecillinam is not known to be teratogenic but is not recommended in pregnancy because of insufficient safety data.

4c   Which antibiotics used to treat UTI should be avoided or are contraindicated during pregnancy?

Quinolones are contraindicated during all stages of pregnancy due to the risk of arthropathy.

5a   How would you counsel the patient on the medication she has been prescribed?

You have been prescribed cefalexin, an antibiotic to treat your infection.

Are you allergic to any antibiotics? (Approximately 10% of patients allergic to penicillins will also be allergic to cephalosporins). Take one capsule three times a day for one week. It is important to take the capsules at regular intervals and finish the week's course.

5b   What nutritional advice could you offer the patient to aid a healthy pregnancy?

A healthy diet during pregnancy helps reduce the risk of having an infant of low birth weight who is at increased risk of poor health. A good diet contains a wide variety of foods including bread, cereals, pasta, rice and potatoes; fruit and vegetables; lean meat; fish and pulses; and reduced fat milk and dairy products. Listeriosis is a rare but serious disease if it occurs in pregnancy. Some cases of listeria have been associated with food. Foods such as Brie, Camembert and blue-veined cheeses, pâté and undercooked meat, eggs and poultry should be avoided. Fruit, vegetables and salads should be washed thoroughly.

Case study level 3 – Pelvic inflammatory disease – see page 152

1a   What is pelvic inflammatory disease (PID)?

This is a general term for the infection of the upper genital tract including uterus, fallopian tubes and ovaries. PID is thought to occur as a result of the spread of organisms from the lower to the upper genital tract.

Sexually transmitted infections are a common cause of PID. The main organisms are *Chlamydia trachomatis* and *Neisseria gonorrhoeae*.

No single symptom, sign or laboratory finding is both sensitive and specific for the diagnosis of PID.

1b   What symptoms may be associated with PID and which apply to Miss AK?

PID can be asymptomatic and so the incidence of PID is unknown. Symptoms include:

- lower abdominal pain (usually most prominent symptom)
- dyspareunia
- abnormal vaginal bleeding
- abnormal vaginal discharge
- dysuria
- nausea and vomiting (rare in acute infection).

2a   Where is the ideal place to manage a case of PID?

Ideally all women with suspected PID should be managed in a GUM (genito urinary medicine) clinic but treatment should not be delayed if they cannot be seen immediately.

2b   In which circumstances would a patient be referred to hospital?

- If the patient is pregnant.
- If the diagnosis is uncertain (e.g. appendicitis or ectopic pregnancy cannot be excluded).
- If patient cannot tolerate oral medication.
- If patient immunosuppressed (e.g. HIV positive).

2c   What are the implications for sexual partners?

Contact tracing of all male sexual partners in the previous six months is recommended. Ideally the GUM clinic would do the contact tracing and manage partners. Test partner for chlamydia and treat. Test partner for gonorrhoea and treat if woman with PID or partner has positive swabs.

3   What are long-term complications if PID is untreated?

- Tubal infertility affects around 10% of women with a history of PID.
- Ectopic pregnancy occurs in 1–5% of women who have had PID and go on to conceive.
- Chronic pelvic pain develops in 30% of women who have had PID.
- Tubo-ovarian abscess is usually associated with anaerobic infection.

4a   Which antibiotics can be used to treat PID and which would you suggest?

Ceftriaxone 250 mg as a single intramuscular dose followed by doxycycline 100 mg orally twice daily and metronidazole 400 mg twice daily both for 14 days.

A suggested alternative is ofloxacin 400 mg orally twice daily plus oral metronidazole 400 mg twice daily, both for 14 days. This regimen is not recommended if the woman is at high risk of gonococcal PID because of increasing quinolone resistance of gonorrhoea infection in the UK.

4b   What adverse effects do the antibiotics prescribed to treat PID commonly cause?

- Broad-spectrum antibiotics all have the potential to cause gastrointestinal side-effects, such as nausea, vomiting and diarrhoea.
- Ceftriaxone is a cephalosporin antibiotic. Consider using a different antibiotic if the person has a true penicillin allergy, as cephalosporins show cross-reactivity to penicillins in about 8% of people.
- Ofloxacin, a quinolone antibiotic, can cause tendon damage or seizures. Treatment should be stopped if pain or inflammation of a tendon occurs. Precipitation of seizures is rare unless the person is already prone to epilepsy or related conditions.

- Metronidazole may cause gastrointestinal effects and react with alcohol. Common adverse effects include a metallic taste and gastrointestinal irritation (in particular nausea and vomiting). These are more common at higher doses. Some people taking oral metronidazole experience disulfiram-like reactions to alcohol (flushing, increased respiratory rate, increased pulse rate). Thus, people taking metronidazole should be advised of the possible consequences of drinking alcohol.
- Doxycycline can cause oesophageal irritation and rarely photosensitivity.

4c   What is the reason for including metronidazole?

Metronidazole is included to improve coverage for anaerobes as initial infection with *Chlamydia* or *Neisseria gonorrhoea* can cause epithelial damage, allowing other organisms to enter the cervix and cause ascending infection.

4d   Which analgesics would be useful?

- Paracetamol is a safe and effective analgesic and antipyretic that is suitable for most patients.
- Ibuprofen is an effective analgesic and antipyretic and has a favourable risk–benefit profile.
- Codeine (alone or in combination with regular paracetamol) can be helpful when paracetamol alone is insufficient. Prescribing it separately offers greater flexibility in dosing and hence pain control.

5   What counselling is essential in this case?

The importance of completing the course of antibiotics in order to reduce the risk of long term complications.

The importance of screening for sexually transmitted diseases.

The need for screening and treatment of sexual partners to prevent reinfection.

The need to avoid intercourse until both they and their partner(s) have completed treatment. The possible long term health implications for their health and the health of their partner(s).

6   Miss AK is on the combined oral contraceptive (COC) pill. What advice would you give her?

Warn the patient that the antibiotics may interfere with the combined oral contraceptive pill (COC), as she is taking this. She should use condoms for one week after completion of the antibiotic course, and the next COC pill pack should be started without a break and thus omitting the pill-free week.

Case study level Ma – Endometriosis management in secondary care – see page 154

1   What is endometriosis and why does it occur?

The endometrium is the tissue that lines the inside of the uterus. Endometriosis is a condition where endometrial tissue is found outside the uterus. It is 'trapped' in the pelvic area and lower abdomen. The exact cause is unknown. A reflux of menstruation occurs in many women but in endometriosis refluxed cells implant in the pelvis, bleed in response to cyclic hormone stimulation and increase in size. Patches of endometriosis can cause adhesions and form into cysts which can fill with thick fluid and are known as 'chocolate' cysts.

2   What are the presenting signs and symptoms? Which does Mrs DS exhibit?

Presentation varies. It is often cyclic and responds to menstruation, but over time pain becomes a chronic pain syndrome which is acyclic and only disappears in pregnancy or menopause. Women can also have advanced lesions with tissue destruction and adhesions and may be asymptomatic. Endometriosis may be detected when investigating causes of infertility.

3   How is it diagnosed and how common is it?

A definitive diagnosis can only be made visually by laparoscopy. Ultrasound or MRI scans can show endometriotic cysts but not minor lesions. The true prevalence is unknown because surgical confirmation is needed. Incidence peaks around 40 years of age. Diagnosis may be delayed if infertility rather than pain is the problem. The condition has a familial tendency. A study has confirmed prevalence among first-, second- and third-degree relatives, which suggests this disorder has a genetic basis. Women with severe chronic pain have a more advanced stage of disease at initial diagnosis.

4   What are the treatment aims/options?

The aims are to improve symptoms (e.g. pain and heavy bleeding), improve fertility and reduce the size of or remove ectopic endometrial deposits.

Options are medical hormonal treatments and/or surgery. Surgical treatment by laparoscopic ablation of endometriotic lesions plus adhesiolysis may improve fertility. Hormonal treatments should not be used for endometriosis in women with fertility problems as they tend to lead to ovarian suppression. Laparoscopic ablation of endometrial deposits may relieve pain in some women. Radical surgery (e.g. total abdominal hysterectomy, salpingo-oophorectomy or both) is reserved for women who have completed their family and in whom other treatments have failed. It is usually curative although endometriosis can recur in women receiving HRT after bilateral salpingo-oophorectomy.

5   What is the theory behind hormonal treatments?

The hypothalamus causes pulsed releases of gonadotrophin-releasing hormone (GnRh). This results in the anterior pituitary producing follicle-stimulating hormone and luteinising hormone, which in the ovaries results in the production of oestrogens and progestogens. The different hormone treatments work by affecting different parts of this cascade. The end-result is to reduce the amount of oestrogen that is made or to block its actions in endometrial cells.

6   What are the range of hormonal treatments available, their limitation and side-effects?

Combined oral contraceptives

Combined oral contraceptives (COCs) are the most commonly used down-regulators of ovaries; although this is an off-licence use. Although oestrogen is present, the progestogen thins the endometrium and results in sparse bleeding at the regular withdrawals. COCs relieve endometriosis-related pain and may be useful if the main symptom is heavy bleeding. Tricycling COCs (using COCs continuously for three months followed by one week without pills) may improve quality of life by reducing frequency of menstrual bleeding. This practice is off-licence but the regimen is safe, well tolerated and acceptable by women.

Adverse effects include nausea, vomiting, headache, breast tenderness, changes in body weight, fluid retention and thrombosis. World Health Organization (WHO) medical eligibility criteria for COC use should be consulted.

Progestogens

Progestogens are the 'oldest' treatment for endometriosis. They induce endometrial atrophy and reduce oestrogen levels by inhibiting ovulation.

- Norethisterone is taken continuously and can be taken long term if required.
- Medroxyprogesterone is taken orally continuously. It is licensed to be taken for 90 days although some clinicians advise continued use if adverse effects are minimal and symptoms are well controlled.

Adverse effects include; irregular bleeding, bloating, skin changes, mood changes and weight gain.

Androgens

Androgens (danazol and gestrinone) inhibit secretion of pituitary gonado-trophins. They have androgenic, anti-oestrogenic and anti-progestogenic activity and usually cause amenorrhoea and induce a postmenopausal state.

- Danazol is licensed to be taken continuously for up to six months but can only be used when other treatments have failed. It does not reduce bone mineral density as its anabolic effects counteract the effect of lowered oestrogen levels.
- Gestrinone is licensed to be taken continuously for up to six months. It has similar actions to danazol but has a longer half-life, allowing twice weekly instead of daily dosing.

Both are poorly tolerated because of androgenic adverse effects, which include weight gain, hirsutism, acne, mood changes and occasionally deepening of the voice, which may be irreversible.

GnRh analogues

GnRh analogues (buserelin, naferelin, goserelin, leuprorelin and triptorelin) initially stimulate pituitary secretion and then rapidly inhibit secretion due to 'pituitary downregulation'. This is followed by anovulation, markedly reduced oestrogen levels and amenorrhoea, inducing a postmenopausal state and regression of endometrial deposits.

- Buserelin and naferelin are available as intranasal preparations. As these need daily dosing they are not commonly prescribed, as psychologically the patient is constantly reminded of the disease.
- Goserelin, leuprorelin and triptorelin are monthly depot injection preparations which are more convenient.

GnRh analogue treatment is only licensed for six months and only a single course of treatment is recommended by the manufacturers. The main concern with GnRh analogues is that they adversely affect bone mineral density, which typically falls by 4–6% during six months' treatment. These adverse effects may be reduced by additional 'add-back' therapy. This is a combination of one or more hormones with GnRh analogues to minimise or eliminate hypo-oestrogenic adverse effects such as bone loss and hot flushes. This is often started at the time of commencing treatment with GnRh analogues. Tibolone 2.5 mg daily is the preferred treatment.

Other adverse effects of GnRh analogues include insomnia, reduced libido, vaginal dryness and headaches.

7   What counselling should be offered for the hormonal treatments?

With progestogens and androgens adequate contraceptive measures (e.g. barrier methods) should be used. With buserelin or naferelin, if a nasal decongestant is required, it should not be administered before or for at least 30 minutes after GnRh analogue use. With naferelin, sneezing during or immediately after dosing may impair absorption. If sneezing occurs, repeating the dose may be advisable.

Case study level Mb – Management of severe pre-eclampsia/ eclampsia – see page 156

1   Define the terms eclampsia/pre-eclampsia and severe pre-eclampsia.

- Eclampsia is defined as the occurrence of one or more convulsions superimposed on pre-eclampsia.
- Pre-eclampsia is pregnancy-induced hypertension in association with proteinuria (>0.3 g in 24 hours) ± oedema; virtually any organ system may be affected.
- Severe pre-eclampsia is severe hypertension (diastolic blood pressure >110 mmHg on two occasions or systolic blood pressure >170 mmHg on two occasions) together with significant proteinuria (at least 1 g/L).

2   List the clinical features of severe pre-eclampsia (in addition to hypertension and proteinuria).

Clinical features of severe pre-eclampsia include:

- severe headache
- visual disturbance
- epigastric pain and/or vomiting
- signs of clonus
- papilloedema
- liver tenderness
- platelet count falling to below 100×10^6/L
- abnormal liver enzymes (ALT or AST rising to above 70 IU/L)
- HELLP syndrome (haemolysis, elevated liver enzymes, low platelets).

3a   Comment on the significance of Mrs MB's test results.

In pre-eclampsia, a rise in uric acid correlates with poorer outcome for both mother and baby. If creatinine is found to be elevated early in the disease process, underlying renal disease should be suspected. Falling platelet count is associated with worsening disease and is itself a risk to the mother. If count is less than 100×10^6/L there may be associated coagulation abnormalities, and delivery should be considered. An AST level >75 IU/L is significant and >150 IU/L is associated with increased morbidity to the mother.

3b   What is HELLP syndrome and how is this diagnosis confirmed?

HELLP syndrome is a group of symptoms used to characterise pre-eclampsia or eclampsia in pregnant women who also show signs of liver damage and abnormalities in blood clotting. It is characterised by:

- H aemolysis
- EL (elevated) liver enzymes
- LP (low platelet) count.

A diagnosis of HELLP syndrome needs confirmation of haemolysis by blood film to look for fragmented cells.

4a   What are the treatments used in the management of hypertension during pregnancy? Critically appraise the evidence for options available.

Antihypertensive treatment should be started if systolic blood pressure >160 mmHg or diastolic >110 mmHg. If a woman has other markers of potentially severe disease (e.g. heavy proteinuria) treatment can be considered at lower degrees of hypertension. The drug with which there is most experience in the treatment of hypertension in pregnancy is methyldopa. Other drugs with which there is experience include prazosin, hydralazine and nifedipine. ACE inhibitors and angiotensin II antagonists are contraindicated in pregnancy as they have multiple adverse effects in the fetus. Administration of certain beta-blockers, such as atenolol, during pregnancy may result in an increase in fetal growth retardation, although labetalol may be reasonably safe. Labetalol should be avoided in women with known asthma.

Diuretics are no longer used in pregnancy and are usually reserved for women with renal or cardiac problems.

4b   What would you recommend for Mrs MB?

Labetalol can be given orally or intravenously. Nifedipine can be given orally; in general the SR preparation is used and it is never used sublingually so as not to drop the blood pressure too quickly.

4c   Mrs MB's condition worsens – now what treatment would you suggest?

The Magpie Study demonstrated that administration of magnesium sulphate to women with pre-eclampsia reduces the risk of an eclamptic seizure. If given, it should be continued for 24 hours following delivery or 24 hours after the last dose, whichever is the later.

5   What signs and symptoms should be monitored if a woman is prescribed magnesium sulphate and what is prescribed if signs of magnesium toxicity are observed?

- Regular assessment of urine output, maternal reflexes, respiratory rate and oxygen saturation is important.

- Magnesium sulphate is mostly excreted in urine; if urine output falls to below 20 mL/h, the infusion should be stopped.
- Magnesium toxicity can be assessed clinically as it causes loss of deep tendon reflexes and respiratory depression.
- Calcium gluconate 1 g (10 mL) is given by slow intravenous injection (over 10 min) for magnesium toxicity.

6   How should fluid balance be managed in a patient with pre-eclampsia?

Fluid restriction is advisable to reduce the risk of fluid overload in the intrapartum and postpartum periods. Total fluids should be limited to 80 mL/h or 1 mL/kg per hour. Pulmonary oedema has been associated with inappropriate fluid management. There is no benefit of fluid expansion; it may increase the risk of caesarean section. The regimen of fluid restriction should be maintained until there is a postpartum diuresis as oliguria is common with severe pre-eclampsia.

7   How should Mrs MB be managed post delivery?

- She should be carefully reviewed before discharge as there is a risk of late seizures.
- Continue antihypertensives as dictated by blood pressure monitoring. Treatment may need to continue for up to three months.
- If there is persistent hypertension and proteinuria at six weeks she may need further investigation for renal disease.
- Currently there is insufficient evidence to recommend any particular antihypertensive. Good practice is to avoid methyldopa postnatally due to its adverse side-effect profile, especially depression.
- In breastfeeding women, labetalol, atenolol, nifedipine and enalapril are in use either singly or in combination.

8

Malignant diseases case studies

Michael Powell

Case study level 1 – Non-small cell lung cancer

Learning outcomes

Level 1 case study: You will be able to:

- describe the risk factors
- describe the disease
- describe the pharmacology of the drug
- outline the formulation including drug molecule, excipients, etc. for the medicines
- summarise basic social pharmacy issues (e.g. opening containers, large labels).

Scenario

Mr AP, a 56-year-old former coal miner, presents to your hospital pharmacy from the oncology outpatients department with a prescription for the following medications:

- ondansetron 4 mg p.o. b.d. for 5 days
- dexamethasone 2 mg p.o. b.d. for 5 days
- ranitidine 150 mg p.o. b.d. for 2 weeks.

On questioning the patient, you discover that he suffers from the 'more common' type of lung cancer and is undergoing 'irradiation' treatment currently. At this point you also notice that his right index and middle fingers as well as his teeth are stained yellow.

Questions

1   What are the main types of lung cancer?
2a   What are the risk factors associated with the development of lung cancer?
2b   Is it possible that Mr AP has any of the risk factors for developing lung cancer?
3   Briefly describe the class of drugs that ondansetron, dexamethasone and ranitidine belong to and: (a) how ondansetron and dexamethasone work in the management of nausea and vomiting; (b) how ranitidine works in the management of dyspepsia; and (c) the rationale for co-prescribing ranitidine and dexamethasone.
4a   Mr AP states that he readily suffers from bouts of constipation and is concerned that these new tablets may worsen this. What would you advise?
4b   What are the other typical side-effects of the drugs prescribed for Mr AP?
5   Mr AP also states that due to the large tumour 'pressing on my food pipe', he is currently having difficulty swallowing tablets. What alternative formulations could you suggest in order to facilitate medication compliance in this case?

Reference

Cancer Research UK (2004) Chapter Seven: Lung cancer and smoking – UK. In: Toms JR (ed.) *CancerStats Monograph 2004*. London: Cancer Research UK, pp. 45–53.

General references

Joint Formulary Committee (2008) *British National Formulary 55*. London: British Medical Association and Royal Pharmaceutical Society of Great Britain, March.
Lee J, McKenna R *et al.* (2001) Non-small cell lung cancer, mesothelioma and thymoma. In: Pazdur R, Coia L, Hoskins W, Wagman L (eds) *Cancer Management: A Multi-disciplinary Approach – Medical, Surgical and Radiation Oncology*. Melville, NY: PRR Inc., pp. 87–125.
Summary of Product Characteristics (2008) Zofran tablets. Available at http://emc.medicines.org.uk/emc/assets/c/html/displayDocPrinterFriendly.asp?documentid =17653 [Accessed 7 July 2008].

Case study level 2 – Treatment of advanced colorectal cancer

Learning outcomes

Level 2 case study: You will be able to:

- interpret relevant lab and clinical data
- identify monitoring and referral criteria
- explain treatment choices
- describe goals of therapy including monitoring and the role of the pharmacist/clinician
- describe issues – counselling points, adverse drug reactions, drug interactions, complementary/alternative therapies and lifestyle advice.

Scenario

Mrs KT, a 52-year-old hospital cleaner, is admitted as an inpatient to your oncology ward with symptoms from advanced colon cancer. Her GP referred her to the hospital oncology team three weeks ago for investigations (including colonoscopy and subsequent biopsy of a colonic mass, as well as whole body computerised tomography (CT) scan) that revealed stage IV metastatic colon cancer. Her consultant oncologist has now admitted her for FOLFOX systemic cytotoxic chemotherapy treatment.

At the time of admission, her laboratory results from blood analysis were as follows:

Full blood count	
Hb	8.8 g/dL (12.0–14.7 g/dL)
White blood cells	7.2×10^9/L (3.9–10.1×10^9/L)
Neutrophils	4.6×10^9/L (1.9–6.8×10^9/L)
Platelets	346×10^9/L (150–400×10^9/L)
Biochemistry	
Na$^+$	139 mmol/L (137–145 mmol/L)
K$^+$	2.6 mmol/L (3.6–5.0 mmol/L)
Urea	10.7 mmol/L (2.5–6.1 mmol/L)
Creatinine	126 micromol/L (62–106 micromol/L)
Liver function tests	
Total bilirubin	17 micromol/L (3–22 micromol/L)
ALT	30 units/L (0–52 units/L)
ALP	101 IU/L (38–126 IU/L)
GGT	42 units/L (12–43 units/L)

She has no significant past medical history and is currently not taking any regular medications.

Mrs KT's consultant oncologist decides to commence her on the FOLFOX chemotherapy regimen as follows:

- oxaliplatin 85 mg/m^2 i.v. infusion over 2 hours Day 1 only
- folinic acid 200 mg/m^2 i.v. infusion over 2 hours Days 1 and 2
- 5-fluorouracil 400 mg/m^2 i.v. bolus Days 1 and 2
- 5-fluorouracil 600 mg/m^2 i.v. infusion over 22 hours Days 1 and 2
- repeated every 14 days for up to six cycles.

The oncologist also prescribes intravenous hydration for the first 24 hours, in order to correct Mrs KT's hypokalaemia and dehydration, as follows:

- sodium chloride 0.9% 1000 mL i.v. infusion + potassium chloride 40 mmol over 12 hours
- sodium chloride 0.9% 500 mL i.v. infusion + potassium chloride 20 mmol over 12 hours.

Mrs KT's height is 174 cm and weight is 53 kg (body surface area = 1.63 m^2). She refuses to have a central line placed so will be receiving her chemotherapy through a peripheral intravenous catheter.

Questions

1 What are the typical signs and symptoms of bowel cancer that should alert a healthcare professional to refer to a specialist?
2 Comment on Mrs KT's laboratory results – what do they indicate?
3a What doses of chemotherapy drugs should Mrs KT receive, assuming normal haematological, renal and hepatic function?
3b What are the typical side-effects of the FOLFOX regimen?
3c How can these side-effects be managed?
4 What patient parameters can be followed to monitor for treatment effectiveness and toxicity?
5 What is the overall goal of treatment for Mrs KT? Outline the role of the clinical pharmacist in this.

Reference

Summary of Product Characteristics (2008) Eloxatin injection. Available at http://emc. medicines.org.uk/emc/assets/c/html/displayDocPrinterFriendly.asp?documentid =17367 [Accessed 7 July 2008].

General references

de Gramont A, Figer A, Seymour M *et al.* (2000) Leucovorin and fluorouracil with or without oxaliplatin as first line treatment in advanced colorectal cancer. *Journal of Clinical Oncology* 18: 2938– 2947.

Taylor I, Garcia-Aguilar J and Goldberg S (eds) (1999) Chapter 2: Clinical presentation. In: *Colorectal Cancer Fast Facts.* Oxford: Health Press, pp. 16–20.

Case study level 3 – Treatment of metastatic breast cancer and its complications

Learning outcomes

Level 3 case study: You will be able to:

- interpret clinical signs and symptoms
- evaluate laboratory data
- evaluate treatment options
- state goals of therapy
- describe a pharmaceutical care plan to include advice to a clinician
- describe the prognosis and long-term complications
- describe the social pharmacy issues, which could include supply (e.g. complex treatments at home, concordance and compliance) and lifestyle issues.

Scenario

Mrs CR, 43 years old, has been admitted to the oncology ward at your hospital after being referred by her GP. She presents with a one-week history of drowsiness, nausea and vomiting, loss of appetite and abdominal pain. The consultant oncologist initially reviewed her in his outpatient clinic where a blood sample was taken and she was further examined. Her height and weight were also recorded: height 162 cm and weight 79 kg (body surface area 1.84 m^2).

Her blood results were as follows:

Full blood count	
Hb	12.6 g/dL (12.0–14.7 g/dL)
White blood cells	8.1×10^9/L ($3.9–10.1 \times 10^9$/L)
Neutrophils	3.2×10^9/L ($1.9–6.8 \times 10^9$/L)
Platelets	514×10^9/L ($150–400 \times 10^9$/L)

Biochemistry	
Na$^+$	142 mmol/L (137–145 mmol/L)
K$^+$	4.4 mmol/L (3.6–5.0 mmol/L)
Urea	3.8 mmol/L (2.5–6.1 mmol/L)
Creatinine	97 micromol/L (62–106 micromol/L)
Adjusted serum Ca^{2+}	3.72 mmol/L (2.1–2.55 mmol/L)

Liver function tests	
Total bilirubin	19 micromol/L (3–22 micromol/L)
ALT	181 units/L (0–52 units/L)
ALP	419 IU/L (38–126 IU/L)
GGT	268 units/L (12–43 units/L)

HER-2 status (previously performed)
HER-2 immunohistochemistry   3+ (N/A)

Her drugs on admission were:

- MST tablets 30 mg p.o. b.d.
- Oramorph liquid 20 mg p.o. 4 hourly p.r.n.
- senna 2 tablets p.o. q.d.s.
- tramadol 50 mg p.o. q.d.s.
- metoclopramide 10 mg p.o. o.d.

Past medical history

Mrs CR first presented 18 months previously with grade 3 invasive breast cancer which was oestrogen receptor negative. She was initially treated with surgery (wide local excision and axillary clearance), adjuvant anthracycline-based chemotherapy and radiotherapy. Mrs CR has no other significant past medical history.

Questions

1a From Mrs CR's presenting complaints, what are the possible causes of her current clinical signs and symptoms?
1b What advice would you give to the clinicians treating Mrs CR regarding her current drug therapy on admission?
2   Comment on Mrs CR's laboratory results – what do they indicate?

The results of Mrs CR's various investigations (chest X-ray, CT scan and bone scan) as well as the laboratory results confirm a diagnosis of advanced breast cancer, with extensive metastatic disease in the liver and bone.

3   What treatment options are now available to Mrs CR and what are the goals of therapy for her with regard to: (a) chemotherapy, (b) management of malignant hypercalcaemia/bone metastases, and (c) management of liver capsule pain?
4   Briefly outline a pharmaceutical care plan for Mrs CR, including advice to the clinician.
5a Her consultant oncologist decides to prescribe the following chemotherapy regimen and supportive medication:

- dexamethasone 8 mg p.o. b.d. for 3 days starting Day 1
- trastuzumab 8 mg/kg i.v. loading dose Day 1 (then 6 mg/kg i.v. for subsequent doses)
- metoclopramide 20 mg i.v. pre-docetaxel chemotherapy Day 2 then 10 mg p.o. q.d.s. for 3 days
- docetaxel 100 mg/m² i.v. Day 2.

(Chemotherapy repeated every three weeks for up to six cycles – trastuzumab continued until disease progression.) Comment on the appropriateness of this chemotherapy regimen as a treatment option. Are the doses appropriate for Mrs CR and if not, what would you advise the clinician to do? How are these drugs administered? What acute patient monitoring would you advise Mrs CR's nurse to undertake during and just after administration of trastuzumab?

5b   Based on your advice to the clinician, what should be the total doses of chemotherapy administered to Mrs CR?

6   Outline the specific toxicities associated with trastuzumab and docetaxel therapy, including any longer term complications.

7   How should Mrs CR's chemotherapy be monitored?

Mrs CR is discharged home one week later, having received her first cycle of chemotherapy and having recovered from her presenting symptoms on admission. Her discharge medication is:

- MST tablets 10 mg p.o. b.d.
- Oramorph liquid 2.5 mg p.o. 4 hourly p.r.n.
- senna 2 tablets p.o. b.d.
- metoclopramide 10 mg p.o. q.d.s. p.r.n.
- dexamethasone 2 mg p.o. daily until 2 days before her next cycle of chemotherapy, then increase to 8 mg p.o. b.d. for 3 days to start the day before her next cycle of chemotherapy.

8   Outline the major counselling points you would make to Mrs CR on her discharge medication and any other non-drug related issues. What other aspects of her treatment would you discuss with her?

References

Marty M, Cognetti F, Maraninchi D *et al.* (2005) Randomized phase II trial of the efficacy and safety of trastuzumab combined with docetaxel in patients with human epidermal growth factor 2-positive metastatic breast cancer administered as first line treatment: the M77001 study group. *Journal of Clinical Oncology* 23: 4247–4250.

NICE (National Institute for Health and Clinical Excellence) (2002a) Improving outcomes in breast cancer – manual update. Available at http://www.nice.org.uk/nice media/pdf/Improving_outcomes_breast cancer_manual.pdf [Accessed 4 July 2008].

NICE (2002a) Guidance on the use of trastuzumab for the treatment of advanced breast cancer. Technology Appraisal 34. Available at http://www.nice.org.uk/guidance/index.jsp?action=article&o=32314 [Accessed 4 July 2008].

General references

Summary of Product Characteristics (2008a) Herceptin injection. Available at http://emc.medicines.org.uk/emc/assets/c/html/displayDocPrinterFriendly.asp?documentid=3567 [Accessed 7 July 2008].

Summary of Product Characteristics (2008b) Taxotere injection, Available at http://emc.medicines.org.uk/emc/assets/c/html/displayDocPrinterFriendly.asp?documentid=4594 [Accessed 7 July 2008].

Watson M, Lucas C, Hoy A (2006) Chapter One: Pain. In: *Adult Palliative Care Guidance*, 2nd edn. South West London, Surrey, West Sussex and Hampshire and Sussex Cancer Networks and Northern Ireland Palliative Medicine Group.

Case study level Ma – Management of testicular cancer

Learning outcomes

Level M case study: You will be able to:

- interpret clinical signs and symptoms
- evaluate laboratory data
- critically appraise treatment options
- state goals of therapy
- describe a pharmaceutical care plan to include advice to a clinician
- describe the prognosis and long-term complications
- describe the social pharmacy issues, which could include supply (e.g. complex treatments at home, concordance and compliance) and lifestyle issues
- describe the monitoring of therapy.

Scenario

Day 1

Mr AC, a 22-year-old accountant, presents as an emergency admission to your oncology ward for investigations and consideration for urgent chemotherapy treatment. He presents with a two-week history of malaise and lethargy, dyspnoea, right testicular swelling and difficulty in passing urine. He is not on any medications currently. An urgent blood sample is taken and the results show the following:

Full blood count	
Hb	16.1 g/dL (13.1–16.5 g/dL)
WBC	6.6×10^9/L (3.49–9.21×10^9/L)
Neutrophils	3.0×10^9/L (1.6–5.6×10^9/L)
Platelets	355×10^9/L (150–400×10^9/L

Biochemistry	
Na+	140 mmol/L (137–145 mmol/L)
K+	3.9 mmol/L (3.6–5 mmol/L)

Urea	12.9 mmol/L (3.2–7.1 mmol/L)
Creatinine	215 micromol/L (71–133 micromol/L)

Renal function	
EDTA clearance	57 mL/min (80–120 mL/min)

Liver function tests	
Total bilirubin	16 micromol/L (3–22 micromol/L)
ALT	45 units/L (0–72 units/L)
ALP	122 IU/L (38–126 IU/L)
GGT	20 units/L (15–73 units/L)

Tumour markers	
β-HCG	3275 IU/L (0–4 IU/L)
AFP	614 ng/mL (0–13 ng/mL)
LDH	751 IU/L (313–618 IU/L)

On examination, Mr AC is found to have a mass in his right testicle. A CT scan confirms the presence of bilateral pulmonary metastases and a large retroperitoneal mass.

An orchidectomy was arranged and histology confirmed a diagnosis of non-seminomatous germ cell tumour. Based on the levels of β-HCG and AFP and other prognostic factors, the disease is classed as 'good prognosis' stage IV teratoma.

Questions

1. Comment on the clinical signs and symptoms and initial laboratory results – what do they indicate?
2. Outline a pharmaceutical care plan for Mr AC at this stage.
3. Outline and critically appraise the possible treatment options available at this stage. What are the goals of therapy?

In view of his extensive metastatic disease classed as good prognosis, the treating oncologist has decided to prescribe the BEP regimen as follows:

- bleomycin 30 000 IU i.v. infusion Day 1, 8, 15
- etoposide 165 mg/m^2 i.v. infusion Day 1, 2, 3
- cisplatin 50 mg/m^2 i.v. infusion Day 1 and 2.

Repeated every three weeks, for three cycles.

Height 182 cm, weight 88 kg, body surface area 2.1 m^2.

4. Should any adjustment be made to the chemotherapy doses based on Mr AC's laboratory results?
5. What antiemetics should Mr AC be prescribed and why?

Day 5

Mr AC was tolerating his chemotherapy well. He suffered only occasional bouts of slight nausea and was already finding it easier to breathe and pass urine. He was discharged home that evening with the following medication:

- ondansetron 8 mg p.o. b.d. for 1 day
- dexamethasone 8 mg p.o. b.d. for 3 days
- metoclopramide 10 mg p.o. q.d.s. for 3 days
- domperidone suppositories 30 mg PR q.d.s. p.r.n.

Day 24

Mr AC was readmitted for his second cycle of BEP chemotherapy. On discussion he reports suffering from severe nausea and two or three episodes of vomiting over a 4-day period just after being discharged following his first cycle. Further questioning also reveals considerable non-compliance with his prescribed antiemetic regimen. He had decided that as he felt reasonably well while an inpatient, he thought he 'could do without taking any tablets at home'. He also explained that he did not 'like the idea of using suppositories' to manage the vomiting. The junior doctor on the ward asks you to discuss the importance of treatment compliance with Mr AC.

6   Outline what you would discuss with Mr AC. How would you try to ensure patient concordance with the management of his nausea and vomiting?

7   What other issues would you counsel Mr AC on (e.g. non-pharmacological issues)?

Day 45

Mr AC was treated with his third cycle of BEP chemotherapy and reported few side-effects from the second cycle.

Day 69

Mr AC was seen in clinic where response to treatment was confirmed as excellent, with his β-HCG and AFP levels returning to normal and a repeat CT scan after a third cycle confirming complete resolution of disease.

References

American Society of Clinical Oncology, Kris M, Hesketh PJ *et al.* (2006) American Society of Clinical Oncology guideline for antiemetics in oncology: update 2006. *Journal of Clinical Oncology* 24: 2932–2947.

De Wit R, Roberts JT, Wilkinson PM *et al.* (2001) Equivalence of three or four cycles of bleomycin, etoposide and cisplatin chemotherapy and of a 3- or 5-day schedule in good prognosis germ cell cancer: a randomised study of the European Organization for Research and Treatment of Cancer Genitourinary Tract Cooperative Group and the Medical Research Council. *Journal of Clinical Oncology* 19: 1629–1640.

Schmoll H, Souchon R, Krege S *et al.* (2004) European consensus on diagnosis and treatment of germ cell cancer: a report of the European Germ Cell Cancer Consensus Group (EGCCCG). *Annals of Oncology* 15: 1377–1399.

General reference

Summerhayes M and Daniels S (2003) Appendix 2: Dosage adjustment for cytotoxics in renal impairment. In: *Practical Chemotherapy: A Multidisciplinary Guide.* Oxford: Radcliffe Medical Press, pp. 375–389.

Case study level Mb – Oral chemotherapy

Learning outcomes

Level M case study: You will be able to:

- interpret clinical signs and symptoms
- evaluate laboratory data
- critically appraise treatment options
- state goals of therapy
- describe a pharmaceutical care plan to include advice to a clinician
- describe the prognosis and long-term complications
- describe the social pharmacy issues, which could include supply (e.g. complex treatments at home, concordance and compliance) and lifestyle issues
- describe the monitoring of therapy.

Scenario

Every Monday in your oncology outpatient department, you run a pharmacist/nurse-led oral capecitabine clinic, where patients are referred to you by oncologists for pretreatment counselling, drug history-taking and supplementary chemotherapy prescribing (under set clinical management plans) for the adjuvant treatment of colon cancer or treatment of metastatic colorectal cancer.

Today Mrs RP, a 74-year-old former receptionist, has been referred to you for the first time. Two years ago she was diagnosed with Dukes' C (Stage 3) colon cancer. After undergoing a surgical resection of her tumour (right hemicolectomy) she received adjuvant folinic acid/5-fluorouracil chemotherapy for six months. During a routine follow-up appointment two weeks ago, it was noticed that she had a rising tumour marker (CEA) and she was also complaining of a three-week history of abdominal pain, flatulence, nausea, loss of appetite and had lost 7 kg in weight.

Further investigation had confirmed a recurrence of her colon cancer, with metastatic spread to the lungs and liver.

Mrs RP also had an extensive past medical history:

- deep vein thrombosis (diagnosed 1 month ago)
- ischaemic heart disease (for 12 years)
- congestive heart failure (for 5 years)
- depression.

Questions

1   What are the treatment options for the first-line therapy of metastatic colorectal cancer? Critically appraise these options in relation to the most appropriate therapy for Mrs RP.

2   Briefly describe some of the key principles in the prescribing and dispensing of oral chemotherapy.

Mrs RP arrives at your clinic. You introduce yourself and explain to her how the capecitabine clinic works. You then discuss what medication she is currently taking, which are as follows:

- co-amilofruse 5/40 one tablet p.o. daily
- ramipril 5 mg p.o. daily
- digoxin 125 micrograms p.o. daily
- co-danthramer 10 mL p.o. nocte
- sertraline 50 mg p.o. daily
- warfarin – variable dose according to INR (currently 4 mg alternating with 5 mg daily).

You explain to her that her consultant oncologist has decided that she should commence single-agent oral capecitabine chemotherapy.

3a   What patient parameters need to be checked prior to prescribing capecitabine?

3b   Apart from performing a formal EDTA clearance or 24-hour urine collection, how else may Mrs RP's renal function be estimated?

Mrs RP's laboratory results from a blood analysis performed the previous day reveal the following:

Full blood count
Haemoglobin   13.1 g/dL (12.0–14.7 g/dL)
White blood cells 4.3×10^9/L ($3.9–10.1 \times 10^9$/L)
Neutrophils 3.3×10^9/L ($1.9–6.8 \times 10^9$/L)
Platelets 199×10^9/L ($150–400 \times 10^9$/L)

Biochemistry
Na^+ 137 mmol/L (137–145 mmol/L)
K^+ 5.5 mmol/L (3.6–5.0 mmol/L)
Urea   3.7 mmol/L (2.5–6.1 mmol/L)
Creatinine   47 micromol/L (62–106 micromol/L)

Liver function tests
Total bilirubin   13 micromol/L (3–22 micromol/L)
ALT   33 units/L (0–52 units/L)
ALP   87 IU/L (38–126 IU/L)
GGT   43 units/L (12–43 units/L)

Her height is 154 cm and weight is 51 kg. Her body surface area is 1.47 m^2.

4a Evaluate Mrs RP's laboratory results – what do they indicate? Calculate Mrs RP's current estimated creatinine clearance.

4b What change to therapy would you recommend to her clinician based on these results?

5 Outline a pharmaceutical care plan for Mrs RP, including advice to the clinician.

6 One of your tasks in your clinic is to emphasise the way in which treatment will be monitored and to outline the goal of therapy. What would you say to Mrs RP?

7 Part of your review also includes checking for any potential drug interactions with capecitabine. Briefly outline the major known drug interactions with capecitabine. Which one is relevant to Mrs RP and what would you advise both the clinician and Mrs RP?

Mrs RP returns to your clinic three weeks later for her second cycle, having completed her two-week course of capecitabine with a week's break. She states that she tolerated the chemotherapy very well apart from some diarrhoea – she suffered from nocturnal episodes on three consecutive nights during treatment. You also notice that she has brought back empty boxes of capecitabine from her first cycle, indicating that she finished her treatment as prescribed.

8 What might have caused her diarrhoea? What should Mrs RP have done when the diarrhoea occurred?

9 Mrs RP wonders why her GP cannot prescribe her chemotherapy as she lives just around the corner from him. What do you say to her?

References

BOPA (British Oncology Pharmacy Association) (2004) Position Statement on Safe Practice and the Pharmaceutical Care of Patients Receiving Oral Anti-cancer Chemotherapy. January.

Department of Health (2004) Building a safer NHS for patients: improving medication safety (A Report by the Chief Pharmaceutical Officer). January.

Hoff P (2003) Practical considerations in the use of oral fluoropyrimidines. *Seminars in Oncology* 30(Suppl 6): 88–92.

Hoff P, Ansari R, Batist G *et al.* (2001) Comparison of oral capecitabine with intravenous fluorouracil plus leucovorin as first-line treatment of 605 patients with metastatic colorectal cancer: results of a randomised phase III study. *Journal of Clinical Oncology* 19: 2282–2292.

National Patient Safety Agency (2008) Rapid Response Report (NPSA/2008/ RRR001): Risks of incorrect dosing of oral anti-cancer medicines, 22 January.

NICE (National Institute for Health and Clinical Excellence) (2003) Guidance on the use of capecitabine and tegafur with uracil for metastatic colorectal cancer. Technology Appraisal 61. Available at http://www.nice.org.uk/nicemedia/pdf/61Capecitabine CRCfullguidance.pdf [Accessed 4 July 2008].

Summary of Product Characteristics (2008) Xeloda tablets. Available at http://emc. medicines.org.uk/emc/assets/c/html/displayDocPrinterFriendly.asp?documentid =4619 [Accessed 7 July 2008].

Van Cutsem E, Verslype C, Yejpar S (2001) Oral capecitabine compared with intravenous fluorouracil plus leucovorin in patients with metastatic colorectal cancer: results of a large phase III study. *Journal of Clinical Oncology* 19: 4097–4106.

General references

Allwood M, Stanley A and Wright P (eds) (2002) *The Cytotoxics Handbook*. Oxford: Radcliffe Medical Press.

Baxter K (ed.) (2007) *Stockley's Drug Interactions*, 8th edn. London: Pharmaceutical Press.

Neal A and Hoskin P (1997) *Clinical Oncology: Basic Principles and Practice*. London: Arnold.

Pazdur R, Coia L, Hoskins W and Wagman L (eds) (2003) *Cancer Management: A Multidisciplinary Approach – Medical, Surgical and Radiation Oncology*. Huntington, NY: PRR, Inc.

Solimondo D, Bressler L, Kintzel P and Geraci M (2007) *Drug Information Handbook for Oncology*. Hudson, OH: Lexi-Comp Inc.

Summerhayes M and Daniels S (2003) *Practical Chemotherapy: A Multidisciplinary Guide*. Oxford: Radcliffe Medical Press.

Answers

Case study level 1 – Non-small cell lung cancer – see page 171

1   What are the main types of lung cancer?

Based on therapeutic approach, there are two main subdivisions of lung cancer: small cell lung cancer (SCLC) and non-small cell lung cancer (NSCLC). NSCLC is by far the most common type, accounting for approximately 80% of all lung cancers. Within NSCLC, there are three main tumour subdivisions: adeno-carcinoma, squamous cell carcinoma and large cell carcinoma.

2a   What are the risk factors associated with the development of lung cancer?

By far the biggest risk factor for the development of lung cancer is smoking – approximately 90% of all cases of lung cancer are related to cigarette smoking. An individual who smokes one packet of cigarettes daily has a 20-fold increased risk of lung cancer compared with a non-smoker. Smoking cessation decreases the risk of lung cancer, but a significant decrease in risk does not occur until approximately 5 years after stopping. Other risk factors associated with lung cancer include environmental factors such as passive smoking ('second hand' smoking) and radon exposure (radioactive gas released from granite rock) and occupational factors such as asbestos exposure, silicosis (a respiratory disease caused by inhalation of silica dust) and exposure to hydrocarbon fumes in coal-gas plants, arsenic and chromium.

2b   Is it possible that Mr AP has any of the risk factors for developing lung cancer?

From the observation that Mr AP's fingers and teeth are stained yellow, it appears likely that he is either a smoker or an ex-smoker. Also as a former coal miner, he may have been exposed to other occupational hazards; it has been suggested that up to 15% of lung cancer cases in men may be attributable to occupational factors in conjunction with smoking (Cancer Research UK, 2004).

3   Briefly describe the class of drugs that ondansetron, dexamethasone and ranitidine belong to and: (a) how ondansetron and dexamethasone work in the management of nausea and vomiting; (b) how ranitidine works in the management of dyspepsia; and (c) the rationale for co-prescribing ranitidine and dexamethasone.

Ondansetron is one of a group of $5HT_3$-receptor antagonists currently available in the UK, which also includes granisetron, tropisetron, dolasetron and palonosetron. Dexamethasone is a corticosteroid. Ranitidine is a histamine-2 (H_2)-receptor antagonist.

   The combination of a $5HT_3$-receptor antagonist and corticosteroid is very effective in the management of both chemotherapy- and radiotherapy-induced nausea and vomiting. Ondansetron acts by inhibiting $5HT_3$ (serotonin) receptor stimulation in the chemoreceptor trigger zone (CTZ), vomiting centre and gastrointestinal tract. Dexamethasone is thought to act synergistically with $5HT_3$-receptor antagonists to potentiate the antiemetic effect, although the exact mechanism of action is unclear. Numerous clinical trials have proven this benefit, and the use of both drugs together is now accepted practice.

Ranitidine acts by inhibiting the stimulation of H_2 receptors, resulting in a reduction in acid secretion from the gastrointestinal mucosa and subsequent relief from dyspeptic symptoms.

Many oncologists co-prescribe ranitidine and dexamethasone due to the gastric irritant effect of corticosteroids which can lead to dyspepsia, particularly if a patient is also concurrently receiving other gastrointestinal irritants such as non-steroidal anti-inflammatory drugs (NSAIDs).

4a   Mr AP states that he readily suffers from bouts of constipation and is concerned that these new tablets may worsen this. What would you advise?

One of the most commonly reported unwanted effects of $5HT_3$-receptor antagonists is constipation. This can occur in up to 10% of patients and is generally mild to moderate in nature. Constipation caused by $5HT_3$-receptor antagonists may be exacerbated in those cancer patients on opiate analgesics or other constipating drugs and can lead to serious problems for patients with cancer, for example, when underlying disease puts the patient at risk of intestinal obstruction.

In advising Mr AP on reducing the risk of this it would be important to enquire as to what other medications he is currently on, in order to identify any other constipating drugs. This information could be supported by checking the pharmacy electronic computer records for his drug history.

In addition, it would be important to advise Mr AP:

- not to take ondansetron for any longer than prescribed, unless advised by his doctor;
- not to take any spare ondansetron left over at the end of his treatment period of 5 days to empirically treat any episodes of nausea or vomiting that may be unrelated to chemotherapy or radiotherapy;
- of the importance of a healthy diet with plenty of fibre to contribute to a regular bowel habit;
- of the importance of maintaining mobility and taking exercise; and
- if he does become constipated during the period of treatment with ondansetron, to seek advice from his GP or pharmacist on medications to treat constipation, such as docusate or bisacodyl.

4b   What are the other typical side-effects of the drugs prescribed for Mr AP?

Ondansetron also commonly causes headache that is typically of a mild to moderate nature and may be treated with simple analgesics such as paracetamol. Other unwanted effects are generally mild and transient and include light-headedness, abdominal discomfort, hiccups, fatigue and asymptomatic rises in liver transaminases. ECG changes, including prolongation of the QTc interval, have been reported with $5HT_3$-receptor antagonists, so caution is needed before prescribing these drugs to patients with pre-existing cardiac conduction defects or a history of cardiac rhythm disturbance.

Dexamethasone may cause side-effects typical of corticosteroid administration. Many of its more serious adverse effects occur on long-term treatment, while other generally less serious effects may become apparent during short-term treatment periods. These may include:

- *insomnia* – minimised by advising patients to take the second daily dose in the early afternoon rather than in the evening;
- *gastrointestinal irritation including dyspepsia* – minimised by advising patients to take with or immediately after food;
- *weight gain* – which may manifest as fluid retention in the legs and face, causing a puffy 'moon-shape' appearance that may be particularly prevalent with longer term treatment;
- *increased appetite* – often used to beneficial effect in cancer patients;
- *increased blood glucose levels* (therefore caution in diabetics); and
- occasionally *psychological disturbances* such as euphoria or depression.

Ranitidine is generally well tolerated but may occasionally cause diarrhoea and other gastrointestinal disturbances, altered liver function tests, headache, dizziness, rash and tiredness. Other rare side-effects include acute pancreatitis, bradycardia, atrioventricular block, confusion, depression and hallucinations, particularly in the very ill or elderly.

5   Mr AP also states that due to the large tumour 'pressing on my food pipe', he is currently having difficulty swallowing tablets. What alternative formulations could you suggest in order to facilitate medication compliance in this case?

To ensure Mr AP benefits from the medication that has been prescribed to him it is imperative that he is able to efficiently take his oral medication. Cancer patients often have mechanical obstructions caused by tumours, particularly of the head and neck, oesophagus or lung. These tumours can either grow into the oesophagus or compress it, thus making eating difficult and, as in Mr AP's case, causing difficulty in swallowing tablets or capsules (known as dysphagia). A successful outcome of Mr AP's radiotherapy treatment will likely involve an improvement in his ability to swallow.

It is therefore important for the pharmacist to advise on and provide alternative formulations of medications to facilitate patient compliance. Specifically:

- Ondansetron is available in a liquid form (4 mg/5 mL syrup), oral lyophilisates (tablets which are placed on the tongue, allowed to disperse and then swallowed) or suppositories (although these can cause rectal irritation).
- Dexamethasone is available in a liquid form (2 mg/5 mL oral solution).
- Ranitidine is available either in a liquid form (75 mg/5 mL syrup) or as effervescent tablets that may be dissolved in water.

Again it will be important to seek information from Mr AP about any other concurrent medications he may be taking and whether he is having difficulty swallowing them. Further advice on what to do if his dysphagia is preventing him from fully complying with his concomitant medications may be necessary.

It should also be emphasised to Mr AP that it is important to maintain a healthy diet during the period of dysphagia. A referral to a dietitian by his clinician may be advisable to enable an assessment of diet requirements to be made and advice to be given on alternative nutritional supplements (in liquid form) if required.

Case study level 2 – Treatment of advanced colorectal cancer – see page 173

1   What are the typical signs and symptoms of bowel cancer that should alert a healthcare professional to refer to a specialist?

Patients with colorectal cancer can develop a myriad of symptoms including:

- *Abdominal pain and discomfort*: This is frequently non-specific and may present as a vague, dull pain. Persistent and colicky pain is most likely to represent obstructive symptoms and be caused by a lesion in the descending colon.
- *Change in bowel habit*: Patients over the age of 45 should be further investigated if they present with an alteration in bowel habit that lasts for two weeks or more. Diarrhoea may be bloody and could be associated with a sense of incomplete defecation.
- *Rectal bleeding*: This is relatively common and frequently associated with haemorrhoids. This type of bleeding is usually bright red with anal discomfort also a common feature. Blood from the rectum that is darker in colour and mixed in with stool is more likely to be due to an underlying cancer. Rectal bleeding associated with tenesmus (painful spasm of the anal sphincter along with an urgent desire to defecate without the significant production of faeces) should be investigated promptly.
- *Anaemia*: This is due to bleeding that may be overt (frank rectal bleeding as above) or occult (bleeding otherwise not apparent to the patient and usually only identified by tests that detect faecal blood or, if bleeding is sufficient, it manifests as iron deficiency). The onset of non-specific anaemia of unknown origin is not uncommon in patients with an ascending colon carcinoma. Due to the fact that these patients rarely present with abdominal pain, they often present with advanced disease. Bleeding is occult and may be recognised on faecal occult blood testing of the stools.
- *Anorexia and unexplained weight loss*: These symptoms often accompany colorectal cancer and are frequently associated with advanced disease.

Any combination of these symptoms should prompt the healthcare professional, including the pharmacist, to refer the patient to their GP or hospital doctor for further investigations.

2   Comment on Mrs KT's laboratory results – what do they indicate?

From Mrs KT's laboratory results, four significant abnormalities can be seen and may indicate the following:

- Haemoglobin 8.8 g/dL (normal range 12.0–14.7 g/dL): This result indicates anaemia and as already described, is a typical non-specific symptom of colorectal cancer. It may have resulted from either frank or occult bleeding.
- Potassium 2.6 mmol/L (normal range 3.6–5.0 mmol/L): This result indicates a low serum potassium level or hypokalaemia. The development of hypokalaemia in patients with advanced colorectal cancer may often occur due to diarrhoea or vomiting caused by abdominal pain and discomfort (causing an excessive loss of potassium). It may also occur due to a reduction in the intake of a normal diet leading to a drop in the intake of dietary potassium. Another cause of hypokalaemia may be as a side-effect of certain medications such as diuretics, so it would be important to obtain a full drug history from Mrs KT to determine the likelihood of this (in this case she is not currently taking any regular medications).
- Urea 10.7 mmol/L (normal range 2.5–6.1 mmol/L) and creatinine 126 micromol/L (normal range 62–106 micromol/L): These results indicate a high serum urea and creatinine. This may have occurred as a result of dehydration from excessive fluid loss (e.g. diarrhoea, vomiting), inadequate fluid intake and bleeding. Renal impairment in patients with metastatic cancer may also be due to disease compressing the ureters or spreading to the kidney.

3a　What doses of chemotherapy drugs should Mrs KT receive, assuming normal haematological, renal and hepatic function?

The following doses should be prescribed by the clinician for Mrs KT, based on a body surface area of 1.63 m^2:

- oxaliplatin 139 mg i.v. infusion Day 1 only (85 mg/m^2 × 1.63 m^2)
- folinic acid 326 mg i.v. infusion Day 1 and 2 (200 mg/m^2 × 1.63 m^2)
- 5-fluorouracil 652 mg i.v. bolus Day 1 and 2 (400 mg/m^2 × 1.63 m^2)
- 5-fluorouracil 978 mg i.v. infusion Day 1 and 2 (600 mg/m^2 × 1.63 m^2).

These doses may be rounded off, according to the local hospital pharmacy practice.

3b　What are the typical side-effects of the FOLFOX regimen?

In common with most cytotoxic chemotherapy regimens, general side-effects include bone marrow suppression (causing reductions in white cell count, platelets and haemoglobin in particular), nausea and vomiting, diarrhoea, stomatitis and alopecia.

Oxaliplatin also produces a specific neurological toxicity requiring careful monitoring. This is the principal dose-limiting side-effect of the drug. It involves a sensory peripheral neuropathy characterised by dysaesthesia (impairment of any of the senses, especially of touch) and/or paraesthesia (abnormal skin sensations usually associated with peripheral nerve damage) of the extremities with or without cramps and often triggered by the cold. These symptoms occur in up to 95% of patients treated. The duration of these symptoms, which usually regress between courses of treatment, increases with the number of treatment cycles. In the majority of cases these neurological signs and symptoms improve or totally recover when treatment is discontinued.

Acute neurosensory manifestations due to oxaliplatin can also occur during or within hours of drug administration and are often triggered by exposure to the cold. If this occurs, often the most distressing symptom for the patient is an acute pharyngolaryngeal dysaesthesia that manifests as an extremely uncomfortable sensation of dysphagia (difficulty in swallowing), laryngospasm or bronchospasm, jaw spasm, abnormal tongue sensation and a feeling of chest pressure.

Allergic reactions may also occur due to oxaliplatin, although only rarely are these of a serious nature (<1% of patients).

5-Fluorouracil may produce the 'hand–foot syndrome' (known as palmar–plantar erythrodysaesthesia) that results in a dry, reddened and painful area on the extremities of the hands and feet.

3c   How can these side-effects be managed?

The general side-effects of cytotoxic chemotherapy can be managed as follows:

Bone marrow suppression

The management of this side-effect is imperative as the onset of neutropenic sepsis (lowered neutrophil count with infection) and less commonly thrombocytopenia (lowered platelet count) can be life threatening if left untreated. Patients should receive both written and verbal counselling on the possible signs and symptoms to watch out for. These include fever, sore throat, chills or rigors, and flu-like symptoms. The onset of these symptoms (at about 5–7 days after chemotherapy administration began) should prompt the patient to seek urgent medical attention and often these patients are requested to attend their local hospital accident and emergency department. The development of neutropenic sepsis will require immediate hospital admission and commencement of intravenous antibiotics. Severe manifestations may have to be managed by delay and/or dose modification of the patient's next cycle of chemotherapy.

Nausea and vomiting

Prophylactic administration of antiemetics is essential in any patient receiving FOLFOX chemotherapy. The combination of oxaliplatin and 5-fluorouracil results in a moderate level of emetogenicity and requires the administration of $5HT_3$-receptor antagonists and corticosteroid treatment, generally with a dopamine antagonist such as metoclopramide or domperidone. Severe manifestations may have to be managed by delay and/or dose modification of the patient's next cycle of chemotherapy.

Diarrhoea

This can be controlled with the co-administration of standard antidiarrhoeal agents such as loperamide. All patients on FOLFOX chemotherapy (or any 5-fluorouracil-containing regimen) should be co-prescribed an antidiarrhoeal medication to use on an 'as required' basis. The onset of diarrhoea should also indicate to the patient that they must increase their fluid intake to prevent dehydration. Patients must be warned that if the diarrhoea is not controlled (for example, within 48 hours of onset) then dehydration is a danger and they should be advised to contact their treating hospital or GP for advice. Severe manifestations may have to be managed by delay and/or dose modification of the patient's next cycle of chemotherapy.

Stomatitis

Oral mucositis/stomatitis can be relieved by the administration of mouth care products such as antiseptic and local analgesic preparations. Severe manifestations may have to be managed by delay and/or dose modification of the patient's next cycle of chemotherapy.

Neurological symptoms due to oxaliplatin

The onset of pain and/or a functional disorder (for example, inability to do up buttons on a shirt) are indications, depending on the duration of the symptoms, for dose adjustment or even treatment discontinuation (refer to the Summary of Product Characteristics (2008) for oxaliplatin). In particular, patients who develop acute pharyngolaryngeal dysaesthesia during or within the hours following the 2-hour infusion should receive their future infusions over a 6-hour period as prolonged infusion may minimise this reaction. Patients should also be advised to avoid the main trigger for these reactions – cold (e.g. cold foods/drinks, environments).

Hand–foot syndrome

Many clinicians prescribe pyridoxine tablets or cream to manage this side-effect, however the evidence for this treatment is scarce. Severe manifestations may have to be managed by delay and/or dose modification of the patient's next cycle of chemotherapy (only the 5-fluorouracil component need be dose modified).

4   What patient parameters can be followed to monitor for treatment effectiveness and toxicity?

In assessing treatment effectiveness, the following parameters should be monitored:

- *Subjective measures of disease – reduction in symptoms of cancer.* It is important to record the symptoms that the patient is suffering from as a result of their cancer prior to their first cycle of treatment, in order to allow a measurement of improvement in those symptoms as treatment progresses.
- *Objective measures of disease.* The clinical team will monitor the patient's response to treatment by CT scan or other objective measure of tumour size in any original sites of disease (ie. primary tumour in the colon or sites of metastases). This is typically done every 6–8 weeks during treatment.
- *Tumour markers.* Specific types of cancer may produce so-called 'tumour' markers. These markers can be monitored by serum samples that will show the amount of the marker in the blood. Again it is essential to have a baseline measurement of the specific tumour marker in order to monitor any change during treatment. In the case of Mrs KT, a baseline measurement of the CEA (carcinoembryonic antigen) marker should be taken and then monitored at each cycle of treatment. Response to treatment should be demonstrated by a progressive reduction in tumour marker levels.

In assessing treatment toxicity, the following parameters should be monitored:

- *Haematological parameters.* Full blood count must be analysed prior to administration of FOLFOX chemotherapy to check for persistent bone marrow suppression as previously described. Low neutrophil or platelet counts (typically neutrophils $<1.5 \times 10^9$/L or platelets $<80 \times 10^9$/L) will necessitate a delay in chemotherapy administration, usually by one week.
- *Neurological toxicity.* Patients receiving oxaliplatin must be questioned prior to each cycle of chemotherapy about neurological symptoms and doses should be adjusted according to severity of any functional impairment and duration of symptoms. Refer to the oxaliplatin Summary of Product Characteristics (2008).
- *Other toxicities.* The patient should be methodically questioned about the development of any other side-effects of treatment. Severe grades of toxicity may again necessitate dose adjustment (e.g. severe diarrhoea).
- *Hepatic and renal function.* Patients with advanced cancer may have impaired liver function due to the presence of liver metastases. In this case drug doses may need to be adjusted. In the case of the FOLFOX regimen, 5-fluorouracil dose may need to be reduced if the impairment is moderate or severe. Mrs KT's baseline liver function tests indicate a normal liver function, but these parameters should be monitored carefully throughout treatment. Reduced renal function may also necessitate a decrease in drug dosage. In the case of the FOLFOX regimen, oxaliplatin is contraindicated in patients with severe renal impairment (creatinine clearance <30 mL/min).

5   What is the overall goal of treatment for Mrs KT? Outline the role of the clinical pharmacist in this.

As Mrs KT has advanced metastatic cancer, the goal of treatment is palliative. The objectives must therefore be to prolong her life by controlling her tumour growth in both the primary site and sites of metastases, in parallel with maintaining or improving her quality of life. It is imperative not to impair her quality of life with intolerable side-effects of treatment. The role of the clinical oncology pharmacist is therefore important and should involve:

- checking chemotherapy prescribing by verifying dosage calculations;
- advising medical and nursing staff on correct administration of the chemotherapy drugs to Mrs KT;
- monitoring Mrs KT for chemotherapy toxicity and advising the clinician on dosage adjustments or chemotherapy delay if necessary;
- monitoring serum potassium levels and renal function (serum urea and creatinine) to ensure resolution of her hypokalaemia and renal impairment;
- educating and counselling Mrs KT on the treatment she is receiving and the possible side-effects, as well as how to manage them (as previously described) – it is imperative to ensure that any communication from the clinical pharmacist is in line with that provided by other health professionals, especially clinicians and nurses;
- ensuring that appropriate supportive medication, such as prophylactic antiemetics, are prescribed in line with hospital policies and guidelines;
- counselling Mrs KT on any discharge medication she may be sent home with.

Case study level 3 – Treatment of metastatic breast cancer and its complications – see page 175

1a From Mrs CR's presenting complaints, what are the possible causes of her current clinical signs and symptoms?

Mrs CR presents with a one-week history of drowsiness, nausea and vomiting, loss of appetite and abdominal pain. There are a number of possible reasons why she could be displaying these signs and symptoms.

Drowsiness/nausea and vomiting

These symptoms may be the result of a number of factors:

- *Drug-induced*: Mrs CR is currently taking two potent analgesics, morphine and tramadol. First, as she is on MST (morphine sulphate slow-release preparation) 30 mg twice daily, her dose of Oramorph (morphine sulphate immediate-release preparation) is too high and will almost certainly be contributing to her drowsiness and nausea and vomiting. Oramorph preparations are commonly used to treat 'breakthrough' pain (i.e. pain that 'breaks' through in between her 12-hourly doses of slow-acting morphine) and the dosage should be based on her MST dosage as follows: MST daily dosage = 60 mg daily (30 mg b.d.). So, breakthrough dose of Oramorph = 60 mg divided by 6 (number of 4-hourly doses given in a 24-hour period) = 10 mg per dose. Second, the use of tramadol in addition to morphine is not recommended. It is poor practice to use more than one opiate analgesic drug at any one time, as there may be an exacerbation of opiate toxicity without added efficacy – therefore this is likely to be exacerbating Mrs CR's drowsiness and nausea and vomiting.
- *Hypercalcaemia*: One of the symptoms produced by a raised serum calcium level is that of drowsiness. Hypercalcaemia results from increased

osteoclastic activity (which releases calcium from bone) and decreased excretion of urinary calcium. It occurs in about 10% of the cancer population. An adjusted serum calcium level of 3.72 mmol/L represents severe hypercalcaemia requiring immediate treatment.

■ *Inadequate antiemetic dosage*: Mrs CR is currently taking metoclopramide as a once-daily dosage. However, this drug has a relatively short duration of action (6–8 hours) so should be administered at least 8-hourly on a regular basis to be optimally effective.

Loss of appetite

This could be as a result of Mrs CR's underlying nausea and vomiting as well as her abdominal pain. There could also be a degree of anxiety or depression associated with the possibility of her symptoms representing cancer recurrence, which may also contribute to a loss of appetite.

Abdominal pain

This may be due to liver capsular pain from liver metastases. Mrs CR's abnormal liver function tests may indicate this. If metastatic cancer has spread to her liver, the resultant disease within the liver capsule may cause pain. Another possible cause could be the high dosage of senna that she is taking (8 tablets a day) – excessive dosages of stimulant laxatives such as senna can cause abdominal cramp and pain due to their effect of increasing intestinal motility.

This myriad of symptoms means that it seems likely Mrs CR is suffering from recurrent breast cancer.

1b What advice would you give to the clinicians treating Mrs CR regarding her current drug therapy on admission?

Based on both her blood results and presenting symptoms, the treating medical team should be asked to review her current drug therapy as follows:

■ As her drowsiness and nausea may be being exacerbated by inappropriate opiate analgesic use and as her pain is currently not well controlled, stop tramadol and change the MST to regular immediate-release morphine in order to titrate more appropriately against her analgesic requirements. At this point it would be necessary to question Mrs CR as to her approximate daily usage of Oramorph on a 'p.r.n.' basis in order to estimate her average daily dose of morphine (MST + Oramorph) prior to admission. An initial regular immediate-release morphine dosage of 10 mg p.o. regularly 4 hourly may be suggested.

■ Another option that could be considered if Mrs CR's vomiting is still present is to change oral morphine to a parenteral opiate until such time as her vomiting is controlled. One suggestion would be to convert to continuous subcutaneous diamorphine, for example. The equivalent daily dose of subcutaneous diamorphine is one-third the daily dose of oral morphine (i.e.

60 mg daily oral morphine is equivalent to 20 mg daily of subcutaneous diamorphine).

- Reduce the senna dosage to 1–2 tablets once daily initially (also check Mrs CR's current bowel habits; if diarrhoea then senna should be stopped. However, as Mrs CR will continue to receive opiate analgesia then it is likely that prophylactic laxative therapy will need to be continued, due to opiates causing constipation in almost all patients). Monitor Mrs CR's bowel habits during her inpatient stay in order to ensure the appropriateness of the laxative therapy.
- Increase the metoclopramide dose to 10 mg four times a day and consider changing to the intravenous route, particularly if Mrs CR is continuing to vomit. The administration of metoclopramide orally will be inappropriate if she is unable to retain oral medications due to sickness.

2   Comment on Mrs CR's laboratory results – what do they indicate?

From Mrs CR's laboratory results, the following abnormalities can be observed:

- Increased adjusted serum calcium – this indicates hypercalcaemia which is likely to be caused by cancer progression, possibly to the bones.
- Increased liver function tests – Mrs CR's alanine aminotransferase (ALT), alkaline phosphatase (ALP) and gamma-glutamyl transferase (GGT) levels are all increased above the normal ranges and indicate moderate liver impairment. This may have implications on the ability of the liver to metabolise drugs and must be borne in mind when prescribing any drugs that are metabolised by it.

3   What treatment options are now available to Mrs CR and what are the goals of therapy for her with regard to: (a) chemotherapy, (b) management of malignant hypercalcaemia/bone metastases, and (c) management of liver capsule pain?

As most, if not all, of Mrs CR's symptoms are the result of metastatic breast cancer, it will be necessary to consider treatment of the underlying cancer with systemic therapy. Metastatic breast cancer is incurable. Systemic treatment with chemotherapeutic and/or hormone-modifying agents may produce modest improvements in survival time, but the primary aim of any form of treatment at this stage should be to relieve symptoms and optimise quality of life. The National Institute for Health and Clinical Excellence (NICE) Guidance on improving outcomes in breast cancer (2002a) clearly states that both types of therapy should be considered with the optimum treatment depending on various factors such as previous treatment, the patient's general fitness, the site and extent of recurrence and tumour characteristics.

The treatment options for Mrs CR are therefore as follows:

Chemotherapy

Chemotherapy can produce useful palliation, particularly in patients with rapidly progressing disease, which appears to be occurring in Mrs CR's case. It is also the most appropriate systemic therapy for Mrs CR as the other option for systemic treatment, hormone-modifying agents, are not appropriate in her case as her tumour is oestrogen-receptor negative and therefore very unlikely to respond to hormonal manipulation.

First-line chemotherapy for the treatment of metastatic breast cancer is now largely dependent on the patient's HER-2 antigen status. The HER-2 (human epidermal growth factor receptor 2) protein is overexpressed on the surface of breast cancer cells in approximately 15–25% of patients. The measurement of this protein can be performed by immunohistochemistry methods, where the degree of protein expression is denoted by negative, 1+, 2+ or 3+. As Mrs CR's has HER-2,3+ disease, this denotes strong protein overexpression.

First-line treatment of her metastatic breast cancer should therefore incorporate the monoclonal antibody trastuzumab (Herceptin). NICE (2002b) have issued a technology appraisal on the use of trastuzumab in metastatic breast cancer which states that 'trastuzumab be used in combination with paclitaxel for women with tumours with excessive human epidermal growth factor receptor 2 (HER2) at levels of 3+ who have not had chemotherapy for metastatic breast cancer and for whom anthracycline treatment is inappropriate.'

This guidance is relevant to Mrs CR as she has HER-2,3+ disease, she has not had any previous treatment for metastatic breast cancer (she has only received adjuvant treatment for early stage breast cancer) and she is not suitable for anthracycline-based chemotherapy as she has already received this in the adjuvant setting less than 2 years ago.

Many clinicians now prefer to use docetaxel (licensed to be used in combination with trastuzumab for metastatic breast cancer) instead of paclitaxel as it is more convenient to administer (1 hour infusion for docetaxel instead of 3 hours for paclitaxel) and clinicians generally have more experience of using this agent in breast cancer therapy. The pivotal trial of this combination shows superiority of docetaxel and trastuzumab over docetaxel alone in terms of overall survival, response rate and time to disease progression with little additional toxicity (Marty *et al.*, 2005).

Management of malignant hypercalcaemia/bone metastases

The treatment of Mrs CR's hypercalcaemia is urgent and requires immediate administration of bisphosphonate therapy, the first choice therapy in cases of severe hypercalcaemia. Currently four bisphosphonates are available in the UK for the treatment of malignant hypercalcaemia – sodium clodronate, disodium pamidronate, zoledronic acid and ibandronic acid. The choice of which bisphosphonate to recommend will depend on which one is on the local hospital formulary.

It would also seem appropriate to recommend administration of intravenous hydration as this will help correct any underlying dehydration (caused by Mrs CR's vomiting) and reverse hypercalcaemia. An example i.v. hydration regimen may be: sodium chloride 0.9% 1000 mL over 8 hours ($\times$ 3 infusions over 24 hours).

It is important to note that normalisation of serum calcium may take 3–4 days following bisphosphonate administration so further dosing should not occur before this time.

Continued treatment with bisphosphonate may also be appropriate to not only reduce the likelihood of recurrent hypercalcaemia but also to manage Mrs CR's bone metastases. Many guidelines (including the NICE Improving outcomes guidance for breast cancer, 2002a) recommend the use of bisphosphonates to reduce the onset of skeletal complications such as skeletal fractures. An appropriate suggestion would be to continue one of the bisphosphonates previously outlined at three-weekly intervals (to coincide with chemotherapy administration).

Management of liver capsule pain

The most beneficial treatment of this syndrome should be systemic chemotherapy to cause reduction of the metastases within the liver. However this may take some time to become apparent so other symptomatic measures could be utilised in the interim. The use of opiates may be helpful, but often the use of co-analgesics will be necessary. In the case of liver capsular pain, corticosteroids seem to be reasonably useful in providing relief. A dosage of dexamethasone of 2–4 mg p.o. once daily is often sufficient. This will also potentially have the added benefit of improving Mrs CR's appetite by acting as an appetite stimulant.

Overall the goal of therapy for Mrs CR is to provide palliation of her current symptoms as any systemic therapy will not be curative due to the advanced nature of her disease, and to control the progression of her cancer.

4   Briefly outline a pharmaceutical care plan for Mrs CR, including advice to the clinician.

A pharmaceutical care plan for Mrs CR should:

- identify her current treatment needs,
- define how these needs are to be met and the action required,
- state the endpoints of treatment,
- identify the parameters to be monitored and the frequency of monitoring required (to follow response to treatment and detect side-effects), and
- identify points to be covered when counselling her about her medication.

Identify her current treatment needs

Mrs CR's current treatment needs are to:

- correct her hypercalcaemia,
- control her presenting symptoms including drowsiness, nausea and vomiting and abdominal pain, and
- control progression of her underlying malignancy.

Define how these needs are to be met and the action required

For these treatment needs to be met the following should be undertaken:

- An evaluation of treatment options for her hypercalcaemia.
- A review of her existing medication and consideration of alternative agents (where appropriate).
- An evaluation of treatment options for her metastatic breast cancer.
- Provision of advice to clinicians on any changes and additional agents indicated.

State the endpoints of treatment

The endpoints of treatment for Mrs CR are broadly:

- normocalcaemia (a normalisation of serum calcium levels),
- effective symptom control, and
- optimum control of progression of her underlying malignancy.

For each individual medication prescribed, more specific treatment endpoints could also be included.

Identify the parameters to be monitored and the frequency of monitoring required (to follow response to treatment and detect side-effects).

The parameters to be followed for monitoring treatment response and side-effects for Mrs CR's metastatic breast cancer are outlined in the answer to question 7. For the treatment of hypercalcaemia:

- monitor adjusted serum calcium (check level 3–4 days after bisphosphonate treatment and then check regularly e.g. weekly),
- monitor patient for resolution of the symptoms of malignant hypercalcaemia.

Identify points to be covered when counselling her about her medication.

Points to be covered when counselling Mrs CR on her medication will depend on the agents chosen to treat her. Counselling should provide basic information about the medication, including its name and purpose, and provide clear instructions on how it should be used and any precautions that need to be observed.

5a   Her consultant oncologist decides to prescribe the following chemotherapy regimen and supportive medication:

- dexamethasone 8 mg p.o. b.d. for 3 days starting Day 1
- trastuzumab 8 mg/kg i.v. loading dose Day 1 (then 6 mg/kg i.v. for subsequent doses)
- metoclopramide 20 mg i.v. pre-docetaxel chemotherapy Day 2 then 10 mg p.o. q.d.s. for 3 days
- docetaxel 100 mg/m^2 i.v. Day 2.

(Chemotherapy repeated every three weeks for up to six cycles – trastuzumab continued until disease progression.) Comment on the appropriateness of this chemotherapy regimen as a treatment option. Are the doses appropriate for Mrs CR and if not, what would you advise the clinician to do? How are these drugs administered? What acute patient monitoring would you advise Mrs CR's nurse to undertake during and just after administration of trastuzumab?

The prescribing of trastuzumab and docetaxel therapy for Mrs CR seems entirely appropriate. First-line treatment of HER-2-positive metastatic breast cancer should include trastuzumab plus a taxane, unless there is a contraindication to taxane therapy. However, the dosage of docetaxel is not appropriate due to Mrs CR's liver impairment. Docetaxel is extensively metabolised by the liver into inactive metabolites and deranged liver function can lead to elevated levels of docetaxel and potentially cause severe toxicity (e.g. neutropenic sepsis, infections and stomatitis). Based on pharmacokinetic data with docetaxel at 100 mg/m^2 as a single agent, patients who have both elevations of transaminase (ALT and/or AST) greater than 1.5 times the upper limit of the normal range (ULN) and alkaline phosphatase greater than 2.5 times the ULN should have their dose of docetaxel reduced to 75 mg/m^2. Mrs CR's ALT is 181 units/L and ALP is 419 IU/L so it is appropriate for her docetaxel dosage to be reduced by 25%.

The dose of trastuzumab is appropriate – no dose modifications are considered necessary in liver impairment. Although trastuzumab given as a weekly dose is the licensed schedule in combination with docetaxel, it is now relatively common practice in the UK for oncologists to prescribe it as a three-weekly dosage based on published pharmacokinetic data suggesting the drug has a sufficiently long half-life for dosing at the longer interval.

The recommendations for administration of this combination of drugs is as follows:

- trastuzumab: diluted in 250 mL sodium chloride 0.9% and infused intravenously over 90 minutes on Day 1, followed by:
- docetaxel: diluted in 250 mL glucose 5% and infused intravenously over 60 minutes on Day 2.

Docetaxel should be administered the day after trastuzumab for the first cycle because of the potential for infusion-related reactions to trastuzumab, particularly during or after the first administration. Serious adverse reactions to trastuzumab infusion that have been reported infrequently include dyspnoea (shortness of breath), hypotension, wheezing, hypertension, bronchospasm, supraventricular tachyarrhythmia, reduced oxygen saturation, anaphylaxis, respiratory distress and urticaria (itching). The majority of these events occur during or within 2.5 hours of the start of the first infusion. Should an infusion reaction occur, the infusion should be discontinued and the patient monitored until resolution of any observed symptoms – the infusion may be resumed when symptoms abate. If the first cycle is well tolerated then dosing of the drugs in future cycles may occur on the same day.

In terms of nurse monitoring of the patient during and immediately after the administration of chemotherapy, patients should be observed for at least 6 hours after the start of the first trastuzumab infusion (and for 2 hours after the start of the subsequent three weekly infusions) to monitor for symptoms like fever and chills or other infusion-related symptoms. Vital observations should be monitored routinely during this period also (e.g. blood pressure, temperature) at least during and after the first infusion.

5b Based on your advice to the clinician, what should be the total doses of chemotherapy administered to Mrs CR?

The patient should receive the following doses of chemotherapy drugs:

- trastuzumab 8 mg/kg × 79 kg = 632 mg loading dose week 1 (subsequent doses 6 mg/kg × 79 kg = 474 mg)
- docetaxel 75 mg/m^2 × 1.84 m^2 = 138 mg.

These doses may be rounded off according to the local hospital pharmacy practice.

6 Outline the specific toxicities associated with trastuzumab and docetaxel therapy, including any longer term complications.

Apart from the standard general toxicities associated with cytotoxic chemotherapy such as bone marrow suppression, nausea, diarrhoea, stomatitis and alopecia, other drug-specific toxicities may occur, including the following.

Trastuzumab

- Infusion-related reactions (see answer to Question 5a). The most common adverse reactions are infusion-related symptoms, such as fever and chills, usually following the first infusion.
- Cardiotoxicity: Heart failure has been observed in patients receiving trastuzumab therapy alone or in combination with paclitaxel or docetaxel,

particularly following anthracycline containing chemotherapy. This may be moderate to severe and has been associated with death.

■ Other relatively common side-effects include abdominal pain, asthenia, chest pain, headache, pain, diarrhoea, nausea and vomiting, arthralgia, myalgia and rash.

Docetaxel

■ Immune system disorders: Hypersensitivity reactions generally occur within a few minutes following the start of the infusion of docetaxel and are usually mild to moderate. The most frequently reported symptoms were flushing, rash with or without pruritus, chest tightness, back pain, dyspnoea and drug fever or chills. Severe reactions were characterised by hypotension and/or bronchospasm or generalised rash/erythema.

■ Nervous system disorders: The development of severe peripheral neurotoxicity requires a reduction of dose. Mild to moderate neurosensory signs are characterised by paraesthesia, dysaesthesia or pain including burning. Neuromotor events are mainly characterised by weakness.

■ Skin and subcutaneous tissue disorders: Reversible cutaneous reactions have been observed and are generally mild to moderate. Reactions are characterised by a rash including localised eruptions mainly on the feet and hands (including severe hand and foot syndrome), but also on the arms, face or thorax, and frequently associated with pruritus. Eruptions generally occur within one week after the docetaxel infusion. Severe nail disorders are characterised by hypo- or hyperpigmentation and sometimes pain and onycholysis.

■ Fluid retention includes events such as peripheral oedema and less frequently pleural effusion, pericardial effusion, ascites and weight gain. The peripheral oedema usually starts at the lower extremities and may become generalised with a weight gain of 3 kg or more. Fluid retention is cumulative in incidence and severity. However the incidence of this is markedly reduced by the administration of corticosteroid therapy starting the day before treatment and continued for 3 days.

7   How should Mrs CR's chemotherapy be monitored?

In assessing treatment effectiveness, the following parameters should be monitored:

■ *Subjective measures of disease* – reduction in symptoms of cancer. It is important to record the symptoms that the patient is suffering from as a result of her cancer prior to her first cycle of treatment, in order to allow a measurement of improvement in those symptoms as treatment progresses.

■ *Objective measures of disease*. The clinical team will monitor the patient's response to treatment by CT scan or other objective measure of tumour size in any original sites of disease (i.e. primary tumour in the breast or sites of metastases). This is typically done every 6–8 weeks during treatment. Monitoring of liver function tests is appropriate as an improvement in Mrs CR's transaminase and GGT levels may indicate disease response; conversely a worsening of these parameters may indicate unresponsiveness to treatment.

In monitoring for treatment toxicity, the following parameters may be monitored:

- *Haematological parameters.* Full blood count must be analysed prior to administration of trastuzumab/docetaxel chemotherapy to check for persistent bone marrow suppression. Low neutrophil or platelet counts (typically neutrophils $<1.5 \times 10^9$/L or platelets $<100 \times 10^9$/L) will necessitate a delay in docetaxel administration, usually by one week (although trastuzumab could be continued as bone marrow suppression is not considered to be a contraindication to treatment with this agent). The occurrence of febrile neutropenia between treatment cycles may also necessitate dose reduction of docetaxel.
- *Cardiac function.* All candidates for treatment with trastuzumab, but especially those with prior anthracycline exposure, should undergo baseline cardiac assessment including history and physical examination, ECG, echocardiogram, or MUGA scan or magnetic resonance imaging. Cardiac function should be further monitored during treatment (e.g. every three months). Monitoring may help to identify patients who develop cardiac dysfunction. If patients have a continued decrease in left ventricular function, but remain asymptomatic, the clinician should consider discontinuing therapy if no clinical benefit of trastuzumab therapy has been seen. Caution should be exercised in treating patients with symptomatic heart failure, a history of hypertension or documented coronary artery disease. Generally a minimum baseline left ventricular ejection fraction of 55% is used as a prerequisite for commencement of treatment (this may vary from centre to centre).
- *Other toxicities.* The patient should be methodically questioned about the development of any other side-effects of treatment. Severe grades of toxicity may again necessitate dose adjustment (e.g. severe neurotoxicity, cutaneous toxicity).
- *Hepatic function.* As Mrs CR has baseline liver impairment, it will be essential to monitor her liver function tests closely, not only to assess disease response (as previously discussed) but also to check for deterioration that may preclude further use of docetaxel (e.g. if serum bilirubin were to rise outside the normal range).

8   Outline the major counselling points you would make to Mrs CR on her discharge medication and any other non-drug related issues. What other aspects of her treatment would you discuss with her?

The major counselling points to make to Mrs CR on discharge would include the following:

MST tablets/Oramorph liquid

Apart from basic information such as name of drug, its purpose (pain relief) and the dose and frequency it should be taken, it will be important to educate Mrs CR on the need to take MST tablets regularly at approximately 12-hourly intervals and the need to swallow the tablets whole, as it is a sustained-release preparation. She must also be counselled on the correct use of Oramorph liquid for breakthrough pain – it must only be taken should recurrence of pain occur before her next scheduled dose of MST, and only up to a maximum frequency of 4 hourly. She should also be counselled on the potential side-effects such as constipation, which require the use of prophylactic laxative therapy (in this case, senna).

Senna tablets

Apart from basic information such as name of drug, its purpose (laxative) and the dose and frequency it should be taken, it is important to impress on Mrs CR the necessity to not increase the dose beyond that prescribed unless recommended by her GP or hospital doctor. Unless she was to develop diarrhoea (which is possible while on chemotherapy treatment), she should be counselled to continue taking senna while on morphine treatment.

Metoclopramide tablets

Apart from basic information such as name of drug, its purpose (anti-nausea) and the dose and frequency it should be taken, it is important to educate Mrs CR to take the tablets regularly at the prescribed dosage.

Dexamethasone tablets

Apart from basic information such as name of drug, its purpose (appetite stimulant) and the dose and frequency it should be taken, it will be important to carefully explain that the dosage and frequency is to be increased to 8 mg (4 tablets) twice daily starting from the morning before her next scheduled chemotherapy treatment in order to reduce the likelihood of both allergic type reactions and fluid retention. The doses should also be taken with or immediately after food to reduce the likelihood of dyspeptic symptoms and, for the higher dosage regimen to be taken from the day before chemotherapy treatment, to take the twice daily doses in the morning and by early afternoon, to reduce the likelihood of insomnia at night.

Chemotherapy

It is also important to educate and counsel Mrs CR on the chemotherapy treatment she is receiving and the possible side-effects, as well as how to manage them. It is imperative, however, to ensure that any communication from the clinical pharmacist is in line with that already provided by other health professionals, especially clinicians and nurses. Briefly, this advice should include:

- What to do if she suffers from a fever, sore throat or other non-specific 'flu-like' symptoms – which may indicate neutropenic infection requiring hospital treatment.
- What to do if she suffers from other side-effects such as nausea, diarrhoea or stomatitis.

Often this information will have been provided already to patients undergoing chemotherapy treatment.

The importance of a well-balanced diet and exercise (with plenty of rest) should be reinforced to Mrs CR in order to help her cope with the demands of her treatment.

Case study Level Ma – Management of testicular cancer – see page 178

1   Comment on the clinical signs and symptoms and initial laboratory results – what do they indicate?

Mr AC has presented with the following clinical symptoms: malaise, lethargy, right testicular swelling and difficulty in passing urine. These symptoms taken together with the results of the clinician's examination, CT scan and laboratory results indicate probable metastatic testicular cancer. Right testicular swelling is a common presenting complaint in these patients and the examining clinician has confirmed the presence of a mass independently. Lung metastases are also a common feature of advanced testicular cancer and their presence explains Mr AC's complaint of shortness of breath (dyspnoea). Of real concern is the reduction in urine output and difficulty in passing urine; this indicates possible compression of the ureters by tumour, which is a likely explanation given the presence of a large retroperitoneal mass.

The laboratory results support the clinical signs and symptoms. A raised serum urea and creatinine are likely to be the result of ureteric obstruction caused by the retroperitoneal mass. The reduction in renal function is confirmed by the low EDTA clearance (an approximation of glomerular filtration rate) of 57 mL/min.

The elevations of the germ cell tumour markers β-human chorionic gonadotrophin (β-HCG), α-fetoprotein (AFP) and lactate dehydrogenase (LDH) further support the working diagnosis of testicular cancer. The levels of β-HCG and AFP in particular are negligible in males in normal circumstances, but they are raised in patients with testicular cancers as the tumours secrete these substances in large quantities.

2   Outline a pharmaceutical care plan for Mr AC at this stage.

A pharmaceutical care plan for Mr AC should:

- identify his current treatment needs,
- define how these are to be met and the action required,
- state the endpoints of treatment,
- identify the parameters to be monitored and the frequency of monitoring required (to follow response to treatment and detect side-effects), and
- identify points to be covered when counselling him about his medication.

Identify his current treatment needs

Mr AC's current treatment needs are to:

- minimise/eradicate Mr AC's symptoms of malaise, lethargy, dyspnoea and dysuria,
- improve Mr AC's renal function, and
- treat his underlying testicular cancer.

Define how these are to be met and the action required

For these treatment needs to be met the following should be undertaken:

- an evaluation of treatment options for his testicular cancer,
- consideration of alternative agents (where appropriate), and
- provision of advice to clinicians on any changes and additional agents indicated, such as supportive therapy to prevent the side-effects of treatment.

State the endpoints of treatment

The endpoints of treatment for Mr AC are broadly:

- normalised renal function (reduction in serum urea and creatinine, increase in EDTA clearance),
- effective symptom control, and
- eradication of his underlying malignancy.

For each individual medication prescribed, more specific treatment endpoints could also be included.

Identify the parameters to be monitored and the frequency of monitoring required (to follow response to treatment and detect side-effects)

To monitor for efficacy of treatment and disease response:

- serum β-HCG and AFP (at each cycle),
- CT scan to objectively measure disease response (retroperitoneal mass and lung metastases) after the last cycle (cycle 3),
- renal function (serum urea and creatinine, EDTA clearance) prior to each cycle, and
- improvement in symptoms – prior to each cycle.

To monitor for toxicity:

- haematological parameters – full blood count prior to each cycle,
- gastrointestinal toxicity – nausea and vomiting, mucositis, diarrhoea prior to each cycle,
- neurological toxicity (due to cisplatin) – prior to each cycle,
- renal and liver function – prior to each cycle,
- pulmonary function (bleomycin can rarely cause pulmonary fibrosis) – prior to each cycle, and
- ototoxicity (due to cisplatin) – prior to each cycle.

Identify points to be covered when counselling him about his medication

Points to be covered when counselling Mr AC on his medication will depend on the agents chosen to treat him. Counselling should provide basic information about the medication, including its name and purpose, and provide clear instructions on how it should be used and any precautions that need to be observed.

3   Outline and critically appraise the possible treatment options available at this stage. What are the goals of therapy?

Cytotoxic chemotherapy is the cornerstone of therapy for metastatic testicular cancer. This type of cancer (known as a type of 'germ cell' tumour as it is thought to be derived from cells in the germ cell lineage that are blocked in maturation) has been found to be extremely responsive to chemotherapeutic agents, in particular cisplatin and etoposide. There is no role for radiotherapy at this stage due to the advanced nature of the disease.

Once the diagnosis of a testicular germ cell tumour has been made, staging investigations should be performed to assess the extent of disease and to make an assessment of the prognostic group the patient is in. The International Germ Cell Consensus Classification (IGCCC) prognostic grouping is now used as the standard, and divides testicular cancer into good, intermediate and poor prognosis categories (Schmoll *et al.*, 2004).

Mr AC has been classified as good prognosis.

The BEP regimen (bleomycin, etoposide and cisplatin) has become a gold standard treatment that has been utilised since the mid-1980s. Different versions of the regimen have been tested in the clinical setting, with both a 5-day and a 3-day BEP being commonly used. A recent MRC/EORTC study considered the use of 3-day BEP for three or four cycles versus 5-day BEP for three or four cycles (De Wit *et al.*, 2001). It concluded that the efficacy of 3-day BEP for three cycles was equivalent to the other schedules. This regimen is now the standard treatment for patients with good-prognosis advanced testicular cancer, whereas more intensive regimens (e.g. 5-day BEP for four cycles, VIP, POMB/ACE) are used for the intermediate- and poor-prognosis groups. It would therefore be appropriate for Mr AC to be prescribed three cycles of 3-day BEP as he fits into the good-prognosis group.

The outcome of therapy for patients with good-prognosis testicular cancer is extremely good – the 5-year overall survival rate is 92% (compared with only 48% for poor-prognosis disease). Therefore the goal of therapy for Mr AC must be to aim for cure of his disease by instituting BEP chemotherapy as soon as possible, while minimising as far as possible the side-effects of treatment – by ensuring appropriate doses are prescribed and that supportive medication is optimised.

4   Should any adjustment be made to the chemotherapy doses based on Mr AC's laboratory results?

Mr AC's renal function is reduced, as can be observed from the high serum urea and creatinine levels and low EDTA clearance. Each of the three drugs used in the BEP regimen are renally excreted. In particular the excretion of cisplatin is largely dependant on the kidneys and deterioration in renal function is directly related to the development of acute toxicity (e.g. nephrotoxicity, ototoxicity).

The dose of cisplatin should be reduced by 25% due to the lowered EDTA clearance (which approximates creatinine clearance, a marker of renal function). The doses of etoposide and bleomycin can be maintained at 100% as the EDTA clearance is above 50 mL/min.

Due to the curative intent of the treatment however, it is essential for any consideration of a dose reduction to be first discussed with the senior members of the patient's medical team (preferably the consultant).

If it is agreed that the dose should be reduced at this cycle, a review should occur immediately prior to the next cycle of chemotherapy before the next dose is prescribed. As the renal impairment is likely to be due to the presence of tumour compressing the ureters, a significant improvement in renal function would be expected should the disease respond to treatment and the dose of cisplatin should therefore be able to be increased back to 100%. Close monitoring of the renal function (serum urea, creatinine and EDTA clearance) is therefore essential.

Based on the oncology pharmacist's advice, the dose of cisplatin is reduced to 75% so that the following regimen is prescribed:

- bleomycin 30 000 IU i.v. infusion Day 1 (and 8 and 15)
- etoposide 346 mg i.v. infusion Days 1, 2, 3
- cisplatin 79 mg i.v. infusion Days 1 and 2.

These doses may be rounded off according to the local hospital pharmacy practice.

5 What antiemetics should Mr AC be prescribed and why?

One of the major side-effects of cytotoxic chemotherapy is nausea and vomiting. It is essential therefore to control this with prophylactic antiemetic therapy. A number of agents are currently available and are effective at controlling chemotherapy-induced emesis. The most potent of these are $5HT_3$-receptor antagonists that include ondansetron, granisetron and palonosetron.

There are several important principles to consider when prescribing antiemetics:

- Different cytotoxic agents cause differing levels of emetogenicity.
- Antiemetics must be used at optimal dosage and frequency for maximum effect and be taken regularly.
- The use of cytotoxic drugs with a high level of emetogenicity requires the prophylactic administration of a combination of a $5HT_3$-receptor antagonist and a corticosteroid to prevent the onset of acute nausea and vomiting (i.e. within the first 24 hours).
- Ineffective control of nausea and vomiting in the delayed setting (i.e. beyond the first 24 hours) is more likely if sickness occurs in the acute setting.
- There is little evidence supporting the use of $5HT_3$-receptor antagonists beyond the first 24 hours, and corticosteroids appear to be the most effective component of antiemetic regimens used to prevent delayed nausea and vomiting (American Society of Clinical Oncology et al., 2006).

Of all the many cytotoxic agents available, cisplatin is the most emetogenic drug currently used for cancer patients and any chemotherapy regimen containing this drug would therefore be considered highly emetogenic. Because of this it is imperative to prescribe a $5HT_3$-receptor antagonist plus corticosteroid in the acute phase (first 24 hours) and a corticosteroid combination in the delayed phase (24–96 hours). Most cancer centres and units will have local antiemetic guidelines in place, and these should be adhered to.

It is also imperative that nausea and vomiting are minimised as much as possible to ensure that excessive fluid loss does not lead to dehydration. If this were to occur, Mr AC's renal function could deteriorate even further, therefore predisposing him to toxicity from his cytotoxic therapy, especially cisplatin.

6 Outline what you would discuss with Mr AC. How would you try to ensure patient concordance with the management of his nausea and vomiting?

The oncology pharmacist is ideally placed to provide advice and guidance to oncology patients on their supportive medication. The pharmacist should have an underlying knowledge and understanding of the type of treatment the patient is receiving as well as the adverse effects it can produce. For this reason the pharmacist can provide a key pharmaceutical component to the patient's holistic care and complement the roles of the oncology doctor and nurse.

It is essential to ask Mr AC to outline the timelines for the problems he suffered after his first cycle of BEP and to try to describe the exact nature of the problems he had.

The pharmacist must then outline, in lay language:

- Why antiemetics are necessary for preventing nausea and vomiting.
- Why it is necessary to take them on a regular basis after chemotherapy to prevent the 'delayed' type of sickness that the drugs, in particular cisplatin, can cause.
- The necessity of utilising different routes of administration for delivering antiemetic medication should oral delivery become unsuitable, in this case due to severe nausea and vomiting. In that type of situation, the rectal route is a useful way of administering a drug. It may be that Mr AC has not been given adequate instructions on the use of suppositories and it would therefore be important to check this and provide instructions if not.

In concluding, the pharmacist should then ask the patient if they have understood the information that has been provided and give him the opportunity to ask questions. The patient must be provided with as much relevant information as possible as a patient's understanding of how and why they are taking their supportive medication is essential to them actually carrying out the instructions that they have been given.

7   What other issues would you counsel Mr AC on (e.g. non-pharmacological issues)?

Apart from the usual medication counselling at discharge, it would be prudent to discuss with Mr AC other issues including:

- The importance of maintaining a balanced diet.
- The importance of avoiding foods or other triggers that may cause nausea and vomiting.
- The importance of regular exercise.
- The risk of bone marrow suppression. Mr AC should be warned to avoid people with colds and other infections particularly between days 7 and 14, when his white blood cell counts will be lowest and he will be most prone to infection.
- The importance of adequate mouthcare to avoid mucositis and possible infective complications (e.g. teeth brushing/mouthwashes).

Case study level Mb – Oral chemotherapy – see page 181

1   What are the treatment options for the first-line therapy of metastatic colorectal cancer? Critically appraise these options in relation to the most appropriate therapy for Mrs RP.

The mainstay of treatment for the treatment of metastatic colorectal cancer for the last 40 years has been intravenous 5-fluorouracil (5-FU). It has been investigated as part of numerous regimens, including bolus as a single agent, in combination with modulators such as folinic acid, and as part of continuous infusion schedules. Several studies have shown that prolonged exposure to 5-FU is associated with better antitumour activity and decreased toxicity when compared with bolus regimens.

Oral formulations of 5-FU would allow a protracted exposure without the need for a central venous catheter or costly infusion pump. However oral 5-FU is unreliably absorbed from the gastrointestinal tract, leading to incomplete and erratic bioavailability. This has led to the development of oral prodrugs of 5-FU such as capecitabine (Hoff, 2003) and uracil/tegafur (UFT).

In May 2003, NICE issued a technology appraisal recommending that oral therapy with either capecitabine or UFT be considered as an option for the first-line treatment of metastatic colorectal cancer. This recommendation was based on the evidence from two large phase III clinical trials, both comparing capecitabine against a standard treatment arm of bolus folinic acid and 5-FU (the 'MAYO' regimen). Both studies concluded that capecitabine produced a significantly higher response rate than the 5-FU regimen, although the major endpoints of time to disease progression and overall survival were similar in the two arms (Hoff et al., 2001; Van Cutsem et al., 2001). However chemotherapy-related toxicities were, on the whole, significantly lower in patients treated with capecitabine (including mucositis, diarrhoea, neutropenia, alopecia and nausea). There was a higher incidence of hand–foot syndrome and hyperbilirubinaemia in the capecitabine arm, however.

In recent years, combining 5-FU with newer agents has become common. Studies have shown a higher response rate and better time to disease progression for combinations of oxaliplatin and irinotecan with 5-FU-based regimens, but only in the case of irinotecan plus an infusional 5-FU regimen was a significant overall survival benefit seen. However these regimens are associated with higher levels of toxicity than single agent 5-FU and for that reason it is reasonable to still offer the single-agent 5-FU regimens (as well as single-agent oral 5-FU prodrugs) to some patients who are not expected to tolerate combination chemotherapy very well. The NICE technology appraisal for capecitabine (2003) states clearly that the choice of therapy must be a joint decision of both the clinician and the patient, taking into account such factors as contraindications and side-effects of treatment as well as the clinical condition and preferences of the patient.

Based on Mrs RP's extensive co-morbidities, including cardiovascular disease, plus her advanced age, it would seem entirely reasonable to consider the use of single-agent 5-FU-based chemotherapy in this situation, either administered intravenously or as an oral prodrug formulation.

2   Briefly describe some of the key principles in the prescribing and dispensing of oral chemotherapy.

The standards to which oral chemotherapy agents are prescribed and dispensed are becoming increasingly important due to their increasing availability across a wide range of tumours. All anti-cancer drugs should be regarded as potentially hazardous regardless of the route of administration. For this reason it is essential that the prescribing and dispensing of oral chemotherapy is carried out to the same standards as those in place for intravenous chemotherapy.

The British Oncology Pharmacy Association (BOPA) (2004) produced a position statement on the safe practice and pharmaceutical care of patients receiving oral anti-cancer chemotherapy. Within this document, there are numerous principles that should be adhered to including:

- Other than in exceptional and clearly defined and mutually agreed circumstances, prescribing and dispensing should remain the sole responsibility of the hospital-based oncologist/haematologist and pharmacy respectively.
- Prescribing should be done within the context of written protocols.
- Electronic systems, or prescription proformas/templates, similar to those for parenteral chemotherapy should be used.
- Prescriptions must state clearly for each course of treatment: the dose, frequency of administration, intended start date, duration of treatment and, where relevant, the intended stop date.
- All intended deviations from protocol, such as dose modifications, should be clearly identified as such.
- An authorised pharmacist must screen prescriptions before dispensing.
- All pharmacy staff that are or could be involved with dispensing oral anti-cancer drugs must have access to full copies of all the relevant protocols and work to detailed operating procedures.
- Label instructions must be clear and unambiguous and include, where relevant, the intended duration of treatment.
- Counselling and education of the patient must include information such as: how and when to take their medication, what to do in the case of missing one or more doses or vomiting after taking a dose, likely adverse effects, principles of safe handling, storage and disposal and patient's access to advice and support when at home.
- General risk management must be considered, including issues such as risks of wastage, inappropriate storage and risks to others in contact with the patient, such as children.

The importance of safety in this area is also reinforced by the Department of Health (2004) publication 'Building a safer NHS for patients: improving medication safety'.

In January 2008, the National Patient Safety Agency issued a rapid response report on the risks of incorrect dosing of oral anti-cancer medicines. This report alerted all healthcare staff involved in the use of these medicines of the potentially fatal outcomes if incorrect doses are used. The report made a number of key recommendations for implementation by the NHS and independent sector by July 2008, including many which re-emphasise the principles outlined in the BOPA position statement.

3a   What patient parameters need to be checked prior to prescribing capecitabine?

The following patient parameters are essential to know prior to first prescribing capecitabine treatment:

- full blood count
- serum biochemistry (urea and electrolytes, creatinine)
- liver function tests (especially as Mrs RP has documented metastatic disease in the liver)
- a measure of her renal function
- height and weight to determine body surface area.

3b   Apart from performing a formal EDTA clearance or 24-hour urine collection, how else may Mrs RP's renal function be estimated?

The most accurate ways in which to estimate renal function currently used in the UK are EDTA clearance and 24-hour urine collection. However these measurements are not always considered necessary and renal function may be estimated by one of a number of equations in use.

These equations make a number of assumptions and may be used to estimate Mrs RP's renal function; this is necessary as toxicity from capecitabine can be increased in individuals with renal impairment (creatinine clearance <50 mL/min).

The most commonly used equation for estimating creatinine clearance is the Cockcroft–Gault equation. This equation requires knowledge of the patient's gender, age, weight and serum creatinine. The equation is:

$$\text{Creatinine clearance (mL/min)} = \frac{X \times (140 - \text{age}) \times \text{weight (kg)}}{\text{Serum creatinine (micromol/L)}}$$

where $X = 1.04$ for females and 1.23 for males.

When using this formula, ideal body weight should be used for patients who are 'obese', often considered to be those individuals with an actual body weight more than 15% over their ideal body weight.

4a   Evaluate Mrs RP's laboratory results – what do they indicate? Calculate Mrs RP's current estimated creatinine clearance.

Mrs RP's laboratory results are uneventful apart from a raised serum potassium (hyperkalaemia). This may be due to a number of factors including renal impairment, and often in elderly patients on numerous medications it may be drug-induced. Possible causes of her hyperkalaemia must be considered and then removed as the development of severe hyperkalaemia (serum potassium >6 mmol/L) can cause cardiac disturbances and death.

It is also important to remember that renal function deteriorates with age and with Mrs RP about to commence capecitabine, it is necessary to estimate her current creatinine clearance. Based on the Cockcroft–Gault formula quoted above:

$$\text{Creatinine clearance} = \frac{1.04 \times (140 - 74) \times 51}{47} = 74 \text{ mL/min}$$

4b What change to therapy would you recommend to her clinician based on these results?

It is possible that Mrs RP's hyperkalaemia is drug-induced. The combination of ramipril, an angiotensin-converting enzyme (ACE) inhibitor that can cause potassium retention with co-amilofruse, a combination diuretic, may be contributing to her high serum potassium levels. It would be prudent to advise the clinician to change her diuretic therapy to a potassium-'losing' diuretic (such as furosemide) to counteract the potassium-sparing effect of the ACE inhibitor. It may also be prudent to advise Mrs RP to avoid foods rich in potassium such as dried fruits and bananas.

Her estimated creatinine clearance is 74 mL/min. This represents a relatively normal renal function, particularly for someone of Mrs RP's age. The Summary of Product Characteristics for capecitabine (Summary of Product Characteristics, 2008) states that the dosage only needs to be reduced if creatinine clearance is between 30 and 50 mL/min, to 75% dosage. If creatinine clearance is <30 mL/min, then capecitabine is contraindicated. This is because the incidence of severe adverse effects is more common in patients with renal impairment compared with the overall population.

No adjustment in the capecitabine starting dosage is therefore required based on renal function.

You prescribe oral capecitabine on an approved preprinted prescription form according to protocol and the appropriate clinical management plan. The dosage prescribed is as follows:

- capecitabine 1250 mg/m² p.o. b.d. for 14 days.

Based on Mrs RP's body surface area, she is prescribed capecitabine 1800 mg p.o. b.d. for 14 days.

5 Outline a pharmaceutical care plan for Mrs RP, including advice to the clinician.

A pharmaceutical care plan for Mrs RP should:

- identify her current treatment needs,
- define how these are to be met and the action required,
- state the endpoints of treatment,
- identify the parameters to be monitored and the frequency of monitoring required (to follow response to treatment and detect side-effects), and
- identify points to be covered when counselling her about her medication.

Identify her current treatment needs

Mrs RP's current treatment needs are to:

- minimise/eradicate her symptoms of abdominal pain, flatulence, nausea, and loss of appetite,
- correct Mrs RP's hyperkalaemia,
- treat her underlying metastatic colorectal cancer.

Define how these are to be met and the action required

For these treatment needs to be met the following should be undertaken:

- an evaluation of treatment options for her metastatic colorectal cancer,
- consideration of alternative agents (where appropriate), and
- provision of advice to clinicians on any changes and additional agents indicated, such as supportive therapy to prevent the side-effects of treatment.

State the endpoints of treatment

The endpoints of treatment for Mrs RP are broadly:

- normal serum potassium,
- effective symptom control, and
- optimum control of progression of her underlying malignancy.

For each individual medication prescribed, more specific treatment endpoints could also be included.

Identify the parameters to be monitored and the frequency of monitoring required (to follow response to treatment and detect side-effects)

To monitor for efficacy of treatment and disease response:

- CT scan to objectively measure disease response (lung and liver metastases) – after three to four cycles of treatment,
- serum CEA tumour marker and LFT's – prior to each cycle, and
- improvement in symptoms – prior to each cycle.

To monitor for toxicity:

- haematological parameters – full blood count prior to each cycle,

- gastrointestinal toxicity – nausea and vomiting, mucositis, diarrhoea prior to each cycle, and
- skin toxicity – hand–foot syndrome prior to each cycle.

Identify points to be covered when counselling her about her medication

Points to be covered when counselling Mrs RP on her medication will depend on the agents chosen to treat her. Counselling should provide basic information about the medication, including its name and purpose, and provide clear instructions on how it should be used and any precautions that need to be observed (see also answer to Question 2).

6 One of your tasks in your clinic is to emphasise the way in which treatment will be monitored and to outline the goal of therapy. What would you say to Mrs RP?

Patient education and counselling is an essential part of ensuring that patients fully understand their treatment and its context in the management of their disease. Patients need to understand the overall objective of the treatment being given as well, in order to have a realistic view of what the treatment is aiming to achieve. In this case, Mrs RP will almost certainly have discussed this first with her clinician who will have explained the palliative intent of treatment and the fact that it is not curative due to the advanced nature of her disease.

The pharmacist should therefore look to reinforce the information already provided to Mrs RP by outlining those parameters being monitored (i.e. tumour marker, symptoms and a CT scan after the third or fourth cycle). It will also be necessary to inform Mrs RP of the need to monitor carefully for side-effects. Often it is useful for patients to be asked to record the side-effects that they suffer from during treatment in a patient diary booklet or similar.

7 Part of your review also includes checking for any potential drug interactions with capecitabine. Briefly outline the major known drug interactions with capecitabine. Which one is relevant to Mrs RP and what would you advise both the clinician and Mrs RP?

A number of drugs have been reported to interact with capecitabine and these include:

- Allopurinol – may reduce the efficacy of capacitabine and concurrent use should be avoided.
- Folinic acid – may enhance the effect of capacitabine and concurrent use should be avoided or dosage adjustments may be necessary.
- Phenytoin – increased serum phenytoin levels may occur leading to phenytoin toxicity. Serum phenytoin levels should be monitored.
- Warfarin – altered coagulation parameters and/or bleeding have been reported in patients taking capecitabine concomitantly with coumarin-derivative anticoagulants such as warfarin. Patients taking warfarin

concomitantly with capecitabine should be monitored regularly for alterations in their coagulation parameters (PT or INR) and the anticoagulant dose adjusted accordingly.

Mrs RP is currently taking warfarin to prevent recurrent thromboembolism after having a deep vein thrombosis a month ago. As Mrs RP is likely to require warfarin treatment for at least another two months, it will be necessary to take the following steps:

- Warn the treating oncologist of the nature of the interaction and the need for close monitoring of the patient's INR during treatment with capecitabine. The warfarin dose may need regular adjustment due to the intermittent nature of the capecitabine dosing schedule (two weeks on treatment, one week off treatment), causing fluctuations in the clotting parameters. It would also be prudent to inform the patient's GP and local anticoagulant clinic of the interaction and its significance.
- Advise Mrs RP of the interaction and the need to more carefully monitor her clotting and adjust her warfarin dosage. Mrs RP should be advised of the signs of enhanced warfarin effect (e.g. bleeding from gums, cuts, unexplained bruising etc.).

8 What might have caused her diarrhoea? What should Mrs RP have done when the diarrhoea occurred?

Her diarrhoea has almost certainly been caused by her capecitabine treatment. Capecitabine is a prodrug of 5-fluorouracil and as such may cause similar side-effects to it. Cytotoxic drugs can cause gastrointestinal toxicity such as diarrhoea due to their effect on the rapidly dividing cells of the body, including the cells of the gastrointestinal mucosa.

Mrs RP should be questioned as to whether she is still taking co-danthramer liquid, and if she had stopped taking this during her episodes of diarrhoea. It would be worth counselling her to do this should her diarrhoea recur after the next cycle.

It would be wise to also question Mrs RP as to whether she had been suffering from any concurrent medical condition such as gastroenteritis, which may have also contributed to the diarrhoea.

It is imperative for patients to manage the side-effects of oral chemotherapy appropriately. This includes knowing when to stop taking the tablets should severe adverse effects occur. There are clear recommendations for stopping capecitabine should certain specific side-effects occur whilst taking the drug and contacting the treatment centre for further advice. These include:

- more than four bowel movements each day and/or night-time diarrhoea,
- more than one vomit in any 24-hour period,
- nausea that is interfering with eating, and
- hand–foot syndrome or mucositis that causes more than mild discomfort.

Based on the grade of toxicity that Mrs RP experienced, it may be necessary for Mrs RP to have a dosage reduction for her second cycle (refer to the Summary of Product Characteristics).

Many centres co-prescribe an antidiarrhoeal drug such as loparmide to use in case of diarrhoea. Mrs RP should be counselled to use this to treat diarrhoea should it occur again.

9   Mrs RP wonders why her GP cannot prescribe her chemotherapy as she lives just around the corner from him. What do you say to her?

As described previously, the management of cytotoxic chemotherapy treatment should be kept under the supervision of hospital oncologists and the hospital pharmacy, where the knowledge and expertise is centred. Only in exceptional and clearly defined and mutually agreed circumstances (e.g. where specific shared care agreements are in place with primary care clinicians) may the responsibility for prescribing be shared (BOPA, 2004).

It should therefore be explained to Mrs RP that despite the chemotherapy being oral, it is still essential that the prescribing and dispensing of the tablets occurs within the hospital.

9

Nutrition and blood case studies

Rebekah Raymond and Anita Rana

Case study level 1 – Iron-deficiency anaemia

Learning outcomes

Level 1 case study: You will be able to:

- describe the risk factors
- describe the disease
- describe the pharmacology of the drug
- outline the formulation, including drug molecule, excipients, etc. for the medicines
- summarise basic social pharmacy issues (e.g. opening containers, large labels).

Scenario

Mrs WL, a 70-year-old Chinese woman, reports to her GP because she has been feeling very tired. Mrs WL informs her GP that she has been getting out of breath when walking up stairs which she never had any problem with in the past. On examination, Mrs WL has pallor of the skin, conjunctiva and nail beds and brittle nails. Mrs WL is a strict vegetarian.

The GP performs a blood count and the results show that she has iron-deficiency anaemia.

Questions

1a What is anaemia?
1b What typical blood results might you expect in a patient with iron-deficiency anaemia?

1c   What symptoms does Mrs WL have that support the diagnosis of iron-deficiency anaemia?

1d   What risk factors does Mrs WL have for developing this condition?

2a   What is erythropoiesis and which human growth factor stimulates this?

2b   Describe the life cycle of a red blood cell, starting from the release of erythropoietin and ending with its destruction.

3a   Should modified-release iron preparations be used in the treatment of anaemia? Justify your answer.

3b   What are the side-effects of iron preparations?

4a   What medication would you recommend for Mrs WL? (Give a preparation, dose and frequency.)

4b   How would you counsel Mrs WL about the medication you have recommended?

4c   What follow-up should Mrs WL receive?

5   Mrs WL tells you that she takes magnesium trisilicate for her indigestion when you ask about any other medicines. Can she continue to take this?

General references

Clinical Knowledge Summaries (2008) Anaemia – Iron deficiency Available at http://www.cks.library.nhs.uk/anaemia_iron_deficiency/view_whole_guidance [Accessed 4 July 2008].

Germann WJ, Stanfield CL (2005) *Principles of Human Physiology*, 2nd edn. San Francisco, CA: Pearson Inc publishing as Benjamin Cummings.

Joint Formulary Committee (2008) *British National Formulary 55.* London: British Medical Association and Royal Pharmaceutical Society of Great Britain, March.

Case study level 2 – Pernicious anaemia

Learning outcomes

Level 2 case study: You will be able to:

- interpret relevant lab and clinical data
- identify monitoring and referral criteria
- explain treatment choices
- describe goals of therapy, including monitoring and the role of the pharmacist/clinician
- describe issues – counselling points, adverse drug reactions, drug interactions, complementary/alternative therapies and lifestyle advice.

Scenario

Mrs HJ, a 60-year-old woman, has been admitted to hospital following a number of falls. She is complaining of numbness and tingling in her legs and is having some difficulty walking. Mrs HJ's daughter also mentions that she has become a little confused recently. When the doctor examines her he observes that she is pale and has glossitis. The doctor performs a blood count and the results are as follows:

WBC	4×10^9/L ($4.0–11.0 \times 10^9$/L)
RBC	2.5×10^9/L ($3.8–4.8 \times 10^9$/L)
Hb	7.2 g/dL (12.0–15.0 g/dL)
Hct	0.28 (0.36–0.46)
MCV	110 fL (83.0–101.0 fL)
MCH	34 pg (27.0–32.0 pg)

A blood film is also done for Mrs HJ and this shows oval macrocytes, hypersegmental neutrophils, megaloblasts, anisocytosis and poikilocytosis.

Questions

1   Which of Mrs HJ's results are out of range? Explain what the deranged results signify.
2   Explain the terms glossitis, megaloblast, anisocytosis and poikilocytosis.
3   Mrs HJ is to undergo a Schilling's test. Explain how this test works, how it is performed and what it is used for?
4   Mrs HJ is diagnosed as suffering from pernicious anaemia – what causes pernicious anaemia?
5   Describe the process by which vitamin B_{12} is absorbed and where in the digestive system absorption occurs.
6   What are the risk factors for developing pernicious anaemia and which of these does Mrs HJ have?
7   What signs and symptoms does Mrs HJ have that could be attributed to her pernicious anaemia?
8   What medication would you recommend for Mrs HJ? (Give preparation, dose and frequency.)
9   What are the side-effects of the treatment you have recommended? Include an explanation for any terms you are not familiar with.
10   How would you counsel Mrs HJ about the medication you have recommended?

General references

Franklin H and Epstein MD (1997) Mechanisms of disease: pernicious anemia. *New England Journal of Medicine* 337: 1441–1448.

Germann WJ, Stanfield CL (2005) *Principles of Human Physiology*, 2nd edn. San Francisco, CA: Pearson Inc publishing as Benjamin Cummings.

GPnotebook (2008) Pernicious anaemia. Available at http://www.gpnotebook.co.uk/simplepage.cfm?ID=1530200072 [Accessed 4 July 2008].

Hoffman V and Provan D (1997) ABC of clinical haematology: Macrocytic anaemias. *British Medical Journal* 314: 430.

Joint Formulary Committee (2008) *British National Formulary 55*. London: British Medical Association and Royal Pharmaceutical Society of Great Britain, March.

MedlinePlus (2008) Anaemia. Available at http://www.nlm.nih.gov/medlineplus/anemia.html [Accessed 04 July 2008].

Case study level 3 – Porphyria

Learning outcomes

Level 3 case study: You will be able to:

- interpret clinical signs and symptoms
- evaluate laboratory data
- evaluate treatment options
- state goals of therapy
- describe a pharmaceutical care plan to include advice to a clinician
- describe the prognosis and long-term complications
- describe social pharmacy issues which could include supply (e.g. complex treatments at home, concordance and compliance) and lifestyle issues.

Scenario

Mrs JC, a 33-year-old woman who presented with acute abdominal pain, has been transferred to your ward for further investigation. Mrs JC's current medications are paracetamol and diazepam, which she has been taking for back pain. After further investigations Mrs JC is diagnosed with acute intermittent porphyria.

Questions

1a   What is porphyria?
1b   What is acute intermittent porphyria?
1c   What are the typical presenting symptoms of acute intermittent porphyria?
1d   What are the risk factors for developing acute intermittent porphyria? Which apply to Mrs JC?

2   How is a diagnosis of acute intermittent porphyria made?

3a Mrs JC has been diagnosed with an acute attack of porphyria – how should this be managed pharmaceutically?

3b How would you go about arranging a supply of the necessary medication?

3c How would you advise on the administration of haem arginate?

4   The medical team caring for Mrs JC prescribes diclofenac and co-codamol 30/500 to help manage her pain. Is this analgesia appropriate?

Reference

Thadani H, Deacon A and Peters T (2000) Regular review. Diagnosis and management of porphyria. *British Medical Journal* 320: 1647–1651.

General references

GPNotebook (2008) Porphyria. Available at http://www.gpnotebook.co.uk/simplepage. cfm?ID=1563754508 [Accessed 04 July 2008].

Joint Formulary Committee (2008) *British National Formulary* 55. London: British Medical Association and Royal Pharmaceutical Society of Great Britain, March.

Summary of Product Characteristics (2008) Normosang Human hemin. Orphan Europe. Available at www.orphan-europe.com [Accessed 30 June 2008].

Case study level Ma – Sickle cell anaemia

Learning outcomes

Level M case study: You will be able to:

- interpret clinical signs and symptoms
- evaluate laboratory data
- critically appraise treatment options
- state goals of therapy
- describe a pharmaceutical care plan to include advice to a clinician
- describe the prognosis and long-term complications
- describe the social pharmacy issues which could include supply (e.g. complex treatments at home, concordance and compliance) and lifestyle issues
- describe the monitoring of therapy.

AW, a 25-year-old Afro-Caribbean man, has been admitted to your ward with a sickle cell crisis. AW has a raised temperature and complains of severe pain in his limbs, chest and lower back. His regular medications are:

- phenoxymethylpenicillin 500 mg twice a day
- folic acid 5 mg daily.

AW's blood results are as follows:

WBC	$13.1 \times 10^9/L$ $(4.0–11.0 \times 10^9/L)$
RBC	$3.5 \times 10^9/L$ $(3.8–4.8 \times 10^9/L)$
Hb	8.5 g/dL (12.0–15.0 g/dL)
Hct	0.33 (0.36–0.46)
Bilirubin	45 micromol/L (3–17 micromol/L)

Blood film showed increased reticulocytes, sickle cells and presence of target cells.

1a   What is the cause of sickle cell anaemia?
1b   Which groups of people are at the highest risk of having sickle cell anaemia?
2a   What is a sickle cell crisis? What situations may precipitate a sickle cell crisis?
2b   What do you think may have precipitated AW's crisis?
3   The doctor caring for AW asks your advice regarding analgesia. So far he has prescribed regular paracetamol and full-dose dihydrocodeine but AW is still in severe pain. What recommendations can you make regarding analgesia for AW?
4   Comment on AW's blood results.
5   What other acute management may be necessary for AW?
6a   Why is AW taking phenoxymethylpenicillin and folic acid?
6b   AW has frequent crises and is concerned because he is due to go on holiday shortly. What advice could you give AW to help reduce the risk of further crises?
7   What are the prognosis and long-term complications for patients with sickle cell anaemia?
8a   Due to AW's frequent crises the medical team caring for him is considering initiating hydroxycarbamide (hydroxyurea). What evidence is there to support the use of hydroxycarbamide in the management of sickle cell anaemia?
8b   How is hydroxycarbamide thought to work in the management of sickle cell anaemia?
8c   The medical team ask what dose of hydroxycarbamide should be prescribed and what monitoring they should undertake. What do you advise?
8d   How would you counsel AW regarding his new medication?
8e   Hydroxycarbamide is not licensed for the management of sickle cell anaemia. What implications does this have? What should you do?

Reference

Platt OS, Brambilla DJ, Rosse WF *et al.* (1994) Mortality in sickle cell disease – life expectancy and risk factors for early death. *New England Journal of Medicine* 330: 1639–1644. Available at http://content.nejm.org/cgi/content/full/330/23/1639 [Accessed 4 July 2008].

General references

Allen S (2005) Understanding sickle cell anaemia. *Pharmaceutical Journal* 275: 25–28.

Charache S, Terrin ML, Moore RD *et al.* (1995) Effect of hydroxyurea on the frequency of painful crises in sickle cell anaemia. *New England Journal of Medicine* 332: 1317–1322.

Claster S and Vichinsky EP (2003) Managing sickle cell disease. *British Medical Journal* 327: 1151–1155.

Davies SC and Oni L (1997) Fortnightly review: Management of patients with sickle cell disease *British Medical Journal* 315: 656–660.

Electronic Medicines Compendium (2008) Patient information leaflet for Hydrea. Available at http://www.emc.medicines.org.uk/ [Accessed 4 July 2008].

Electronic Medicines Compendium (2008) Summary of Product Characteristics for Hydrea. Available at http://www.emc. medicines.org.uk/ [Accessed 4 July 2008].

GPNotebook (2008) Sickle cell anaemia. Available at http://www.gpnotebook.co.uk/simplepage.cfm?ID=1087373317 [Accessed 4 July 2008].

Oteng-Ntim E, Okpala IE and Anionwu EN (2003) Sickle cell disease in pregnancy. *Current Opinion in Obstetrics and Gynaecology* 13: 362–368.

Royal Pharmaceutical Society of Great Britain (RPSGB) (2007) Fitness to Practice and Legal Affairs Directorate Fact Sheet: Five. The use of unlicensed medicines in pharmacy. http://www.rpsgb.org/pdfs/factsheet5. pdf [Accessed 4 July 2008].

Case study level Mb – Peri-operative nutrition

Learning outcomes

Level M case study: You will be able to:

- interpret clinical signs and symptoms
- evaluate laboratory data
- critically appraise treatment options
- state goals of therapy
- describe a pharmaceutical care plan to include advice to a clinician
- describe the prognosis and long-term complications
- describe the social pharmacy issues which could include supply (e.g. complex treatments at home, concordance and compliance) and lifestyle issues
- describe the monitoring of therapy.

SC is a 30-year-old woman who is due to undergo surgery for severe Crohn's disease. She has been admitted to the surgical ward for nutritional care prior to her surgery. On examination SC is 165 cm in height and weighs 50 kg.

SC takes the following regular medications:

- mesalazine 500 mg tds
- paracetamol 1 g q.d.s. p.r.n.
- azathioprine 100 mg o.d.
- prednisolone 20 mg o.m.
- Calcichew-D_3 Forte ii o.d.
- alendronic acid 70 mg once a week
- ranitidine 150 mg b.d.
- Ensure Plus 1 carton three times a day
- phenytoin 100 mg t.d.s.
- sodium valproate MR 200 mg b.d.

Prior to her admission, SC was prescribed Ensure Plus cartons three times daily in addition to her usual diet. However, despite the additional nutrition provided by the Ensure Plus, SC has failed to gain sufficient weight. The surgical team caring for SC have decided they need to increase her nutritional intake and plan to commence tube feeding. SC has developed a sore throat and painful mouth due to oral thrush and she is unable to swallow her medication. SC's medications will now need to be administered via an NG tube.

1a Calculate SC's body mass index (BMI).
1b What does this signify?
2a What sort of feed is Ensure Plus?
2b SC confesses to you that she has not been taking the Ensure Plus three times daily as she dislikes the taste. What suggestions can you give her?
3a What is an NG tube?
3b What are the risks associated with the use of an NG tube?
4 What nutritional support options are available to SC now that an NG tube has been inserted?
5a What approach should the pharmacist have in decision-making about SC's regular medications?
5b List and rationalise the medication SC will need to continue while she has an NG tube inserted?
5c For each medication, state how you can administer that drug via an NG tube?
5d Will any of the drug doses need to be changed due to a formulation change?
5e Are there any significant drug–nutrition interactions and how would you manage them?

6   If there is no suitable preparation, can the nurses crush tablets or open capsules?

It is decided that SC will receive her usual diet plus enteral feeding overnight prior to surgery to optimise her condition. Post surgery the team plan to pre-scribe total parenteral nutrition (TPN) and stop the enteral feeding.

7a   In what post-operative situations are the use of parenteral nutrition indicated?
7b   The surgical team have planned for the parenteral nutrition to be for a short period. What type of access is required?
7c   The team caring for SC decide to start her on parenteral nutrition at half of her daily requirements. Why is this?
7d   What is refeeding syndrome?
8   As SC will be 'nil by mouth' postoperatively, her medication will have to be administered intravenously. What advice will you give the nurse on the administration of the drugs?

References

Crook MA, Hally V and Panteli JV (2001) The importance of the refeeding syndrome. *Nutrition* 17: 632–637.

NICE (National Institute for Health and Clinical Excellence) (2006) Nutrition support in adults: Full guideline, appendices. Available at http://guidance.nice.org.uk/page.aspx?o=293220 [Accessed 4 July 2008].

General references

ABPI, Medicines Compendium. Available at www.medicines.org.uk.

Joint Formulary Committee (2008) *British National Formulary 55*. London: British Medical Association and Royal Pharmaceutical Society of Great Britain, March.

Murphy P (2001) Enteral feeds explained. *The Pharmaceutical Journal* September 267: 297–300.

Rahman MH and Beattie J (2004) Medication in the peri-operative period. *The Pharmaceutical Journal* 272: 287–289.

Schulman R, Drayan S, Harries *et al.* (eds) (1998) *UCL Hospitals Injectable Drug Administration Guide*. Oxford: WileyBlackwell.

Singer M and Webb A (2000) *Oxford Handbook of Critical Care*. Oxford: Oxford University Press.

Sweetman S (ed.) (2007) *Martindale The Complete Drug Reference*, 35th edn. London: Pharmaceutical Press.

White R (2006) Peri-operative nutrition – the role of the pharmacist. *Hospital Pharmacist* 13: 361–363.

Case study level 1 – Iron-deficiency anaemia – see page 218

1a   What is anaemia?

Anaemia, defined as a decrease in the oxygen-carrying capacity of the blood, is generally associated with a low haematocrit which can result from either a decrease in the number of erythrocytes or a decrease in the size of the erythrocytes. However, a person can also have anaemia if the haematocrit is normal but each red cell contains less than the normal concentration of haemoglobin. Because most of the oxygen transported in blood is bound to haemoglobin in erythrocytes, a decrease in erythrocyte abundance or size is associated with low levels of haemoglobin.

1b   What typical blood results might you expect in a patient with iron-deficiency anaemia?

- Hb is low – generally due to reduced iron intake or possibly excessive iron loss
- MCV is reduced – small 'microcytic' red blood cells are typical of iron deficiency
- MCH is low – each red blood cell contains less haemoglobin than normal
- MCHC is low – the amount of haemoglobin in the sample is reduced.

Diagnosis would be confirmed by a low serum ferritin.

1c   What symptoms does Mrs WL have that support the diagnosis of iron-deficiency anaemia?

Symptoms are:

- tiredness
- pallor
- shortness of breath on exertion.
- brittle nails

1d   What risk factors does Mrs WL have for developing this condition?

- Diet (poor/vegetarian/vegan diet increases risk of iron-deficiency anaemia).

Other risk factors which may warrant investigation include:

- Bleeding from the gastrointestinal tract
- Malignancy
- Hookworm infestation (a major source of blood loss in many parts of the world, but not northern Europe).

2a   What is erythropoiesis and which human growth factor stimulates this?

Erythropoiesis describes the process of production of red blood cells. Erythropoietin is the human growth factor that stimulates the production of red blood cells.

2b   Describe the life cycle of a red blood cell, starting from the release of erythropoietin and ending with its destruction.

The following points should be included:

- Erythropoietin is released from cells in the kidney in response to low oxygen levels.
- This triggers differentiation of cells in the bone marrow to produce erythrocytes.
- Differentiation results in the loss of nuclei and organelles and the production of haemoglobin.
- The last stage of erythrocyte development in the bone marrow is known as a late normoblast and is released into the bloodstream as a reticulocyte (immature erythrocyte).
- An erythrocyte enters the bloodstream and circulates for around 120 days.
- Erythrocytes are broken down in the reticuloendothelial system to components: iron, bilirubin and amino acids which are released into the bloodstream.

3a   Should modified-release iron preparations be used in the treatment of anaemia? Justify your answer.

Many patients prefer to have a different type of iron preparation to ferrous sulphate tablets – they find they cause them fewer side-effects. The reason for this is generally that the product they prefer either contains less iron to start with or is a modified-release preparation.

Modified-release preparations release iron gradually so less iron is present in the gastrointestinal tract at any one time. However, because they are modified-release, these preparations are likely to carry the iron past the first part of the duodenum into an area of the gut where iron absorption may be poor. The low incidence of side-effects may reflect the small amounts of iron available for absorption under these conditions and so the preparations have no therapeutic advantage and should not be used.

3b   What are the side-effects of iron preparations?

Iron preparations tend to cause gastrointestinal irritation resulting in nausea, epigastric pain and altered bowel habit (constipation or diarrhoea). In older patients there is a risk that constipation may lead to faecal impaction. Side-effects tend to be dose related.

4a   What medication would you recommend for Mrs WL? (Give a preparation, dose and frequency.)

Iron salts should be given by mouth unless there are good reasons for using another route. The *BNF* recommends a treatment dose of 100–200 mg elemental iron per day. This should be given as ferrous sulphate 200 mg three times daily. Dividing the doses gives a greater availability for absorption.

4b   How would you counsel Mrs WL about the medication you have recommended?

Allergies and any other medicines should be enquired about before explaining that Mrs WL should take one tablet three times a day. Explain what side-effects she may experience as above and inform her that she can take the tablets with food if the side-effects are troublesome. It is very important to warn patients that their stools may be darkened (almost black). Compliance is often an issue with iron tablets and good counselling can aid this.

4c   What follow-up should Mrs WL receive?

Mrs WL should have a repeat blood test in 2–4 weeks' time to check her response to iron therapy and another after 2–4 months to confirm replenishment of iron stores.

5   Mrs WL tells you that she takes magnesium trisilicate for her indigestion when you ask about any other medicines. Can she continue to take this?

Magnesium salts reduce the oral absorption of iron. As long as Mrs WL avoids taking her iron tablets at the same time as her indigestion remedy the interaction will be avoided. Mrs WL should be recommended to leave at least 1 hour between taking the two medications to allow her stomach to empty. The fact that Mrs WL needs an indigestion remedy is a concern; she could be suffering from gastric bleeding; unless her GP is already aware that she is taking this she should be referred back to them.

Case study level 2 – Pernicious anaemia – see page 219

1   Which of Mrs HJ's results are out of range? Explain what the deranged results signify.

- Hb, Hct and RBC are low which signifies anaemia
- MCV and MCH are high, which suggests a megaloblastic anaemia

2   Explain the terms glossitis, anisocytosis and poikilocytosis.

- Glossitis: inflammation of the tongue.

- Anisocytosis: abnormal variation in size of the red blood cells (as in pernicious anaemia).
- Poikilocytosis: characteristic of various anaemias; the presence of poikilocytes (abnormally shaped red blood cells) in the blood.

3   Mrs HJ is to undergo a Schilling's test. Explain how this test works, how it is performed and what it is used for?

Schilling's test assesses the oral absorption of vitamin B_{12} and is used to diagnose pernicious anaemia. The patient is injected intramuscularly with non-labelled vitamin B_{12}, to saturate body stores. An oral dose of vitamin B_{12} labelled with cobalt-58 is administered, followed by a second dose labelled with cobalt-57 bound to intrinsic factor. Prior saturation of body stores ensures any absorbed radiolabelled vitamin B_{12} is rapidly excreted in the urine. Urinary excretion of orally administered vitamin B_{12} is low in patients with pernicious anaemia due to poor absorption. Absorption is increased when it is administered with intrinsic factor. The ratio of cobalt-57 to cobalt-58 is thus raised in patients with pernicious anaemia. Intrinsic factor antibody testing is now generally used to diagnose pernicious anaemia, though the Schilling's test may occasionally be used.

4   Mrs HJ is diagnosed as suffering from pernicious anaemia – what causes pernicious anaemia?

Pernicious anaemia is caused by a deficiency of intrinsic factor, which is required for the absorption of vitamin B_{12} in the intestinal tract.

5   Describe the process by which vitamin B_{12} is absorbed and where in the digestive system absorption occurs.

Water-soluble vitamins are absorbed by special transport proteins, some require active transport, others facilitated diffusion in order to cross the gastric lumen. Vitamin B_{12} cannot be absorbed by itself; it has to be bound to intrinsic factor which is secreted into the lumen of the stomach by the parietal cells. Intrinsic factor binds to vitamin B_{12} to form a complex that is subsequently absorbed in the ileum.

6   What are the risk factors for developing pernicious anaemia and which of these does Mrs HJ have?

Risk factors include:

- age – incidence peaks at age 60
- sex – female to male incidence ratio of 1.6:1.0
- early greying of hair
- blue eyes
- blood group A
- veganism/poor-quality diet

- family history of:
  - pernicious anaemia
  - vitiligo
  - myxoedema
  - Hashimoto's disease
  - Addison's disease of the adrenals
  - hypoparathyroidism.

The risk factors that Mrs HJ has are her age and her sex.

7   What signs and symptoms does Mrs HJ have that could be attributed to her pernicious anaemia?

Signs and symptoms are:

- numbness and tingling in her legs and consequent difficulty walking and
- glossitis.

8   What medication would you recommend for Mrs HJ? (Give preparation, dose and frequency.)

As per *BNF*: Hydroxocobalamin injection. Dose: by intramuscular injection, pernicious anaemia and other macrocytic anaemias without neurological involvement, initially 1 mg three times a week for two weeks then 1 mg every three months. Pernicious anaemia and other macrocytic anaemias with neurological involvement, initially 1 mg on alternate days until no further improvement, then 1 mg every two months.

Mrs HJ has symptoms suggestive of neurological involvement – numbness and tingling in the legs, difficulty in walking and confusion – so the dose for pernicious anaemia with neurological involvement should be administered.

9   What are the side-effects of the treatment you have recommended? Include an explanation for any terms you are not familiar with.

As per BNF, side-effects of hydroxocobalamin are nausea, headache, dizziness, fever, hypersensitivity reactions including rash and pruritus, injection-site pain, and hypokalaemia during initial treatment.

10   How would you counsel Mrs HJ about the medication you have recommended?

It should be explained:

- that she has low levels of vitamin B_{12},
- that she is not absorbing it properly from her intestine which is why it has to be administered as an injection,
- that her levels are very low so she is receiving the injection every other day until her symptoms improve, and
- that after she goes home she will need to have the same injection every three months to keep her vitamin B_{12} levels up. Her GP will be able to arrange this for her.

Case study level 3 – Porphyria – see page 221

1a   What is porphyria?

The porphyrias are a heterogeneous group of inherited disorders of haem biosynthesis. Figure A9.1 shows the pathway of haem synthesis. A deficiency in one of the enzymes results in a specific porphyria.

1b   What is acute intermittent porphyria?

Acute intermittent porphyria is a severe form of porphyria which is due to a deficiency of porphobilinogen deaminase (hydroxymethylbilanesynthase).

1c   What are the typical presenting symptoms of acute intermittent porphyria?

The most common presenting symptoms are acute abdominal pain, tachycardia and dark urine. Neurological and psychological symptoms may also be present. Muscular weakness including a proximal myopathy of the arms is also common and can progress to quadraparesis, respiratory paralysis and arrest.

1d   What are the risk factors for developing acute intermittent porphyria? Which apply to Mrs JC?

Porphyria presents most commonly in people in their thirties, it is 4–5 times more common in females. Acute attacks are often triggered by exposure to drugs as well as by fasting, stress or infection. Mrs JC is a woman in her thirties with recent exposure to medications, one of which (diazepam) is a known precipitant of porphyric attacks.

2   How is a diagnosis of acute intermittent porphyria made?

During an acute attack, a fresh urine sample which has been protected from light should be sent to a specialist laboratory to be tested for aminolaevulinic acid and porphobilinogen concentrations. If urinalysis confirms raised urinary excretion of aminolaevulinic acid and porphobilinogen, an analysis of faecal porphyrins can be used to identify the specific porphyria. In acute intermittent porphyria faecal porphyrin levels are generally normal.

Ehrlich's aldehyde test can be used to confirm a diagnosis of acute intermittent porphyria. Equal volumes of urine and Ehrlich's reagent are mixed; a pink colour indicates raised urinary concentration of either porphobilinogen or urobilinogen. In acute intermittent porphyria, raised porphobilinogen is present and the pink precipitate formed is insoluble in chloroform.

However, between attacks urinary levels of aminolaevulinic acid and porphobilinogen may be normal. In this case the demonstration of reduced

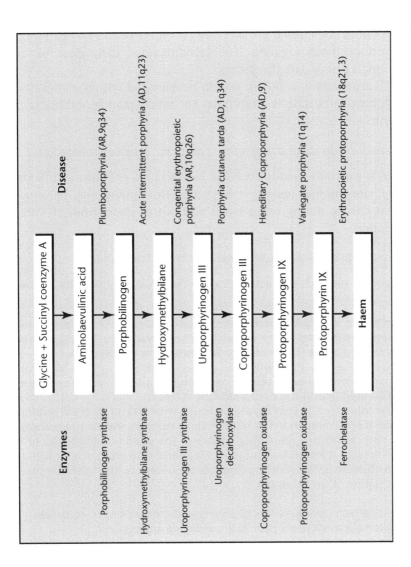

Figure A9.1 Pathway of haem synthesis. Blocks at various parts of the pathway result in different porphyrias (numbers in parentheses show inheritance). AR, autosomal recessive; AD, autosomal dominant. (From Thadani et al., 2000, reproduced with permission.)

hydroxymethylbilane synthetase activity in erythrocytes can be used to confirm a diagnosis of acute intermittent porphyria.

3a   Mrs JC has been diagnosed with an acute attack of porphyria – how should this be managed pharmaceutically?

Oral and intravenous glucose and haem arginate are the mainstay of treatment. Glucose 10% should be infused intravenously for mild attacks and pending the administration of haem arginate. The recommended daily dose of haem arginate is 3 mg/kg once daily for 4 days.

Mrs JC's acute abdominal pain should be managed symptomatically with analgesics known to be safe in porphyria. For severe pain morphine is non-porphyrogenic.

3b   How would you go about arranging a supply of the necessary medication?

Glucose 10% is generally readily available in a hospital environment. Supplies of haem arginate (human hemin), trade name Normosang may be obtained from Orphan Europe during office hours and out of hours from St Thomas' Hospital, London.

3c   How would you advise on the administration of haem arginate?

The summary of product characteristics for Normosang gives the following advice:

- Human hemin should be administered once daily in a dose of 3 mg/kg (up to a maximum of 250 mg or one ampoule). The relevant dose should be drawn up and diluted immediately prior to administration in 100 mL of 0.9% sodium chloride in a glass bottle and infused intravenously over 30 minutes into a large antebrachial or central vein using an inline filter. The solution should be used within the hour following dilution.
- After the infusion, the vein should be rinsed with 100 mL of 0.9% sodium chloride. It is recommended to initially flush the vein with 3 or 4 boluses of 10 mL, after which the remaining volume of the sodium chloride can be infused over 10–15 minutes. (Infusion via a large vein and flushing with sodium chloride 0.9% following infusion are necessary due to the highly irritant nature of the product.)

4   The medical team caring for Mrs JC prescribes diclofenac and co-codamol 30/500 to help manage her pain. Is this analgesia appropriate?

Paracetamol and opioid analgesics are safe to use in porphyria, however diclofenac is one of the drugs known to be unsafe to prescribe in porphyria. There are other NSAIDs such as ibuprofen or naproxen which are not listed as unsafe and the medical team should be advised to amend the prescription accordingly. However if Mrs JC is in severe pain it may be necessary to prescribe a strong opiate. These are safe in porphyria.

Case study level Ma – Sickle cell anaemia – see page 222

1a   What is the cause of sickle cell anaemia?

Sickle cell anaemia is the result of the homozygotic inheritance of the gene for haemoglobin S. The sickle haemoglobin gene shows autosomal recessive inheritance, thus both parents must be carriers of the gene in order for it to be inherited. The red blood cells of individuals with sickle cell anaemia are capable of carrying oxygen. However when they give up oxygen to the tissues the haemoglobin S molecules can crystallise, causing the deformation or sickle shape. The cells regain their original shape when they are reoxygenated but as this process is repeated the cells become irreversibly sickled. It is these sickled cells which produce the symptoms and complications seen in the disease as they occlude the blood vessels.

1b   Which groups of people are at the highest risk of having sickle cell anaemia?

The frequency of sickle cell disease is:

- 1 in 4 in West Africans
- 1 in 10 in Afro-Caribbeans.

It is estimated that 100 000 homozygotes are born each year in Africa, 1500 in the USA, 700 in the Caribbean, and 140 in the UK. Haemoglobin S is also common in Cyprus, Greece, Italy, the Middle East and in populations who originate from these areas.

2a   What is a sickle cell crisis? What situations may precipitate a sickle cell crisis?

A crisis occurs when the sickled cells clog together and occlude the blood vessels causing tissue ischaemia, pain and eventually organ damage. This may be precipitated by: hypoxia, sudden changes in temperature, physical activity (causing tissue anoxia), extreme fatigue, acidosis, infection, stress and anxiety, pregnancy or physical trauma.

2b   What do you think may have precipitated AW's crisis?

AW has a raised temperature and white cell count thus his current crisis is likely to have been precipitated by infection.

3   The doctor caring for AW asks your advice regarding analgesia. So far he has prescribed regular paracetamol and full-dose dihydrocodeine but AW is still in severe pain. What recommendations can you make regarding analgesia for AW?

AW should be prescribed a full dose of NSAID such as diclofenac to be taken regularly (unless contraindicated). Non-steroidal analgesia can be an excellent adjunct to narcotics. The majority of patients admitted to hospital during a sickle cell crisis also require strong opioid analgesia for pain management. This is usually given in the form of intravenous morphine either as an infusion or a patient-controlled analgesia system. Morphine can be given with a loading dose of 0.1 mg/kg followed by an infusion of 10 micrograms/kg per hour.

4   Comment on AW's blood results.

AW's white cell count is raised, probably due to an infection which may well have precipitated this crisis. The low haemoglobin and haematocrit are due to the excessive destruction of red cells that occurs in this haemolytic form of anaemia and the raised bilirubin is due to the rapid breakdown of the cells. Raised reticulocytes are seen in sickle cell anaemia as the body compensates for the increased cell breakdown by increasing production of red cells. Target cells are blood cells which resemble a shooting target and are found in patients with sickle cell anaemia as well as in a number of other conditions.

5   What other acute management may be necessary for AW?

Broad-spectrum antibiotics may be required to treat infection, 24% oxygen should be given at 4 L/min. Fluids should be given to maintain hydration, orally if possible. Blood transfusion may be considered.

6a   Why is AW taking phenoxymethylpenicillin and folic acid?

Sickle cell patients are hyposplenic and receive prophylactic phenoxymethyl-penicillin to help prevent pneumococcal infection. Folic acid is supplementation may be given as the high red cell turnover increases requirements – though many prescribers find this unnecessary as they consider the UK diet contains sufficient folic acid.

6b   AW has frequent crises and is concerned because he is due to go on holiday shortly. What advice could you give AW to help reduce the risk of further crises?

AW should be counselled regarding the importance of taking his prophylactic antibiotics as well as his folic acid.
    It is recommended that sickle cell patients receive vaccination to help prevent infection, the *BNF* recommends the following vaccines for those with splenic dysfunction: *Haemophilus influenzae* type b, meningococcal group C, pneumococcal, influenza.
Sickle cell patients should also be advised to:

- ensure sufficient fluid intake
- keep warm
- maintain a healthy diet rich in folates; regular supplements of folic acid should be taken, especially during pregnancy. All women with sickle cell disease should be advised to take 5 mg folic acid daily
- take enough rest

- obtain prompt treatment of any infection
- avoid vascular stasis (not to wear tight clothing).

Patients travelling abroad should be advised to:

- obtain medical insurance
- increase fluid intake
- abstain from alcohol
- move around during travel, including flights
- take appropriate antimalarial prophylaxis when travelling to malarious areas (unlike sickle cell trait, sickle cell anaemia offers no protection against malaria)
- ensure a bacteriologically clean drinking water supply
- increase oral fluid intake above the standard 3 L/day for adults when they are in hot climates to compensate for the increased insensible losses.

7 What are the prognosis and long-term complications for patients with sickle cell anaemia?

Among children and adults with sickle cell anemia (homozygous for sickle haemoglobin), the median age at death was 42 years for males and 48 years for females (Platt *et al.*, 1994). Complications include:

- painful crises
- infection
- haemolytic anaemia
- jaundice
- stroke
- priapism
- eye problems
- hand–foot syndrome
- acute chest syndrome
- bone and joint problems
- splenomegaly
- end-stage organ disease
- leg ulcers.

8a Due to AW's frequent crises the medical team caring for him is considering initiating hydroxycarbamide (hydroxyurea). What evidence is there to support the use of hydroxycarbamide in the management of sickle cell anaemia?

Several paediatric and adult trials have reported decreases in pain, the incidence of acute chest syndrome and overall mortality with the use of hydroxy-carbamide.

8b How is hydroxycarbamide thought to work in the management of sickle cell anaemia?

Hydroxycarbamide has been shown to restimulate fetal haemoglobin production, reducing organ damage and maintaining splenic function.

8c   The medical team ask what dose of hydroxycarbamide should be prescribed and what monitoring they should undertake. What do you advise?

Starting doses of 15 mg/kg per day may be increased by 5 mg/kg per day until crises are controlled or the dose is not tolerated.

Regular blood tests are required to check for cytopenia, especially neutropenia. The Summary of Product Characteristics for hydroxycarbamide states: The complete status of the blood, including bone marrow examination, if indicated, as well as kidney function and liver function should be determined prior to, and repeatedly during, treatment. The determination of haemoglobin level, total leukocyte counts, and platelet counts should be performed at least once a week throughout the course of hydroxycarbamide therapy. If white blood cell count falls below 2.5×10^9/L or platelet count to $<100 \times 10^9$/L, therapy should be interrupted. Counts should be rechecked after 3 days and treatment resumed when they rise significantly towards normal.

8d   How would you counsel AW regarding his new medication?

AW should be told the dose and frequency of his new medication and the need to store it safely should be emphasised. The importance of regular blood tests should be explained and AW should also be made aware of symptoms that may indicate neutropenia such as unexplained fever, chills or sore throat and should be advised to report to his doctor immediately if this occurs. AW should also be informed that both males and females must stop taking hydroxycarbamide for six months before a planned pregnancy.

8e   Hydroxycarbamide is not licensed for the management of sickle cell anaemia. What implications does this have? What should you do?

Although hydroxycarbamide is a licensed medication, it is not licensed for the management of sickle cell anaemia; use in this case is unlicensed or 'off-licence'. As every pharmacist assumes a duty of care to a patient when supplying a medicine, this means that if an adverse reaction is suffered, the supplying pharmacist may assume some liability along with the doctor who prescribed it.

As a pharmacist you are expected to take the steps that a reasonably competent pharmacist would take to ensure that a supply of medication is made in the best interests of the patient. The Royal Pharmaceutical Society of Great Britain (RPSGB) (2007) would expect these steps to include:

- weighing up the potential risks of making the supply against those of not doing so;
- taking reasonable steps to ensure the prescriber knew that he was using the product outside its marketing authorisation and the possible consequences; and

- checking that there are some data available to support the use of the medication in the manner that it has been prescribed, either from the manufacturer, a drug information service or from the prescriber if he or she has substantial experience of using the product in this way.

The RPSGB (2007) also advises that 'generally speaking it is not appropriate to deviate from a prescriber's directions, but this must be balanced against the pharmacist's professional duty to ensure that every prescription is appropriate for the patient. If the pharmacist feels that a significant risk to the patient's health is likely if the supply is made, then the option of refusing to supply should be given due consideration.'

As well as ensuring that the prescriber is aware of the unlicensed use of the medication it is important to bring this to the attention of the patient. This should be done without undermining the patient's confidence in either the prescriber or the prescribed medicine. This is also necessary because the patient information leaflet which you are supplying with the medication will not include anything to suggest that the product can be used in sickle cell anaemia.

Case study level Mb – Peri-operative nutrition – see page 224

1a Calculate SC's body mass index (BMI).

BMI is weight in kilograms divided by height in metres squared. Thus SC has a BMI of 18.36 kg/m^2.

1b What does this signify?

A BMI of less than 18.5 kg/m^2 indicates that the patient is malnourished. Malnutrition can lead to poor wound-healing, post-operative complications and sepsis.

2a What sort of feed is Ensure Plus?

Ensure Plus is milk-based ready-to-drink sip feed.

2b SC confesses to you that she has not been taking the Ensure Plus three times daily as she dislikes the taste. What suggestions can you give her?

First check whether SC is aware of the range of flavours of Ensure that are available. An alternative flavour or variety of flavours may be all that is needed. Feeds are also often more palatable when chilled. Ensure Plus is a milk-based sip feed; an alternative that may be more appealing to SC is a fruit juice-based feed, for example, Enlive.

If neither of the above options is appropriate it may be useful to make SC aware that neutral-flavoured feeds can be used in sauces and fruit juice ones in jellies, instant whips or pudding mixes. SC should be referred to a dietician for further advice.

3a   What is an NG tube?

An NG tube is a nasogastric tube – a fine tube that is inserted through the nose and fed down through the oesophagus into the stomach. The tube has a radio-opaque tip and an X-ray should confirm the position.

3b   What are the risks associated with the use of an NG tube?

The risks include:

- regurgitation and aspiration into the bronchus,
- tube placement: tracheobronchial intubation, nasopharyngeal perforation, oesophageal perforation, and
- blockage of the NG tube.

4   What nutritional support options are available to SC now that an NG tube has been inserted?

There are ranges of enteral tube feeds available, most of which are nutritionally complete. These include standard feeds, fibre-enriched, high-energy and disease-specific feeds. These feeds provide protein, fat, carbohydrate, vitamins, minerals, trace elements and water. Carbohydrates are provided as sucrose or glucose polymers. Protein may be whole protein or oligopeptides. Fats may be provided as medium-chain or long-chain triglycerides. A standard feed provides 1 kcal/mL and are based on whole protein. Special feeds are available for special purpose. For example, Nepro is a suitable feed for a patient with renal disease who are on haemodialysis or continuous ambulatory peritoneal dialysis because it contains lower nitrogen content than standard feed.

5a   What approach should the pharmacist have in decision-making about SC's regular medications?

A systematic approach should be taken. The pharmacist should consider the following:

- Is the drug needed at all?
- Can the drug be administered via any other route?
- Does the drug come in a suitable formulation for administering via a tube?

5b   List and rationalise the medication SC will need to continue while she has an NG tube inserted?

- Medicines used to control life-threatening conditions should be continued.

- Phenytoin and sodium valproate – SC's anti-epilepsy medicines will need to continue.
- Prednisolone – The stress of surgery causes an increase in plasma adrenocorticotrophic hormone and cortisol concentrations. Cortisol secretion can rise from 30 mg/day to 50 mg/day following minor surgery and 150 mg/day following major surgery. However, an abrupt withdrawal after a prolonged period may lead to acute adrenal insufficiency, hypotension or shock. Thus it is important to continue SC's corticosteroid therapy and additional intravenous hydrocortisone may be administered peri-operatively.
- Paracetamol – As this is being taken as required, a judgement would have to taken by the clinician whether SC still requires the medication. SC's pain score would need to be assessed.
- Azathioprine and mesalazine will be withheld prior to the procedure. These medications are not used to control a life-threatening condition and her surgery may remove the need for these medicines.
- Alendronic acid and Calcichew D_3 Forte can be withheld prior to the procedure as they are for osteoporosis prophylaxis.
- Ranitidine is being used as prophylaxis against steroid-induced gastric or duodenal ulcers. The clinician will need to decide if this needs to continue based on patients previous medical history.

5c   For each medication, state how you can administer that drug via an NG tube?

- Phenytoin – suspension preparation available.
- Sodium valproate – liquid preparation available.
- Prednisolone – dispersible tablets available.
- Paracetamol – dispersible tablets and liquid preparation are available.
- Ranitidine – effervescent and liquid preparations available.

5d   Will any of the drug doses need to be changed due to a formulation change?

There is a difference in bioequivalence between capsules and phenytoin suspension. A 100-mg phenytoin capsule is equivalent to 90 mg of the suspension preparation.

5e   Are there any significant drug–nutrition interactions and how would you manage them?

Enteral feed reduces phenytoin absorption by 75%. The pharmacist can recommend the phenytoin to be given as a single dose, if possible. The enteral feeds should be stopped 2 hours prior to and for 2 hours after the dose. The NG tube should be 'flushed' with 20–50 mL of sterile water before feeds and medication. Phenytoin levels must be monitored as this drug has a narrow therapeutic index.

6   If there is no suitable preparation, can the nurses crush tablets or open capsules?

Crushing tablets and opening capsules should be considered as a last resort as there is a risk to the person administering the medicines. By crushing tablets you are breaking the product licence of that drug. This route would then make this an unlicensed preparation.

Modified-release or slow-release preparations are designed to release the medication over a period of time. Crushing these preparations results in the whole dose being immediately available for absorption. At the least, this will cause an alteration in the patient's drug levels and at the worst it may result in an overdose.

To overcome this, some medications which are soluble can be given more frequently to maintain a steady drug level. For example, dipyridamole 200 mg MR can be changed to 100 mg q.d.s. to have the same effect.

7a   In what post-operative situations is the use of parenteral nutrition indicated?

The most common post-operative indications for parenteral nutrition are an ileus, a perforation or the formation of a fistula.

7b   The surgical team have planned for the parenteral nutrition to be for a short period. What type of access is required?

For short-term feeding (less than 14 days) NICE (2006) recommends parenteral feeding via a peripheral venous catheter for those patients who do not need central access. A GTN patch can be applied above the peripheral venous catheter site to promote vasodilatation of the vein for those patients who have narrow veins. Some TPN is unsuitable for peripheral administration due to the nitrogen and glucose concentration; these must go through a central venous catheter.

7c   The team caring for SC decide to start her on parenteral nutrition at half of her daily requirements. Why is this?

As SC has eaten little for more than 5 days, she is at risk of refeeding syndrome. NICE (2006) recommend that parental nutrition should be introduced at no more than 50% of the requirements for the first 2 days for those at risk of refeeding syndrome.

7d   What is refeeding syndrome?

Refeeding syndrome is defined by Crook et al. (2001) as 'severe electrolyte and fluid shifts associated with metabolic abnormalities in malnourished patients undergoing refeeding, whether orally, enterally or parenterally'.

In a starved patient, the secretion of insulin is decreased in response to the low carbohydrate intake. Catabolised fats and protein are used for energy. This results in an intracellu+1lar loss of electrolytes, in particular phosphates. When the patient starts to feed, a sudden shift from fat to carbohydrate metabolism occurs and secretion of insulin increases. This stimulates cellular uptake of magnesium, phosphate and potassium, which can lead to hypophosphataemia, hypokalaemia, hypomagnesaemia and fluid balance abnormalities. These abnormalities can lead to the clinical features of refeeding syndrome which include cardiac failure, respiratory failure, rhabdomyolysis, arrhythmias and seizures.

8   As SC will be 'nil by mouth' postoperatively, her medication will have to be administered intravenously. What advice will you give the nurse on the administration of the drugs?

■   Phenytoin i.v. 100 mg t.d.s. – Inject slowly undiluted and directly into a large vein through a large-gauge needle or i.v. catheter). Maximum rate: 50 mg/min.

■   Sodium valproate i.v. 200 mg b.d. – To reconstitute, inject the solvent provided (4 mL) into the vial, allow to dissolve and extract the appropriate dose. Due to displacement of solvent by sodium valproate the concentration of reconstituted sodium valproate is 95 mg/mL. Give as a slow intravenous injection over 3–5 minutes.

■   Paracetamol 1000 mg i.v. – Infuse over 15 minutes.

■   Prednisolone 20 mg is changed to hydrocortisone 100 mg t.d.s. i.v. bolus: over at least 30 seconds. Manufacturer recommends over 1–10 minutes.

10

Musculoskeletal and joint disease case studies

Nicola Parr and Tracy Garnier

In this chapter, Case study levels 1 and 2 both explore the management of a single patient with rheumatoid arthritis. Rheumatoid arthritis is a frequently encountered condition with a large number of pharmaceutical treatment options. Creating two cases using the one patient allows a more detailed examination of the management of these patients.

Case study level 1 – Rheumatoid arthritis

Learning outcomes

Level 1 case study: You will be able to:

- describe the risk factors
- describe the disease
- describe the pharmacology of the drug
- outline the formulation including drug molecule, excipients, etc. for the medicines
- summarise basic social pharmacy issues (e.g. opening containers, large labels).

Scenario

Mrs PJ is a 67-year-old woman who has recently attended the hospital's rheumatology clinic. She has been diagnosed with rheumatoid arthritis. She has come to the community pharmacy where you work to collect her new prescription for sulfasalazine and diclofenac.

1a What is rheumatoid arthritis?
1b What are the risk factors for developing rheumatoid arthritis?
1c What are the clinical features of rheumatoid arthritis?
1d What investigations are performed to help confirm a diagnosis of rheumatoid arthritis?
2a The major treatments for rheumatoid arthritis include NSAIDs and DMARDs. What do the abbreviations NSAID and DMARD stand for?
2b Sulfasalazine is a DMARD. Describe its mode of action.
2c Sulfasalazine is comprised of two components – 5-aminosalicylic acid (5-ASA), also known as mesalazine, and its carrier molecule, sulfapyridine. How are these two components chemically linked?
2d When sulfasalazine is taken orally, which enzymes are responsible for cleaving this bond and where does this take place?
2e State the common side-effects of sulfasalazine.
2f Sulfasalazine is known to be a sulfa drug as it contains sulfapyridine. What is a sulfa drug and how does this affect the side-effect profile of sulfasalazine?
3a List the formulations of sulfasalazine that are currently available.
3b Which of these formulations are licensed for rheumatoid arthritis?
3c What other conditions is sulfasalazine licensed for?
4 When you hand Mrs PJ her dispensed prescription, what information or help would you give her to ensure that she knows how to use her medications appropriately?

Reference

Bryant DM and Aldred A (2007) Rheumatoid arthritis and osteoarthritis. In: Walker R and Whittlesea C (eds) *Clinical Pharmacy and Therapeutics*, 4th edn. Edinburgh: Churchill Livingstone.

General references

ABPI Electronic Medicines Compendium. Available at http:/www.medicines.org.uk [Accessed 4 July 2008].

Joint Formulary Committee (2008) *British National Formulary 55*. London: British Medical Association and Royal Pharmaceutical Society of Great Britain, March.

Riley SA and Turnberg LA (1990) Sulphasalazine and the aminosalicylates in the treatment of inflammatory bowel disease. *Quarterly Journal of Medicine, New Series* 75: 551–562.

SIGN (Scottish Intercollegiate Guidelines Network) (2000) Management of early rheumatoid arthritis. SIGN Publication No.48. Available at http://www.sign.ac.uk/guidelines/fulltext/48/section2.html [Accessed 4 July 2008].

Case study level 2 – Rheumatoid arthritis

Learning outcomes

Level 2 case study: You will be able to:

- interpret relevant lab and clinical data
- identify monitoring and referral criteria
- explain treatment choices
- describe goals of therapy, including monitoring and the role of the pharmacist/clinician
- describe issues – counselling points, adverse drug reactions, drug interactions, complementary/alternative therapies and lifestyle advice.

Scenario

Mrs PJ is a 67-year-old woman with rheumatoid arthritis. Her current prescription includes:

- Salazopyrin EN 500 mg twice a day
- diclofenac 50 mg three times a day
- paracetamol 1 g up to four times a day when required.

She collected her first prescription for sulfasalazine two weeks ago. She has returned to the pharmacy and asks to speak to you. She has several problems with her medication which she wishes to discuss. First, she complains that her medication is not working properly and she tells you that she has not noticed any benefit from it. She asks you whether you think she should make an appointment with her GP to discuss this.

Questions

1a How is the dose of sulfasalazine normally initiated and titrated?
1b Why is the dose increased gradually?
1c What advice would you give Mrs PJ in answer to her question?

Mrs PJ also mentions that she has to go to her practice nurse for some blood tests but she's not sure why. The *BNF* recommends that liver function tests, full blood counts and renal function tests are carried out regularly.

2a How often should the above tests be performed?

2b   Why should these tests be performed?

In the course of the conversation, Mrs PJ tells you that since she has started taking her new medication, she has been experiencing stomach discomfort about half an hour after she has taken her tablets.

3a   What do you think could be the cause of this problem?
3b   What suggestions could you offer Mrs PJ to help resolve this problem?
3c   What alternative medication might a doctor prescribe to help Mrs PJ with her upset stomach?

Four months later, Mrs PJ returns to your pharmacy. She says that she still has not had much benefit from her sulfasalazine despite the fact that her dose has been titrated to an appropriate level.

4a   What are the goals of therapy when treating rheumatoid arthritis?
4b   Please list the alternative treatments that may be used in the management of rheumatoid arthritis and briefly discuss when an alternative treatment would be tried.

References

Bryant DM and Alldred A (2007) Rheumatoid arthritis and osteoarthritis. In: Walker R and Whittlesea C (eds) *Clinical Pharmacy and Therapeutics*, 4th edn. Edinburgh: Churchill Livingstone.

Clinical Knowledge Summaries (2008) Dyspepsia. Available at http://cks.library.nhs.uk/dyspepsia_unidentified_cause/management/quick_answers/Scenario_dyspepsia_no_alarm_features_taking_nsaids#-328918 [Accessed 4 July 2008].

General references

ABPI Electronic Medicines Compendium (2008) Available at http://www.medicines.org.uk [Accessed 4 July 2008].

Joint Formulary Committee (2008) *British National Formulary 55*. London: British Medical Association and Royal Pharmaceutical Society of Great Britain, March.

National Institute for Health and Clinical Excellence (2004) Dyspepsia – management of dyspepsia in adults in primary care. Available at http://www.nice.org.uk/guidance/CG17/?c=91507 [Accessed 4 July 2008].

Case study level 3 – Gout

> **Learning outcomes**
>
> Level 3 case study: You will be able to:
>
> - interpret clinical signs and symptoms
> - evaluate laboratory data
> - evaluate treatment options
> - state goals of therapy
> - describe a pharmaceutical care plan to include advice to a clinician
> - describe the prognosis and long-term complications
> - describe the social pharmacy issues which could include supply (e.g. complex treatments at home, concordance and compliance and lifestyle issues).

Scenario

Mr KT is a 58-year-old man who has been admitted to the surgical ward on which you work for a total knee replacement. He lives with his wife and two sons. He smokes 15 cigarettes a day and usually drinks about 35 units of alcohol a week. He is slightly overweight with a BMI of 27 kg/m². His current medication includes

- amlodipine 5 mg daily
- bendroflumethiazide 2.5 mg daily
- paracetamol 1 g four times a day
- codeine phosphate 30 mg four times a day when required.
- enoxaparin 40 mg s.c. daily.

Apart from hypertension, he has no other co-morbidities or relevant past medical history.

His operation was a success and he is recovering well. However, during his stay he develops excruciating pain in the big toe of his right foot and his toe is very swollen. He is subsequently diagnosed with gout.

Questions

1a   What is gout? Briefly discuss the pathophysiology of the condition.
1b   List three ways in which gout can manifest itself.
1c   List the risk factors for developing gout and discuss which risk factors Mr KT potentially may have for developing gout.
1d   Describe the symptoms of gout.

1e What investigations should the doctors carry out to help them confirm whether Mr KT has gout?

2 During your rounds, Mr KT asks you if you could tell him what he could do to avoid another attack of gout. What lifestyle advice would you give him?

3 Mr KT requires treatment for his attack of gout. Please discuss the options available for treating an acute attack. For each option discussed, include the following information:

- dose
- contraindications to use
- cautions for use
- potential side-effects.

Which option would you recommend for Mr KT?

4a When you are clinically checking Mr KT's medication chart, you notice that he is on the following medication:

- amlodipine 5 mg daily
- bendroflumethiazide 2.5 mg daily
- paracetamol 1 g four times a day.

Which of these medications can aggravate gout and why?

4b What advice would you give to the doctor looking after Mr KT?

Mr KT's acute attack of gout resolves and he is discharged home. His GP is aware of his problem with gout and after he experiences a second attack of gout, his GP decides that it would be prudent to start him on some long-term prophylaxis against future attacks.

5a Why wasn't Mr KT prescribed prophylactic treatment after his first attack?

5b What options are available and which one is usually the drug of choice?

References

Alldred A (2005) Gout – Pharmacological management. *Hospital Pharmacist* 12: 395–400.

Alldred A and Capstick T (2007) Gout and hyperuricaemia. In: Walker R and Whittlesea C (eds) *Clinical Pharmacy and Therapeutics*, 4th edn. Edinburgh: Churchill Livingstone.

Johnstone A (2005) Gout – the disease and non-drug treatment. *Hospital Pharmacist* 12: 391–393.

General reference

Joint Formulary Committee (2008) *British National Formulary 55*. London: British Medical Association and Royal Pharmaceutical Society of Great Britain, March.

Case study level Ma – Osteoarthritis

Learning outcomes

Level M case study: You will be able to:

- interpret clinical signs and symptoms
- evaluate laboratory data
- critically appraise treatment options
- state goals of therapy
- describe a pharmaceutical care plan to include advice to a clinician
- describe the prognosis and long-term complications
- describe the social pharmacy issues which could include supply (e.g. complex treatments at home, concordance and compliance) and lifestyle issues
- Describe the monitoring of therapy

Scenario

Mrs KR is a 70-year-old woman who weighs 80 kg and is 162 cm tall. Her BMI is 30 kg/m^2. Mrs KR lives alone and has no immediate family in this country. Her past medical history includes osteoarthritis and hypertension. Her medication includes:

- lercanidipine 10 mg daily
- bendroflumethiazide 2.5 mg daily
- diclofenac 50 mg three times daily
- paracetamol 1 g four times daily.

Her blood pressure is 138/85 mmHg and her haemoglobin level is 13.1 g/dL (reference range 12–18 g/dL).

She has been admitted to hospital complaining of abdominal pain and chest pain. After an ECG, which is normal and various other tests, a cardiac problem is excluded and it is decided that she requires an OGD.

Questions

1 What does OGD stand for? Why do you think it might be being performed?
2 Mrs KR has had her blood pressure and haemoglobin level checked, why might the medical staff do this?
3 Mrs KR is subsequently diagnosed with gastritis. Which of her medicines may have caused this?

4 What advice would you give regarding the management of this problem?

5 Mrs KR is taking lercanidipine to manage her hypertension. Lercanidipine is an asymmetric 1,4-dihydropyridine. Draw the chemical structure and state which enantiomer causes the antihypertensive activity associated with lercanidipine. Indicate the chiral centre(s) within your structure.

6 Mrs KR is taking analgesics to manage the symptoms of her osteoarthritis. What is osteoarthritis?

7 What are the signs and symptoms of osteoarthritis?

8 What risk factors may predispose patients to getting osteoarthritis and which risk factors does Mrs KR have?

9 What non-drug recommendations could you give her regarding the management of osteoarthritis?

10 Mrs KR is using diclofenac, an NSAID to manage the symptoms of her osteoarthritis. How do NSAIDs work in the treatment of osteoarthritis?

11 What are the contraindications and cautions for the use of diclofenac?

12 Critically appraise the alternative treatments available for osteoarthritis?

A year later, the GP refers Mrs KR to her consultant as she has been having difficulty walking and severe pain in her knee joint. The consultant discusses her condition and mentions the possibility of a knee replacement as the joint is badly affected.

13 Knee replacement would involve major surgery. What are the risk factors for Mrs KR?

14 Recovery from a knee replacement can take some time and several healthcare professionals are likely to be involved. Discuss the role for each professional involved in Mrs KR's care plan following hospital discharge.

References

Bryant DM and Alldred A (2007) Rheumatoid arthritis and osteoarthritis. In: Walker R and Whittlesea C (eds) *Clinical Pharmacy and Therapeutics*, 4th edn. Edinburgh: Churchill Livingstone.

NICE (National Institute for Health and Clinical Excellence) (2008) Osteoarthritis. The care and management of osteoarthritis in adults. Available at http://www.nice.org. uk/nicemedia/pdf/CG59NICEguideline.pdf [Accessed 4 July 2008].

General references

Clinical Knowledge Summaries (2008) Osteoarthritis: knee replacement. Patient information leaflet. Available at http://cks.library.nhs.uk/patient_information_leaflet/knee_ replacement# [Accessed 4 July 2008].

Joint Formulary Committee (2008) *British National Formulary 55*. London: British Medical Association and Royal Pharmaceutical Society of Great Britain, March.

NICE (2004) Dyspepsia – management of dyspepsia in adults in primary care. Available at http://www.nice.org.uk/guidance/CG17/?c=91507 [Accessed 4 July 2008].

Wood J (1999) Osteoarthritis and its management. *The Pharmaceutical Journal* 262: 744–746.

Case study level Mb – Osteoporosis

Learning outcomes

Level M case study: You will be able to:

- interpret clinical signs and symptoms
- evaluate laboratory data
- critically appraise treatment options
- state goals of therapy
- describe a pharmaceutical care plan to include advice to a clinician
- describe the prognosis and long-term complications
- describe the social pharmacy issues which could include supply (e.g. complex treatments at home, concordance and compliance) and lifestyle issues
- describe the monitoring of therapy.

Scenario

Mrs TY is a 77-year-old woman who has been admitted to the orthopaedic ward where you work as the clinical pharmacist. She slipped on the wet floor in a supermarket and has been diagnosed with a fractured hip. She is normally fit and well and doesn't take any regular medication or have any relevant past medical history. She is 157 cm tall and weighs 49 kg. She lives alone, has never smoked and drinks a small glass of sherry most nights.

Mrs TY is in considerable pain from her fracture. She is prescribed paracetamol 1 g four times daily and codeine 30 mg four times daily when required. She is still complaining of pain.

Questions

1a What recommendations could you make to help manage her pain?

1b What are the contraindications and cautions for the analgesics you are recommending?

1c Are there any adjunctive treatments you would recommend to the doctor that should be prescribed?

1d   What parameters would you monitor as you consider this woman's pharmaceutical care?

2a   Later in the week Mrs TY has surgery to repair her hip fracture. She is also diagnosed with osteoporosis. What is osteoporosis?

2b   What is the difference between primary and secondary osteoporosis?

2c   Which drugs may be implicated in the development of osteoporosis?

2d   What are the signs and symptoms of osteoporosis?

2e   What are the risk factors for osteoporosis and which does Mrs TY have?

2f   What lifestyle advice could you offer to Mrs TY?

3   Discuss the options for the treatment of osteoporosis and decide which you think would be the most suitable for Mrs TY.

4a   Before Mrs TY is discharged she is prescribed alendronate 70 mg once weekly and a calcium and vitamin D preparation, 1 tablet twice a day. What are the indications for alendronate?

4b   How does alendronate work?

4c   What are the side-effects of alendronate?

4d   List the main drug or food interactions associated with alendronate.

4e   What advice would you give to Mrs TY regarding the taking of her alendronate and the calcium and vitamin D preparation?

4f   What other advice would you give Mrs TY regarding the administration of her alendronate?

4g   Alendronate 70 mg once weekly is available as Fosamax once weekly 70 mg white tablets. What excipients are contained in this formulation and discuss the pharmaceutical role of each excipient.

5   Mrs TY tells you that she has heard of a new treatment called teriparatide from a friend who came to visit her in hospital. She wonders if it would be good for her. Using the NICE guidelines, discuss whether this would be a suitable option for her. How would you answer Mrs TY's question?

Reference

NICE (National Institute for Health and Clinical Excellence) (2008). Osteoporosis – Secondary prevention including strontium ranelate. Available at http://www.nice.org.uk/guidance/TA161/guidance/pdf/English/ [Accessed 4 July 2008].

General references

Ferguson N (2000) Osteoporosis–prophylaxis and treatment. *Hospital Pharmacist* 7: 69–71.

Joint Formulary Committee (2008) *British National Formulary 55*. London: British Medical Association and Royal Pharmaceutical Society of Great Britain, March.

Tanna N (2005a) Osteoporosis and its prevention. *The Pharmaceutical Journal* 275: 521–524.

Tanna N (2005b) Osteoporosis and its treatment. *The Pharmaceutical Journal* 275: 581–584.

Answers

Case study level 1 – Rheumatoid arthritis – see page 244

1a   What is rheumatoid arthritis?

Rheumatoid arthritis (RA) is a progressive disease which mainly affects the joints of the body. It is an inflammatory condition which follows a relapsing, remitting course, which can be very variable. The hands and wrists are most commonly affected although other joints may be involved. It is usual that the disease is found in symmetrical joints, although this is not always the case.

The synovial lining of the joints becomes inflamed and proteolytic enzymes are released which cause the bone and cartilage to be destroyed. This leads to the deformation of joints.

Patients with rheumatoid arthritis may also suffer from wide range of symptoms which affect other parts of the body. These symptoms may include anaemia, dry eyes, osteoporosis and nodules, among other things.

1b   What are the risk factors for developing rheumatoid arthritis?

The cause of rheumatoid arthritis is unknown, but it is thought that a mixture of genetic and environmental factors affect whether someone develops the condition. Some of the factors that have been linked to the development of rheumatoid arthritis include:

- Previous family history – patients with a first-degree relative with rheumatoid arthritis are more likely to have it themselves.
- Gender – women are more likely to have rheumatoid arthritis than men
- Previous infection – the onset of rheumatoid arthritis can occur after an infection. The Epstein–Barr virus, parvoviruses and mycobacteria have been linked to the development of rheumatoid arthritis.

1c   What are the clinical features of rheumatoid arthritis?

The initial symptoms of rheumatoid arthritis are vague. They can include fatigue, malaise, joint pain, swelling of joints and stiffness. Patients will complain of joint pain and a loss of function in the affected joints. Radiographs may show erosion of the joint and a loss of joint space.

The American Rheumatism Association developed a set of criteria by which to diagnose rheumatoid arthritis, although the criteria tend to apply to patients with established disease (Bryant and Alldred, 2007). The criteria state that the patient should have four or more of the following criteria to be diagnosed with rheumatoid arthritis:

- morning stiffness lasting longer than 1 hour for a period of more than six weeks

- arthritis of at least three joints for more than six weeks
- arthritis of hand joints lasting longer than six weeks
- symmetrical arthritis of at least one area for longer than six weeks
- rheumatoid nodules as observed by a physician
- serum rheumatoid factor as assessed by a method positive in less than 5% of control subjects
- radiographic changes as seen on anterioposterior films of wrists and hands.

1d What investigations are performed to help confirm a diagnosis of rheumatoid arthritis?

A diagnosis of rheumatoid arthritis is made by assessing the presenting signs and symptoms. Biochemical investigations are performed and are useful in confirming the diagnosis. The tests carried out include erythrocyte sedimentation rate (ESR), C-reactive protein (CRP), plasma viscosity, liver function tests, full blood count, urea & electrolytes and urinalysis. The patient will also be tested for the presence of rheumatoid factor and antinuclear antibodies. These tests are not specific to rheumatoid arthritis but may help with diagnosis and management of the condition.

2a The major treatments for rheumatoid arthritis include NSAIDs and DMARDs. What do the abbreviations NSAID and DMARD stand for?

- NSAID = non-steroidal anti-inflammatory drug.
- DMARD = disease modifying anti-rheumatic drug.

2b Sulfasalazine is a DMARD. Describe its mode of action.

The precise mode of action is unknown. Sulfasalazine has an immuno-modulatory effect as well as an antibacterial action. It also has influences on the arachidonic cascade and alters the activity of enzymes involved in the inflammatory process.

2c Sulfasalazine is comprised of two components – 5-aminosalicylic acid (5-ASA), also known as mesalazine, and its carrier molecule, sulfapyridine. How are these two components chemically linked?

5-ASA and sulfapyridine are linked by an azo bond.

2d When sulfasalazine is taken orally, which enzymes are responsible for cleaving this bond and where does this take place?

Bacterial azoreductase enzymes in the colon cleave the azo bond between 5-ASA and sulfapyridine, releasing the 5-ASA component.

2e State the common side-effects of sulfasalazine.

Diarrhoea, nausea, vomiting, headache, rash, loss of appetite and raised temperature are the most common side-effects. Potentially fatal leucopenia, neutropenia, agranulocytosis, aplastic anaemia and thrombocytopenia may occur rarely. Hepatitis has been reported rarely.

2f   Sulfasalazine is known to be a sulfa drug as it contains sulfapyridine. What is a sulfa drug and how does this affect the side-effect profile of sulfasalazine?

Sulfa drugs are also known as sulfonamides. These drugs contain a sulfonamide group in their chemical structure. Some patients can be allergic to this group of drugs which also includes sulfamethoxazole (found in Septrin) and some diuretics, as well as other drugs. Allergic reactions to sulfa drugs can include rashes as well as more serious adverse drug reactions such as Stevens–Johnson syndrome and blood dyscrasias.

3a   List the formulations of sulfasalazine that are currently available.

The formulations available are:

- tablets 500 mg
- enteric-coated tablets (including EN-Tabs) 500 mg
- suspension 250 mg/5 mL
- suppositories 500 mg.

3b   Which of these formulations are licensed for rheumatoid arthritis?

Enteric-coated tablets (including EN-Tabs) 500 mg.

3c   What other conditions is sulfasalazine licensed for?

Sulfasalazine is also licensed for treatment of mild to moderate and severe ulcerative colitis and maintenance of remission, and active Crohn's disease.

4   When you hand Mrs PJ her dispensed prescription, what information or help would you give her to ensure that she knows how to use her medications appropriately?

First consider whether Mrs PJ may have problems using her medication due to her rheumatoid arthritis. Many patients with rheumatoid arthritis will have deformed joints, making it difficult for them to open medicine bottles or to use blister packs. Does Mrs PJ require an aid to help her open her bottles?

Sulfasalazine

The prescribed dose should be discussed with Mrs PJ and she should be advised when to take the tablets. The patient should report any unexplained bleeding or bruising, purpura, sore throat, fever or malaise that occurs during the treatment to her doctor as soon as possible. She should be advised that if she wears contact lenses, her lenses may be stained. Further information on the specific types of contact lenses affected can be obtained from the manufacturers. Mrs PJ should be told to avoid taking indigestion remedies at the same time as this drug. She should also be warned that this medication may cause her urine to be coloured orange.

Diclofenac

The patient should be told about the prescribed dose and when to take the tablets. The pharmacist should check whether Mrs PJ suffers from asthma or has a previous history of peptic ulcer or upper gastrointestinal disease. The patient should be advised to take the medication with, or after food as diclofenac may cause stomach irritation.

Case study level 2 – Rheumatoid arthritis – see page 246

1a   How is the dose of sulfasalazine normally initiated and titrated?

The patient should start with one tablet daily, increasing their dosage by a tablet a day each week until one tablet four times a day, or two tablets three times a day are reached, according to tolerance and response.

1b   Why is the dose increased gradually?

Nausea may be a problem for some patients, hence the dose is titrated up gradually to avoid this.

1c   What advice would you give Mrs PJ in answer to her question?

Mrs PJ should be informed that the onset of effect of sulfasalazine is slow and an initial benefit may not be seen for 4–16 weeks.

It would be useful to check what instructions Mrs PJ has been given regarding the titration of her medication. She is currently on a dose at the lower end of the titration scale.

You could ask Mrs PJ when her follow-up appointment with the prescribing doctor is due. If she has an appointment in the very near future, her dose may be increased at that consultation.

If Mrs PJ has not been given a titrating dose, it may be worth suggesting that she contacts her prescribing doctor to confirm the instructions given to her at the initial appointment. It is important to reiterate that the onset of action of the sulfasalazine is slow.

2a   How often should the above tests be performed?

Close monitoring of the full blood count and liver function tests is necessary initially and then at monthly intervals for at least the first three months of treatment. Renal function tests may be performed periodically as recommended by the manufacturers.

2b   Why should these tests be performed?

Side-effects of sulfasalazine include blood dyscrasias which usually occur in the first 3–6 months of treatment. The full blood count should be checked regularly so that any haematological abnormalities can be identified at an early stage.

There have been reports of hepatitis and renal dysfunction in patients taking sulfasalazine, therefore liver function tests and renal function tests should be performed at regular intervals.

3a   What do you think could be the cause of this problem?

As the symptoms initially appear to be related to her medication she may be experiencing gastric irritation as a result of her diclofenac or she may be suffering from nausea due to the sulfasalazine. Ask Mrs PJ whether she is suffering from any alarm symptoms like gastrointestinal bleeding, unintentional weight loss, difficulty swallowing, abdominal swelling or persistent vomiting. If Mrs PJ is experiencing any of these symptoms, she should be referred to her GP urgently.

3b   What suggestions could you offer Mrs PJ to help resolve this problem?

With further questioning, it may be possible to clarify the symptoms and to ascertain whether one of the drugs is likely to be causing the problem. You should check that Mrs PJ is taking her diclofenac with food so as to reduce the risk of gastric irritation. If you decide that the problem is likely to be dyspepsia, in most cases an antacid may help. In this case, however, an antacid could not be taken at the same time as either sulfasalazine or diclofenac. This is because both are enteric-coated tablets and the presence of an antacid may lead to the premature dissolution of the coating due to the presence of an alkaline pH. Therefore, the use of an antacid would not be a suitable suggestion.

As this is a suspected adverse drug reaction, it would be prudent to suggest to Mrs PJ that she returns to her GP to discuss this issue with them.

3c   What alternative medication might a doctor prescribe to help Mrs PJ with her upset stomach?

If the doctor decided that the cause of Mrs PJ's upset stomach may be NSAID-induced dyspepsia, it would be usual to stop NSAID treatment. However in the case of Mrs PJ, this might not be possible due to her concurrent medical history of rheumatoid arthritis.

The doctor may decide to stop the NSAID and see how Mrs PJ manages without the diclofenac or may consider adding in a proton pump inhibitor, in line with Clinical Knowledge Summaries (2008) guidance, to manage the incidence of NSAID-induced dyspepsia. If it is felt that the problem is related to the sulfasalazine and the nausea does not abate, the doctor may try an alternative treatment. As Mrs PJ is currently only on a low dose of sulfasalazine it would not really be possible to reduce the dose and still maintain efficacy.

4a   What are the goals of therapy when treating rheumatoid arthritis?

When treating rheumatoid arthritis, the goals of therapy are to reduce the symptoms of the disease, slow progression of the disease and limit the amount of joint deformation, while improving the patient's quality of life.

4b   Please list the alternative treatments that may be used in the management of rheumatoid arthritis and briefly discuss when an alternative treatment would be tried.

When a drug has been titrated to the maximum dose that can be tolerated and the level of disease control is still unacceptable, therapy may be switched to an alternative agent or another drug may be added in. Other treatments available for managing rheumatoid arthritis include:

- methotrexate
- gold injections
- antimalarials
- leflunomide
- penicillamine
- ciclosporin
- azathioprine
- cyclophosphamide
- cytokine modulators
- corticosteroids.

Case study level 3 – Gout – see page 248

1a   What is gout? Briefly discuss the pathophysiology of the condition.

Gout is a syndrome caused by an inflammatory response to the formation of monosodium urate crystals which develop secondary to hyperuricaemia (Johnstone, 2005).

Patients have a raised level of uric acid in the body either due to increased production of uric acid or decreased excretion of uric acid. This leads to the deposition of monosodium urate crystals in the joints which causes inflammation and pain. Patients suffer from recurrent attacks of gouty arthritis due to these deposits.

1b List three ways in which gout can manifest itself.

There are various stages of gout including:

- asymptomatic hyperuricaemia
- acute gout
- chronic gout
- chronic tophaceous gout
- gouty nephropathy.

1c List the risk factors for developing gout and discuss which risk factors Mr KT potentially may have for developing gout.˜

Possible risk factors include trauma, unusual physical exercise, surgery, severe systemic illness, severe dieting, dietary excess, alcohol, drugs, status epilepticus, psoriasis, renal failure, lead intoxication, Down's syndrome, high purine diet, cytolytic therapy, myeloproliferative and lymphoproliferative disorders. Mr KT has several risk factors which increase his chances of developing gout:

- He has recently undergone a surgical procedure.
- He is overweight, which may indicate dietary excess.
- He drinks 35 units of alcohol a week which is more than the recommended weekly amount.

1d Describe the symptoms of gout.

If a patient is suffering from acute gout they will complain of severe pain in a joint. The great toe is the joint that is most commonly affected. The joint will be red, hot, swollen and very tender. The pain may be so severe that the patient cannot even tolerate bedsheets resting on the joint affected.

1e What investigations should the doctors carry out to help them confirm whether Mr KT has gout?

A definitive diagnosis of gout is made by aspirating synovial fluid from the affected joint. The aspirated fluid is then examined under a microscope for the presence of monosodium urate crystals. Other tests may be used to help with diagnosis of gout, to exclude the presence of an infection and to give a baseline before drugs are started to treat the condition. These tests include measuring the plasma urate or uric acid to confirm the presence of hyperuricaemia. Other tests would include the measuring of urea, creatinine, full blood count, C-reactive protein, blood glucose, fasting lipids and liver function tests.

2   During your rounds, Mr KT asks you if you could tell him what he could do to avoid another attack of gout. What lifestyle advice would you give him?

Mr KT should be advised to reduce his weight and reduce his alcohol intake. He should restrict his intake of red meats and food with a high purine content (e.g. meat extracts, kidney, liver, crab, anchovies, mackerel and sardines) and he should aim to increase his fluid intake to about 2 litres per day (assuming that he is not fluid restricted).

3   Mr KT requires treatment for his attack of gout. Please discuss the options available for treating an acute attack. For each option discussed, include the following information:

- dose
- contraindications to use
- cautions for use
- potential side-effects.

Which option would you recommend for Mr KT?

The drug options for controlling an acute attack of gout include NSAIDs, etoricoxib, colchicine and steroids (Table A10.1).

NSAIDs are the first-line agents for treating an acute attack of gout, providing there are no contraindications. Indometacin and diclofenac are the agents most frequently used. Alldred and Capstick (2007) state that the most important factor determining therapeutic success is not the NSAID chosen but how soon NSAID therapy is initiated. Treatment should continue until all symptoms have resolved.

Etoricoxib is the only COX-2 inhibitor licensed for acute gout. It has a similar efficacy to indometacin. It may be useful in patients who cannot tolerate non-selective NSAIDs due to gastrointestinal irritation. It is a more expensive option than other agents and there are several contraindications and cautions that should be borne in mind before suggesting it for a patient with acute gout.

Colchicine is the second-line agent for treating gout. Its use may be limited by its side-effects and its slower onset of action. As in the case of NSAIDs, it needs to be initiated as quickly as possible. Side-effects include nausea, vomiting and diarrhoea. Colchicine is traditionally given as 1 mg initially then 500 micrograms no more frequently than every 4 hours until pain is relieved or vomiting or diarrhoea occur. The patient should be given no more than 6 mg per course to prevent toxic effects. A course should not be repeated within 3 days. However, a lower dose of 500 micrograms three or four times a day may be used to reduce the risk of toxicity from the drug.

The use of steroids is an alternative to NSAIDs or colchicine. If the gout is only affecting one or two joints then an intra-articular injection may be given (unlicensed indication). A differential diagnosis between septic arthritis and acute gout must be certain because intra-articular steroids will exacerbate an

Table A10.1 Drug options for controlling an acute attack of gout

Drug	Dose	Contraindications	Cautions	Side-effects
Indometacin	150–200 mg daily in divided doses	History of hypersensitivity to aspirin or another NSAID, severe heart failure, patients with previous or active peptic ulceration	Allergic disorders, pregnancy and lactation – manufacturers advise to avoid use, coagulation defects, renal, hepatic and cardiac impairment, the elderly, epilepsy, parkinsonism, psychiatric disturbance	Gastrointestinal discomfort, nausea and diarrhoea, gastrointestinal bleeding and ulceration, hypersensitivity reactions, fluid retention, renal impairment
Diclofenac	150 mg daily in divided doses	History of hypersensitivity to aspirin or another NSAID, severe heart failure, patients with previous or active peptic ulceration, porphyria	Allergic disorders, renal, hepatic and cardiac impairment, the elderly; avoid use in pregnancy, lactation, coagulation defects	Gastrointestinal discomfort, nausea and diarrhoea, gastrointestinal bleeding and ulceration, hypersensitivity reactions, fluid retention, renal impairment

Drug	Dose			
Etoricoxib	120 mg daily for max 8 days	History of hypersensitivity to aspirin or another NSAID, moderate or severe heart failure, patients with active peptic ulceration, ischaemic heart disease, cerebrovascular disease, peripheral arterial disease, inflammatory bowel disease, uncontrolled hypertension, pregnancy, breastfeeding	Renal, hepatic and cardiac impairment including cardiac failure, LV dysfunction. dehydration, hypertension, oedema and patients with risk factors for developing heart disease, the elderly, in coagulation defects	Gastrointestinal discomfort, nausea and diarrhoea, gastrointestinal bleeding and ulceration, hypersensitivity reactions, fluid retention, renal impairment
Colchicine	Initially 1 mg, then 500 micrograms no more frequently than every 4 hours until pain is relieved or vomiting or diarrhoea occur. Max 6 mg per course; course not to be repeated within 3 days	Pregnancy	The elderly, gastrointestinal disease, cardiac impairment, renal impairment or hepatic impairment. Manufacturers advise to avoid use in breastfeeding	Nausea, vomiting and abdominal pain. Excessive doses may cause profuse diarrhoea, gastrointestinal haemorrhage, rashes, renal and hepatic damage

See *BNF* for further information.

infection. (For information on individual intra-articular steroid injections, consult the *BNF* and product literature.)

Systemic steroids (e.g. prednisolone) can also be used. These may be of use in patients with severe or polyarticular attacks or those with renal disease or heart failure which may preclude the use of NSAIDs or colchicine.

Colchicine would be the agent of choice for Mr KT due to his concurrent medical history of hypertension. NSAIDs should be used with caution in patients with a history of cardiac impairment, which includes hypertension.

4a   When you are clinically checking Mr KT's medication chart, you notice that he is on the following medication:

- amlodipine 5 mg daily
- bendroflumethiazide 2.5 mg daily
- paracetamol 1 g four times a day.

Which of these medications can aggravate gout and why?

Bendroflumethiazide can aggravate gout. Its renal actions mean that it can cause a raised plasma level of uric acid, thus precipitating an attack of gout.

4b   What advice would you give to the doctor looking after Mr KT?

You should discuss with the doctor and the patient whether bendroflumethiazide could be stopped. Drugs that aggravate gout should usually be withdrawn, if possible. You would need to check Mr KT's blood pressure and see if an alternative antihypertensive could be given instead.

5a   Why wasn't Mr KT prescribed prophylactic treatment after his first attack?

There are varying opinions on when prophylactic treatment should be initiated after an attack of gout. It is usually recommended that if a patient experiences two or more gouty attacks per year, long-term hypouricaemic agents should be considered.

Long-term hypouricaemic agents that decrease serum uric levels should not be used during an acute attack. This is because these drugs cause the mobilisation of uric acid stores in response to a decreasing serum level. This can then prolong the attack or precipitate another attack of gouty arthritis.

5b   What options are available and which one is usually the drug of choice?

The options available are allopurinol, probenecid (named patient only) and sulfinpyrazone. Allopurinol is the drug usually chosen as a first line agent for the prevention of gout. Colchicine may be given at a dose of 500 micrograms twice or three times daily when allopurinol or uricosuric drugs are initially commenced in order to prevent an attack of gout. NSAIDs may also be used but this would not be an appropriate option for Mr KT.

Case study level Ma – Osteoarthritis – see page 250

1   What does OGD stand for? Why do you think it might be being performed?

OGD stands for oesophago-gastro-duodenoscopy. It involves passing an endo-scope with a camera and a light down the oesophagus to look at the oeso-phagus, stomach and duodenum. It is being performed to decide whether Mrs KR is suffering from gastritis, a gastric ulcer or from another condition affecting the upper gastrointestinal tract which may be causing her current symptoms.

2   Mrs KR has had her blood pressure and haemoglobin level checked, why might the medical staff do this?

If she is anaemic or has low blood pressure, it may indicate that she has had a gastroinstestinal bleed.

3   Mrs KR is subsequently diagnosed with gastritis. Which of her medicines may have caused this?

Diclofenac is the most likely culprit. One of the side-effects of diclofenac is gas-tric irritation.

4   What advice would you give regarding the management of this problem?

The diclofenac should be stopped initially. Mrs KR may be prescribed a proton pump inhibitor to help manage the symptoms. In cases such as this, it may be that in the future the NSAID needs to be restarted to help manage Mrs KR's osteoarthritis. Mrs KR should take a proton pump inhibitor concurrently to pre-vent a return of the gastritis.

5   Mrs KR is taking lercanidipine to manage her hypertension. Lercanidipine is an asymmetric 1,4-dihydropyridine. Draw the chemical structure and state which enantiomer causes the antihypertensive activity associated with lercanidipine. Indicate the chiral centre(s) within your structure.

The chemical structure of lercanidipine is shown in Figure A10.1. The chiral centre is in the carbon, position 4. The antihypertensive activity of lercanidi-pine is mainly due to its (S)-enantiomer.

6   Mrs KR is taking analgesics to manage the symptoms of her osteoarthritis. What is osteoarthritis?

Osteoarthritis is a chronic disease which is characterised by pain and stiffness in the joints. It is not simply a disease caused by wear and tear, many factors can be involved. There is a loss of cartilage and a loss of joint space. There may be bony overgrowths at joint margins. The joints most commonly affected are those of the hands, the knees, hips and spine.

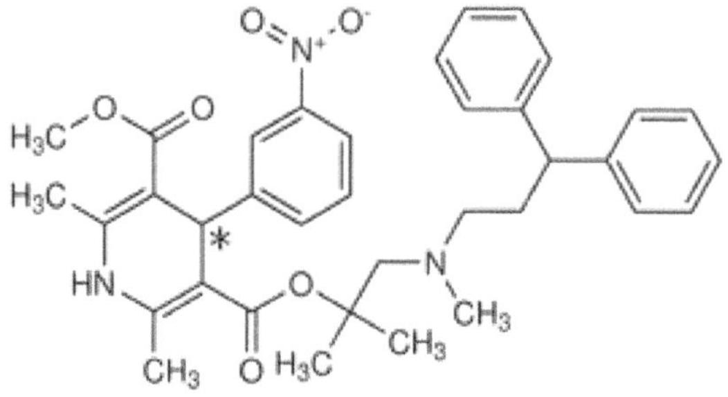

Figure A10.1 Chemical structure of lercanidipine.

7   What are the signs and symptoms of osteoarthritis?

Patients will complain of joint pain. The joint pain is often worsened by movement. The patient will also suffer from stiffness of the joint with a limitation of its movement and sometimes, swelling. Osteoarthritic changes may be visible on an X ray.

8   What risk factors may predispose patients to getting osteoarthritis and which risk factors does Mrs KR have?

Risk factors include age, obesity, gender (under 45 years osteoarthritis is more common in males, over 55 years it is more common in females), systemic disorders, environmental factors, such as jobs which involve abnormal joint loading, and a genetic predisposition. The patient's ethnic group may also be a factor as more hip osteoarthritis is seen in white Europeans than black or Asian populations.

Mrs KR is female, obese and is 70 years of age thus increasing her risk of osteoarthritis.

9   What non-drug recommendations could you give her regarding the management of osteoarthritis?

Mrs KR should be advised to try and lose weight. She may wish to discuss the possibility of physiotherapy treatment with her GP. Patients should be encouraged to exercise gently and that exercise should include local muscle stretching and general aerobic exercise. The use of heat and cold therapy may help, as may ultrasound. Some patients may find a TENS (transcutaneous electrical nerve stimulation) machine is helpful.

10   Mrs KR is using diclofenac, an NSAID to manage the symptoms of her osteoarthritis. How do NSAIDs work in the treatment of osteoarthritis?

NSAIDs help to reduce the pain and inflammation caused by osteoarthritis.

NSAIDs inhibit arachidonate cyclo-oxygenase and therefore reduce the production of prostaglandins and thromboxanes.

The decreased levels of prostaglandins means there is less sensitisation of the nociceptor endings and therefore, less pain is felt.

The reduction in prostaglandin production means that there is less vasodilation and less oedema and thus, less inflammation.

11   What are the contraindications and cautions for the use of diclofenac?

Diclofenac is contraindicated in those with a history of hypersensitivity to aspirin or another NSAID, severe heart failure, patients with previous or active peptic ulceration, or porphyria. It should be avoided in pregnancy. It should be used with caution in patients with allergic disorders, renal, hepatic and cardiac impairment, the elderly, in lactation and in those with coagulation defects.

12   Critically appraise the alternative treatments available for osteoarthritis?

Paracetamol is considered to be first-line treatment for osteoarthritis. It should be taken regularly. Paracetamol is the initial drug of choice because there is only a small inflammatory component to osteoarthritis and paracetamol is usually effective in the early stages of the disease. Compound analgesics like cocodamol may be used although their benefit over paracetamol alone is small and the opioid component may lead to unwanted side-effects.

According to NICE guidance, topical NSAIDs should be considered ahead of oral NSAIDs, COX-2 inhibitors or opioids for patients with osteoarthritis (NICE, 2008). They have not been shown to be any more effective than oral NSAIDs but they appear to have fewer side-effects (Bryant and Alldred, 2007).

Topical capsaicin may be of use in hand or knee osteoarthritis.

If a patient has ineffective or insufficient pain relief from paracetamol and a topical NSAID, then an oral NSAID or COX-2 inhibitor or weak opioid may be substituted or added in. There may be an element of inflammation as part of the disease and in some patients an NSAID may help. NICE recommend that a proton pump inhibitor is co-prescribed if an NSAID is taken regularly in order to reduce the risk of gastrointestinal events (NICE, 2008).

Intra-articular corticosteroids may be useful in some patients, particularly if there is an acute flare of the disease. The joint is injected with a steroid and this can reduce inflammation and joint effusion. The joint should not be injected more than once every three months·

Glucosamine and chondroitin are chondroprotective agents which are used in the treatment of osteoarthritis. There is conflicting evidence regarding their efficacy and their place in the management of osteoarthritis is unclear. They are not recommended by NICE for osteoarthritis (NICE, 2008).

13 Knee replacement would involve major surgery. What are the risk factors for Mrs KR?

Possible risk factors for Mrs KR would include:

- *Age* – Mrs KR is 70 years old and the associated risks are much higher in the elderly.
- *Infection* – a risk associated with any invasive surgery and treatment may range from antibiotic therapy to occasionally a total removal of the knee joint.
- *Fracture* – this may occur to the bone close to the artificial joint, either during surgery or after surgery.
- *Excess bone/scar tissue formation* – this may occur around the artificial knee joint, resulting in restricted joint movement. Removal of the excess bone/scar tissue may necessitate further surgery to restore movement.
- *Kneecap dislocation* – further surgery would be required.
- *Numbness* – surrounding the wound scar.
- *Bleeding* – may occur unexpectedly around the joint.
- *Damage* – to ligament/artery/nerve may occur.
- *Thrombosis* (blood clot) – may occur up to six weeks after surgery. Rarely, a blood clot can pass to the lungs causing a pulmonary embolism and a medical emergency. Treatment may necessitate anticoagulants.

14 Recovery from a knee replacement can take some time and several healthcare professionals are likely to be involved. Discuss the role for each professional involved in Mrs KR's care plan following hospital discharge.

- *Consultant* – would contact the GP for Mrs KR and inform him or her of any changes in medication, along with other care issues. The consultant would also arrange to see Mrs KR for a follow-up visit approximately six weeks following discharge. Further follow-up visits are then arranged usually every 2 years.
- *GP* – would review the care plan for Mrs KR and prescribe any new medications.
- *Social worker* – Mrs KR lives alone and may require home support following her discharge. A social worker would help with her emotional or physical needs, in addition to find her appropriate support services.
- *Nurse* – would provide regular wound dressing until recovery.
- *Physiotherapist* – would oversee and monitor progress for Mrs KR, explaining any knee exercises to aid recovery. A CPM (continuous passive motion) machine may be used to provide support to the knee in addition to decreasing swelling and improving circulation. Initially, Mrs KR is likely to require a walking frame (for approximately one week) and then would be encouraged to just use a walking stick (until the hospital follow-up visit in six weeks).
- *Pharmacist* – would be involved in the medicines management for Mrs KR and would review existing and new medications since her hospital discharge.

Case study level Mb – Osteoporosis – see page 252

1a   What recommendations could you make to help manage her pain?

Mrs TY could have codeine phosphate prescribed four times a day on a regular basis. Elderly patients are prone to experiencing side-effects, including constipation and drowsiness, from large doses of codeine. For this reason, it would be advisable for the dose to remain at 30 mg four times a day for now, rather than increasing to 60 mg four times a day straight away. Once this has been tried, the dose could be further increased if necessary, as the maximum dose is 240 mg per day. Codeine phosphate can be taken every 4 hours if required.

Mrs TY could also be prescribed an NSAID, for example, ibuprofen or diclofenac. As Mrs TY is elderly, this should be used with caution, however, and preferably on a short-term basis. Mrs TY's renal function should be checked before recommending an NSAID. Her renal function should be monitored periodically while in hospital and she should be advised to report symptoms of gastric irritation.

It may be necessary to ask the doctor to prescribe a small dose of morphine on an as-required basis, to be administered if the pain does not abate.

1b   What are the contraindications and cautions for the analgesics you are recommending?

Codeine and morphine are contraindicated in acute respiratory depression, acute alcoholism and where there is a risk of paralytic ileus. They should also be avoided in patients with raised intracranial pressure or head injury and in comatose patients.

Codeine and morphine should be used with caution in hypotension, hypothyroidism, asthma (avoid during an attack) and decreased respiratory reserve, shock, prostatic hypertrophy, obstructive or inflammatory bowel disorders, diseases of the biliary tract, pregnancy and breastfeeding. They may precipitate coma in patients with hepatic impairment and as such, they should be avoided or a reduced dose used. In patients with renal impairment, the dose should be reduced or they should be avoided. If used in the elderly and debilitated, the dose should be reduced.

Codeine and morphine should also be used with caution in convulsive disorders and if a patient is dependent on opioids, they should not be withdrawn abruptly. (See *BNF* for further cautions and contraindications.)

NSAIDs are contraindicated in those with a history of hypersensitivity to aspirin or another NSAID, severe heart failure, patients with previous or active peptic ulceration.

NSAIDs should be used with caution in patients with allergic disorders, renal, hepatic or cardiac impairment, coagulation defects, pregnancy and lactation and also in the elderly. (See *BNF* for further cautions and contraindications.)

1c   Are there any adjunctive treatments you would recommend to the doctor that should be prescribed?

A laxative should be prescribed as Mrs TY is prescribed codeine which can cause constipation. As Mrs TY is immobile and has a fracture of the lower limb, she should have some form of thromboprophylaxis.

1d   What parameters would you monitor as you consider this woman's pharmaceutical care?

- *Pain score* – to ensure adequate pain relief.
- *Bowel movements* – to avoid constipation as a result of immobility and opioids.
- *Full blood count* – to monitor for signs of infection and for signs of thrombocytopenia if a low molecular weight heparin is chosen as a thromboprophylactic agent.
- *Respiratory rate* – to monitor for respiratory depression as a result of codeine or morphine use.
- *Blood pressure* – to ensure that Mrs TY is not hypotensive or hypertensive.
- *Urea and electrolytes* – to monitor renal function if an NSAID is to be initiated.

Also, watch for signs of confusion or drowsiness as a result of the codeine prescription.

2a   Later in the week Mrs TY has surgery to repair her hip fracture. She is also diagnosed with osteoporosis. What is osteoporosis?

Osteoporosis is a disease which affects the bones. Patients have a low bone mineral density and the bone structure has deteriorated. This leads to weakened bones which are more susceptible to breaking. Fractures of the wrist, hip and spine occur most frequently but other bones may be affected.

2b   What is the difference between primary and secondary osteoporosis?

The most common form of osteoporosis is primary osteoporosis. Primary osteoporosis is seen in postmenopausal women and is also caused by advancing age. In some cases it may be idiopathic with no identifiable cause.

In secondary osteoporosis, a specific cause can be identified for the bone loss. It may be a chronic disease like hyperthyroidism, hyperparathyroidism, diabetes mellitus, amenorrhoea or anorexia nervosa, among others, which leads to the condition or in some cases of secondary osteoporosis, a drug may be implicated.

2c   Which drugs may be implicated in the development of osteoporosis?

Corticosteroids, heparin treatment, particularly if used during pregnancy, and anticonvulsants have all been implicated in the development of osteoporosis.

2d   What are the signs and symptoms of osteoporosis?

One of the first signs of osteoporosis is when a patient experiences a non-traumatic fracture. Fractures of the wrist, hip and spine are the most typical of osteoporotic fragility but fractures of other bones are not uncommon.

A person may have difficulty standing or sitting up straight due to weakening of the bones. The fractures that patients sustain can result in severe pain and disability.

Patients can undergo a dual-energy X-ray absorptiometry (DEXA) scan to confirm the diagnosis of osteoporosis. Osteoporosis is defined as having a bone mineral density which is at least 2.5 standard deviations below the peak bone mass when measured by a DEXA scan (e.g. a T-score −2.5 SD or below).

2e   What are the risk factors for osteoporosis and which does Mrs TY have?

Risk factors for osteoporosis include:

- age
- being female
- being caucasian
- having a low BMI (<19 kg/m^2)
- untreated early menopause
- family history of maternal hip fracture before 75 years
- limited exercise
- prolonged immobility
- smoking
- high alcohol intake
- poor nutrition
- long-term use of systemic corticosteroids
- rheumatoid arthritis.

First, Mrs TY is elderly and female which increases her risk of osteoporosis. She is postmenopausal. She drinks a small amount of alcohol but this is within the recommended weekly limits and is unlikely to cause a problem. She lives alone and therefore it is possible that her nutritional intake could be improved but this would need to be investigated further.

2f   What lifestyle advice could you offer to Mrs TY?

Mrs TY should try to maintain a healthy balanced diet with adequate calcium and vitamin D intake, avoid excessive alcohol, reduce her caffeine intake, increase her vegetable consumption and try to take up some weight-bearing exercise. She should also take steps to avoid trips or falls, such as having her eyesight tested regularly and assessing her home environment for risks.

3   Discuss the options for the treatment of osteoporosis and decide which you think would be the most suitable for Mrs TY.

When choosing a treatment for osteoporosis, there are various factors that should be taken into consideration. These include age of the patient, the severity of the disease, any other co-morbidities and, in the case of women, the presence of menopausal symptoms.

Options for treatment include hormone replacement therapy (HRT), bisphosphonates, calcitriol, calcitonin, raloxifene, strontium ranelate, and teriparatide. Hormone replacement therapy is generally indicated for women who are under 50 years and are experiencing a premature menopause. Symptomatic menopausal women may opt to use HRT also, as the benefits outweigh the risks for up to 5 years treatment. They may choose an alternative treatment for osteoporosis if preferred. Hormone replacement therapy is not recommended for first line treatment for long-term prevention of osteoporosis in women over 50 years of age.

Bisphosphonates are licensed for use in postmenopausal osteoporosis and glucocorticoid induced osteoporosis. They are often used in older women with osteoporosis and they are recommended by NICE as the first-line agent for the secondary prevention of osteoporotic fractures in postmenopausal women. Alendronate and etidronate are licensed for men with osteoporosis.

Raloxifene is a selective oestrogen receptor modulator (SERM). Its role in osteoporosis is to slow down bone loss. It has been shown to increase bone density by 0.5–1%. It is licensed for the prevention and treatment of postmenopausal osteoporosis. Its side-effects include a small increase in the frequency of hot flushes, leg cramps, peripheral oedema and thrombosis risk (Tanna 2005).

Calcitriol may be an option, if bisphosphonates are unsuitable. It decreases bone loss and decreases the frequency of vertebral fractures. It is usually only recommended by specialists.

Calcitonin is also another option that may be used if a patient cannot take bisphosphonates. It is administered intranasally or via subcutaneous or intramuscular injection. It is usually only prescribed in specialist clinics.

Strontium ranelate is a relatively new product which has a dual action. It works by reducing bone resorption and by increasing bone formation. It is available in a sachet and is mixed in water.

Teriparatide is a recombinant human parathyroid hormone which promotes bone growth. It is available in the form of an injection and only prescribed by osteoporosis specialists. NICE have issued guidance on who is eligible to receive it.

Mrs TY is an elderly woman with a fractured hip. NICE (2005) recommends that postmenopausal patients who have experienced a fracture should receive bisphosphonates as treatment for secondary prevention of fractures.

In patients who cannot tolerate bisphosphonates and who have a combination of other risk factors, raloxifene or strontium ranelate may be an alternative. See NICE guidance for further information.

As Mrs TY has no contraindications to treatment and has not experienced a previous treatment failure, she should be started on a bisphosphonate. Calcium and vitamin D supplementation should also be initiated to ensure an adequate dietary intake.

4a Before Mrs TY is discharged she is prescribed alendronate 70 mg once weekly and a calcium and vitamin D preparation, 1 tablet twice a day. What are the indications for alendronate?

Alendronate is licensed for the treatment of postmenopausal osteoporosis and osteoporosis in men, prevention of postmenopausal osteoporosis and the prevention and treatment of corticosteroid-induced osteoporosis.

4b How does alendronate work?

Alendronate reduces bone resorption by decreasing osteoclast activity, thereby strengthening the bones.

4c What are the side-effects of alendronate?

The main side-effects of alendronate include oesophageal reactions, abdominal pain and distension, dyspepsia, regurgitation, melaena, diarrhoea or constipation and flatulence.

4d List the main drug or food interactions associated with alendronate.

Alendronate absorption is reduced by antacids, calcium salts and iron. Concurrent use with aminoglycosides may lead to hypocalcaemia. Patients should be told to take alendronate 30 minutes before food and other medication.

4e What advice would you give to Mrs TY regarding the taking of her alendronate and the calcium and vitamin D preparation?

Mrs TY should be advised to take her calcium supplement at a different time of day to her alendronate. Calcium salts can reduce the absorption of alendronate. She should take her alendronate 30 minutes before any medication. She may wish to take her alendronate before breakfast, followed by her first dose of calcium at lunchtime and her second dose of calcium at dinnertime. She should take her alendronate 30 minutes before any medication. She may wish to take her alendronate on rising followed by her first dose of calcium at least half an hour later or she may wish to take her alendronate before breakfast, followed by her first dose of calcium at lunchtime and her second dose of calcium at dinnertime. The options should be discussed with Mrs TY so that she can decide which regimen she would find the easiest to remember.

4f   What other advice would you give Mrs TY regarding the administration of her alendronate?

Mrs TY should be advised to take her alendronate 30 minutes before food and other medication. She should take her tablet with a full glass of water (approximately 200 mL) and she should remain upright for 30 minutes after taking it.

4g   Alendronate 70 mg once weekly is available as Fosamax Once Weekly 70 mg white tablets. What excipients are contained in this formulation and discuss the pharmaceutical role of each excipient.

- Microcrystalline cellulose – mainly used as a binder or diluent in solid oral dose formulations. It also has lubricant and disintegrant properties which make it a useful excipient in tablet manufacture.
- Lactose anhydrous – used as a binding agent.
- Croscarmellose sodium – used as a tablet disintegrant.
- Magnesium stearate – used as a lubricant in tablet formulations.

5   Mrs TY tells you that she has heard of a new treatment called teriparatide from a friend who came to visit her in hospital. She wonders if it would be good for her. Using the NICE guidelines, discuss whether this would be a suitable option for her. How would you answer Mrs TY's question?

First, Mrs TY should be advised that teriparatide is only available as an injection and, therefore, Mrs TY may not find this an acceptable route of administration. Second, the NICE guidelines state that teriparatide should only be used in postmenopausal women who are unable to take bisphosphonates or strontium or who have had an unsatisfactory response bisphosphonates. They must also have experienced more than two fractures and have a T-score which fits into the range specified in the NICE guidance (NICE 2008).

As Mrs TY has only just been recently started on alendronate, she would not be eligible for teriparatide because, as yet, she has not had a treatment failure or experienced any side-effects from alendronate. She also has only one fracture so far.

11

Eyes and ENT case studies

Sandeep Singh Nijjer, Rona Robinson and Nader Siabi

Case study level 1 – Ears

Learning outcomes

Level 1 case study: You will be able to:

- describe the risk factors
- describe the disease
- describe the pharmacology of the drug
- outline the formulation, including drug molecule, excipients, etc. for the medicines
- summarise basic social pharmacy issues (e.g. opening containers, large labels).

Scenario

Mr RI, a middle-aged man, comes into the pharmacy and asks for your advice. Over the last couple of weeks, he feels that his hearing, particularly in his left ear has become 'progressively deaf', and the ears feel 'full up'. He has no other symptoms, has not tried anything already and nor does he take any medication. Upon further discussion, Mr RI mentions that he had his ears 'syringed' a couple of years ago by the nurse at the GP's surgery, and thinks he may need to go again, but wonders whether he should use the ear drops advertised on TV last week as it would save him the trip.

Questions

1a   What is the cause of the symptoms?
1b   What are the risk factors for developing this condition?
2   What is the general management of this condition in a community pharmacy setting?
3   How do the products generally used to treat the condition work?
4   How can a product's formulation affect the outcome of treatment for the condition?
5   What advice can you give to help the patient manage this condition?

General references

Allen S (2006) Outer and middle ear problems. *The Pharmaceutical Journal* 276: 83–86.

Blenkinsopp A, Paxton P and Blenkinsopp J (2005) Common ear problems. In: *Symptoms in the Pharmacy. A Guide to the Management of Common Illness*, 5th edn. Oxford: Blackwell Publishing.

Clinical Knowledge Summaries (2007) Earwax guidance. Available at http://cks.library. nhs.uk/earwax [Accessed 4 July 2008].

Joint Formulary Committee (2008) *British National Formulary 55*. London: British Medical Association and Royal Pharmaceutical Society of Great Britain, March.

Nathan A (2006) Ear problems. In: *Non-prescription Medicines*, 3rd edn. London: Pharmaceutical Press.

Case study level 2 – Conjunctivitis

Learning outcomes

Level 2 case study: You will be able to:

- interpret relevant lab and clinical data
- identify monitoring and referral criteria
- explain treatment choices
- describe goals of therapy, including monitoring and the role of the pharmacist/clinician
- describe issues – counselling points, adverse drug reactions, drug interactions, complementary/alternative therapies and lifestyle advice.

Mr JM, a 45-year-old man, comes into the pharmacy on a Friday evening in June, wishing to speak to you. A couple of days ago, he woke to find that his left eye felt 'gritty' and was 'all stuck together with whitish pus'. When he cleaned the pus away, he saw that his eye was 'reddish' in colour, and noticed a few 'lumpy' patches on the lower part of the white of the eye, which worried him, so he has tried not to touch the other eye.

Upon further discussion, he reveals that his vision is fine and that some-times he gets 'hayfever' in the eyes. He also takes metformin and gliclazide tablets. He states that his wife had 'watery red eyes' last week and is using the 'antibiotic eye drops' recently advertised on the television, and asks if he should use the drops as well.

1   What is the cause of the symptoms?
2   What symptoms would necessitate a referral to a medical practitioner?
3   What is the general management of this condition in a community pharmacy setting?
4   What is the goal of therapy and the role of the pharmacist in the management of this condition? How do the products generally used to treat the condition work? How can a product's formulation affect the outcome of treatment for the condition?
5   What advice can you give to help the patient manage this condition?

General references

Blenkinsopp A., Paxton P. and Blenkinsopp J (2005) Eye problems: the painful red eye. In: *Symptoms in the Pharmacy. A Guide to the Management of Common Illness*, 5th edn. Oxford: Blackwell Publishing.

Clinical Knowledge Summaries (2007a) Conjunctivitis – allergic. Available at http://cks.library.nhs.uk/conjunctivitis_allergic [Accessed 4 July 2008].

Clinical Knowledge Summaries (2007b) Conjunctivitis – infective. Available at http://cks.library.nhs.uk/conjunctivitis_infective [Accessed 4 July 2008].

Elton M (2005) Conjunctivitis and chloramphenicol. *The Pharmaceutical Journal* 274: 725–728.

Epling J and Smucny J (2006) Bacterial conjunctivitis. In: *Clinical Evidence*, Vol. 15. London: BMJ Publishing Group.

Nathan A (2006). Minor eye conditions. In: *Non-prescription Medicines*, 3rd edn. London: Pharmaceutical Press.

Case study level 3 – Hayfever

Learning outcomes

Level 3 case study: You will be able to:

- interpret clinical signs and symptoms
- evaluate laboratory data
- evaluate treatment options
- state goals of therapy
- describe a pharmaceutical care plan to include advice to a clinician
- describe the prognosis and long-term complications
- describe the social pharmacy issues which could include supply (e.g. complex treatments at home, concordance and compliance) and lifestyle issues.

Scenario

It is March and Mr JA, a 20-year-old university student, comes into a community pharmacy to buy something for a runny nose. On questioning he has had symptoms for the last eight weeks which he thought was a head cold and has been self-medicating with Vicks Sinex nasal spray and Sudafed tablets. His runny nose, frequent sneezing and runny eyes are continuing to be troublesome and he is worried about his forthcoming exams.

Mr JA's previous medical history includes porphyria and childhood asthma. His past drug history comprises salbutamol inhaler and beclometasone inhaler for childhood asthma.

Questions

1   What is allergic rhinitis and how does it differ from cold symptoms?
2   What are the trigger factors for hay fever?
3   What are the treatment options for hay fever?
4   What is the management plan for Mr JA's current symptoms?

Four weeks later Mr JA returns to the pharmacy complaining that his eyes are still running and are now itchy and he now cannot wear his contact lenses and although the sneezing has improved he is still suffering from itchy throat and occasional cough.

5   What further treatment options are now available?

6   What are the side-effects of nasal corticosteroids and are there any long-term complications?

7   Mr JA asks about complementary medicines as he does not want to take medications long term. What would you advise?

8   What is the long-term management plan for Mr JA?

General reference

Barnes J, Anderson LA, Phillipson JD (2002) Eyebright. In: *Herbal Medicines*, 2nd edn. London: Pharmaceutical Press.

Joint Formulary Committee (2008) *British National Formulary 55*. London: British Medical Association and Royal Pharmaceutical Society of Great Britain, March.

Schapawal A (2002) Randomised controlled trial of Butterbur and cetirizine for treating seasonal allergic rhinitis. *British Medical Journal* 324: 144.

Case study level Ma – Sinusitis

Learning outcomes

Level M case study: You will be able to:

- interpret clinical signs and symptoms
- evaluate laboratory data
- critically appraise treatment options
- state goals of therapy
- describe a pharmaceutical care plan to include advice to a clinician
- describe the prognosis and long-term complications
- describe the social pharmacy issues which could include supply (e.g. complex treatments at home, concordance and compliance) and lifestyle issues
- describe the monitoring of therapy.

Scenario

Mr JC, age 21, who has recently changed his job to become a painter and decorator, comes into your pharmacy and complains of severe nasal congestion, headache and blurred vision for 3 days. His has recently suffered cold symptoms. He took two paracetamol tablets which helped briefly. A friend has advised that he takes an antihistamine to treat these symptoms. And he asks for your advice and recommendations.

Mr JC tells you he had childhood asthma and is allergic to penicillin.

Questions

1   What other questions do you need to ask this patient to help with a working diagnosis?

2   Mr JC has had a greenish yellow discharge for the last 3 days together with facial pain around the eyes and nose. He complains of a loss of sense of smell and taste since having the cold symptoms last week. He has not developed a temperature. What is the possible diagnosis?

3   Due to the presence of a number of the above symptoms you believe Mr JC has acute sinusitis. What are the predisposing factors for sinusitis?

4   What are the treatment options?

5   Should the patient be given beclometasone nasal spray?

6   A week later Mr JC returns to the pharmacy with a slight improvement of his symptoms until yesterday when he developed fever and dizziness and slight hearing loss and ear pain. What would you now recommend?

7   The new junior GP calls you and asks your advice on which antibiotic to prescribe.

8   Mr JC returns to the pharmacy with a prescription for doxycycline 100 mg 2 stat then 1 daily for 7 days. How would you counsel this patient?

General references

Joint Formulary Committee (2008) *British National Formulary* 55. London: British Medical Association and Royal Pharmaceutical Society of Great Britain, March.

Clinical Knowledge Summaries (2006) Management of sinusitis. Available at http://cks. library.nhs.uk/sinusitis/management [Accessed 4 July 2008].

Case study level Mb – Glaucoma

Learning outcomes

Level M case study: You will be able to:

- interpret clinical signs and symptoms
- evaluate laboratory data
- critically appraise treatment options
- state goals of therapy
- describe a pharmaceutical care plan to include advice to a clinician
- describe the prognosis and long-term complications
- describe the social pharmacy issues which could include supply (e.g. complex treatments at home, concordance and compliance) and lifestyle issues
- describe the monitoring of therapy.

Mr George Smith, 61 years old, presents you with his repeat prescription. He is concerned that one of his medications is affecting his vision and asks you to identify the one that is likely to be causing this.

His present medical history includes chronic obstructive pulmonary disease (COPD) and urinary incontinence. The pharmacy Patient Medication Record (PMR) includes latanoprost drops for glaucoma which was dispensed six months ago.

Mr Smith's current and past drug histories are as follows:

Current drug history::

- Seretide 500 Accuhaler, one puff twice daily
- salbutamol inhaler two puffs p.r.n.
- salbutamol nebuliser solution 5 mg, one 3–4 times daily
- ipratropium bromide nebulising solution 500 micrograms/2 mL, one four times daily
- tolterodine 2 mg twice daily
- tetracycline 250 mg two twice daily
- hypromellose 0.3% drops p.r.n.

Past drug history:

- latanoprost 50 micrograms/mL one drop at night
- tolterodine, first prescribed about six months ago for urinary incontinence by an urologist consultant.

Patient's COPD seems to be controlled on combination of inhalers and nebuliser solution. He would use salbutamol and ipratropium solution 2–3 times a day, but when his COPD got worse, he would increase to 4–6 times daily.

Urinary incontinence appears to be under control at present but he has been experiencing extreme dry mouth and eyes.

In recent weeks, he has noticed significant deterioration in his vision with slight redness in both eyes. He puts this down to 'just getting old'. However he is due to see his eye consultant in six months' time. The last appointment was about six months ago. The consultant decided to stop latanoprost eye drops and told him everything is normal.

1   What is glaucoma, define different types and why is it important to be treated when diagnosed?
2   What are the risk factors for developing glaucoma? Identify the possible causes of worsening of his glaucoma condition.

3   Why are some drugs contraindicated in certain diseases even if they are given as eye drops?

4   How does latanoprost work in the treatment of glaucoma? Discuss the range of drugs and route of administration that can be used to treat this patient's glaucoma.

5   What other treatment options are available for treating this patient's incontinence?

General references

Electronic Medicines Compendium (2006) Ventolin nebules. Available at www.emc.medicines.org.uk [Accessed November 2006].

German WJ and Stanfield CL (2005) *The Principles of Human Physiology*, 2nd edn. San Francisco, CA: Pearson Education, Inc., Benjamin Cummings Publications

Joint Formulary Committee (2008) *British National Formulary 55*. London: British Medical Association and Royal Pharmaceutical Society of Great Britain, March.

Rang HP, Dale MM, Ritter JM and Moore PK (2003) *Pharmacology*, 5th edn. Edinburgh: Churchill Livingstone.

SIGN (Scottish Intercollegiate Guidelines Network) (2004) National Clinical Guideline No: 79, Management of urinary incontinence in primary care, December. Available at http://www.sign.ac.uk/pdf/sign79.pdf [Accessed 4 July 2008].

Walker R and Edwards C (1999) *Clinical Pharmacy and Therapeutics*, 2nd edn. Edinburgh: Churchill Livingstone.

Answers

Case study level 1 – Ears – see page 275

1a   What is the cause of the symptoms?

Earwax is a normal secretion. The main component, cerumen, is a protective wax-like substance with antifungal and antibacterial properties that traps particles and so helps keep the ears clean. Earwax is formed when cerumen secreted by the sebaceous and apocrine glands in the external auditory canal combines with sebum, exfoliated skin cells, sweat, hair and retained dust.

Normally earwax is spontaneously moved out of the ear by jaw movements and removed by washing. The production of excessively cohesive cerumen, or the failure of external auditory canal skin cells to separate and migrate externally, can lead to earwax accumulation, which dries and hardens, forming a solid plug, obstructing the ear canal and resulting in reversible deafness (conductive hearing impairment), discomfort or other problems, such as preventing eardrum inspection.

1b   What are the risk factors for developing this condition?

A risk factor would affect the normal earwax removal process. Examples include wearing a hearing aid or using cotton buds to clean ears which can cause impaction. In older patients, lower levels of sebum secretion can make the wax drier and harder.

2   What is the general management of this condition in a community pharmacy setting?

Generally, within a community pharmacy setting, wax softeners are the mainstay of treatment. NHS Clinical Knowledge Summary (CKS) guidance recommends only to remove symptomatic earwax (discomfort, hearing impairment). Treatment depends upon a patient's preference as no consistent evidence has been found to suggest one wax softener type is more effective than another. Although, aqueous-based preparations are considered first-line options, with CKS guidance recommending plain tap water or sodium bicarbonate BP ear drops as effective wax disintegrators.

3   How do the products generally used to treat the condition work?

Wax softener ear drops (cerumenolytics) are aqueous- or oil-based products which either directly soften, loosen and partially dissolve excess earwax, or indirectly through mechanisms such as aiding water penetration into the wax, or mechanically dispersing the wax. Generally, cerumenolytic preparations take several days to produce a noticeable effect, and are unlikely to completely dissolve and remove severely compacted wax plugs as a monotherapy. However, if ear syringing is required, drop use would facilitate this process.

4   How can a product's formulation affect the outcome of treatment for the condition?

Excipients within cerumenolytic preparations or the solvent base itself may affect the potential effectiveness of a product or the risk of suffering adverse effects with use. An example of the latter is with preparations of an oily base, potentially causing external ear canal irritation and inflammation. An example of the former could be of the use of glycerol as an excipient, which also softens wax (in combination with other cerumenolytics).

Adverse effects associated with cerumenolytic preparations suggested in the literature include:

- irritation
- pain
- itching
- 'buzzing' sensation within the ear.

It has also been advised that people with nut allergy should not use almond oil-based preparations.

5   What advice can you give to help the patient manage this condition?

Pharmacists can advise patients on how best to administer ear drops, therefore reducing the risk of treatment failure through incorrect product usage, and general advice regarding the condition itself.

Adminstration of ear drops

The following has been recommended for effective ear drop use:

- If possible another person should administer the drops.
- Patients should lie their head on a flat surface, with the affected ear up facing.
- The drops should be warmed ideally to body temperature, by holding the container in the hands for a few minutes.
- The ear pinna for adults should be lifted upwards and backwards, or for children downwards and backwards to straighten the ear canal.
- After instilling the required number of drops, the tragus (small projection in front of the external ear canal) should be pressed once gently to help the drops down the ear canal and expel air bubbles.
- The patient should remain with head down and ear uppermost for at least 5 minutes to allow for absorption.

General advice

- Cotton wool buds should not be poked into the ear, as wax is pushed further in and eardrum perforation is possible.
- Ear syringing is made more effective with prior use of drops to soften wax.
- Drop administration may sometimes initially worsen any sensation of deafness, however this should resolve within a few minutes.
- If no symptom improvement is noted after 7 days of recommended treatment use, then the patient should consult their GP.

Case study level 2 – Conjunctivitis – see page 276

1   What is the cause of the symptoms?

The patient has infective conjunctivitis, which usually starts in one eye and can 'spread' to both eyes. Conjunctivitis is inflammation of the conjunctiva, a protective membrane covering the white of the eye and inside surface of eyelids, due to allergy, infection or physical irritation. For infective causes, both bacteria and viruses can be responsible, with staphylococcal species common bacterial causes and adenoviruses for viral cases, with the latter more common in adults.

Symptoms of infective conjunctivitis include conjunctiva hyperaemia, making the sclera of the eye appear red, usually bilaterally for infective and allergy-related cases and an uncomfortable superficial 'gritty' eye sensation. Bacterial infections tend to have the presence of a yellow-white muco-purulent discharge and a papillary reaction (small bumps on the conjunctiva appearing as a fine velvety surface), compared with a more watery discharge for viral or allergy-related causes.

2   What symptoms would necessitate a referral to a medical practitioner?

The presence of the following symptoms and criteria have been identified in the literature as requiring referral to the GP:

- painful red eyes: a 'deep-seated pain' within the eye could relate to a sight-threatening condition such as glaucoma
- affected vision
- recent trauma/eye injury/'foreign' body presence in the eye
- 'cloudy' cornea
- copious yellow-green purulent discharge that re-accumulates after being wiped away
- marked redness of the eye
- photophobia
- irregular/abnormal pupil changes
- marked swelling in and around the eye (possibly glaucoma)
- family history of or suffering presently with a serious eye condition, or has undergone recent surgical procedures of the eye
- failure to respond to treatment after 48 hours
- restricted eye movement
- eye inflammation with associated facial or scalp rash
- associated symptoms of generally feeling unwell
- babies under three months of age (particularly neonates and premature infants)
- 'undiagnosed' dry eyes
- vernal keratoconjunctivitis: a chronic form of allergic conjunctivitis.

In contact lens wearers, poor lens maintenance can lead to sight-threatening microbial keratitis, relating to *Pseudomonas aeruginosa* or *Acanthamoeba* infection, and advice must be sought from their contact lens practitioner or doctor.

3   What is the general management of this condition in a community pharmacy setting?

Infective conjunctivitis is usually a self-limiting, non-harmful condition, with spontaneous symptom resolution within 2–14 days that is not dependent upon treatment. Within a pharmacy setting, it may be appropriate to treat any superficial infective conjunctivitis, in the absence of any requirement to refer a patient to a doctor, with chloramphenicol eye drops, which current clinical opinion suggests as the first-line choice, as sometimes it is difficult clinically to distinguish bacterial from viral conjunctivitis. Other issues regarding empirical treatment include reducing the risk of transmission and secondary infection, balanced against the risk of unnecessary treatment and adverse effects.

The antiseptic compounds propamidine and dibromopropamidine have been used for years within proprietary products for the treatment of bacterial conjunctivitis in adults and children, although with little evidence of any efficacy.

4   What is the goal of therapy and the role of the pharmacist in the management of this condition? How do the products generally used to treat the condition work? How can a product's formulation affect the outcome of treatment for the condition?

Pharmacists play a key role in acting as 'gatekeepers' to other NHS services, through differentiating minor self-treatable symptoms from major disease. If asked to advise on, for example, a minor eye symptom, then choosing the 'right' therapy to meet the patient's needs, with maximal benefit and minimised adverse effect is necessary. In addition to helping patients understand a therapy's posology, the nature of their condition can be explained to help provide greater 'concordance' and a better outcome.

Pharmacists can also promote 'positive' public health. For example, with this case of a diabetic patient, pharmacists can help them manage a normal blood glucose level and reduce the risk of developing diabetic retinopathy and secondary cataracts.

5   What advice can you give to help the patient manage this condition?

Advice should be tailored to allow a patient to gain the maximal benefit from any recommended medication, and can include points relating to correct medication use, general advice regarding the condition and what to do if treatment fails.

Examples of product-related advice include discussing with patients the risk of experiencing mild transient burning sensations after drop administration, with possibly a 'bad' taste sensation at the back of the throat following nasolacrimal duct drainage.

General advice could relate to discussing the contagiousness of infective conjunctivitis and so maintaining good hygiene measures to stop cross-contamination, and if necessary, about not wearing contact lenses during infection and for 24 hours after completing treatment.

In terms of treatment outcome, patients should be advised that if symptoms do not improve within 48 hours of treatment, then to seek medical advice.

Case study level 3 – Hay fever – see page 278

1   What is allergic rhinitis and how does it differ from cold symptoms?

Allergic rhinitis is immunoglobulin E mediated and is characterised by inflammation of the mucous membranes of the nose resulting from exposure to allergens. The classical symptoms are nasal itching, sneezing, watery and often profuse rhinorrhoea and congestion. The symptoms may peak about 6–12 hours after the initial exposure to the allergens which further manifest as nasal obstruction and sneezing.

Cold symptoms are slightly different; runny nose is accompanied by low-grade fever, sore throat, headache, with or without cough. Itchy eyes and sneezing are not usually present.

Mr JA is showing symptoms of seasonal allergic rhinitis (hay fever) but has been using cold remedies for eight weeks which has resulted in rebound nasal congestion, worsening his symptoms and complicating his hay fever.

2   What are the trigger factors for hay fever?

Hay fever is most commonly due to hypersensitivity to pollens (tree pollen in springtime, grass and weed pollen during the summer) and occasionally mould spores (during the late summer and autumn months). There is a strong link between allergic rhinitis and other immune-mediated diseases such as atopic eczema and asthma.

3   What are the treatment options for hay fever?

Advise the person on allergen avoidance and how best to achieve this (e.g. pollen count highest in the evening so advise closing of windows at night). Drug treatment is also usually necessary to help with symptoms. Assess the type and severity of the allergic rhinitis:

■   Is it intermittent or persistent (i.e. symptoms longer than four weeks)?
■   Is it mild, moderate, or severe (i.e. does it interfere with normal daily activity)?

Antihistamines and intranasal corticosteroids are the first-line treatments for allergic rhinitis. Sodium cromoglicate, ipratropium bromide and decongestants, are alternative or add-on treatments. Drug treatment should be selected according to the severity, frequency and duration of symptoms:

■   Mild intermittent: use an oral non-sedating (e.g. cetirizine or loratidine) or intranasal antihistamine (e.g. azelastine) as required. Consider using an intranasal decongestant in the short term (7 days maximum) if blockage is a problem. But this does not apply to Mr AJ as he has used this for a number of weeks and it is already causing rebound symptoms.

- Mild persistent or moderate–severe intermittent: use an oral or intranasal antihistamine, or an intranasal corticosteroid (e.g. beclometasone or fluticasone). Intranasal decongestants and sodium cromoglicate are useful add-on drugs.
- Moderate–severe persistent: intranasal corticosteroids are the drug of choice. Antihistamines, intranasal decongestants, and sodium cromoglicate are alternatives if steroids are contraindicated, or can be used as add-on drugs. Ipratropium bromide is useful for people with persistent watery effusion.

Drug treatment should be tailored to the person's individual needs, as well as the severity, frequency, and duration of their condition. The suitability of each drug for an individual is also dependent on its efficacy for individual symptoms, its onset and length of action, its formulation, and its adverse-effects profile.

4   What is the management plan for Mr JA's current symptoms?

Both Vicks Sinex, which contains oxymetazoline, and Sudafed, which contains pseudoephedrine, should be stopped because these are contributing to some of his symptoms. (rebound effect). Recommend a once-a-day non-sedating anti-histamine. However, only cetirizine is safe – the other antihistamines are contraindicated because of his history of porphyria.

5   What further treatment options are now available?

Topical mast cell stabilisers are best used for prophylaxis of allergic eye symptoms. Sodium cromoglicate is effective in most people. Lodoxamide and nedocromil are more expensive, but may be worth trying in people with inadequate response to sodium cromoglicate. Mr JA cannot use eye drops because he wears contact lenses therefore nasal corticosteroids are recommended.

Intranasal corticosteroids are effective in reducing ocular symptoms as well as nasal symptoms. The mechanism of action is unclear: it may partly be due to a systemic effect resulting from local absorption, although systemically related adverse effects are uncommon. These are used once or twice daily depending on choice and should be used regularly during the hay fever season.

6   What are the side-effects of nasal corticosteroids and are there any long-term complications?

Intranasal corticosteroids are safe if used correctly. Adverse effects are usually localised and include dryness, irritation and nose bleed (which may require stopping treatment for a period). Rarely, ulceration and nasal septal perforation (usually after nose surgery) can occur. Headaches, smell and taste disturbances, and hypersensitivity reactions have been reported.

Systemic effects caused by intranasal corticosteroids are rare. The MHRA

(Medicines and Healthcare products Regulatory Agency) has noted that the risks of systemic corticosteroids are low if used within licensed doses.

7   Mr JA asks about complementary medicines as he does not want to take medications long term. What would you advise?

There is no evidence-based research that any complementary medicines or treatments (e.g. acupuncture, herbal or dietary interventions or homeopathic remedies) are effective to treat hay fever. Butterbur and euphrasia have been used as alternatives to conventional medicines but safety data are lacking.

8   What is the long-term management plan for Mr JA?

Depending on the severity of his symptoms the patient can be referred to his GP for allergy testing with a view to desensitisation injections once the allergen has been identified. Mr JA should be advised to start his hay fever treatment four weeks before the start of the season, depending on which pollen type he is allergic to.

Case study level Ma – Sinusitis – see page 279

1   What other questions do you need to ask this patient to help with a working diagnosis?

- How long have you had the symptoms?
- Can you describe the pain?
- Is there any nasal discharge?
- Do you have temperature?
- Do you have any other symptoms?

2   Mr JC has had a greenish yellow discharge for the last 3 days together with facial pain around the eyes and nose. He complains of a loss of sense of smell and taste since having the cold symptoms last week. He has not developed a temperature. What is the possible diagnosis?

Allergic rhinitis, viral cold, hay fever, acute sinusitis or nasal blockage. Symptoms associated with sinusitis include:

- pain and tenderness of the infected sinus,
- throbbing pain which is worse on moving the head,
- toothache or jaw pain on eating,
- high temperature (fever), and
- a blocked or runny nose.

Infected mucus may produce a greenish or yellowish discharge. If the nose becomes blocked with mucus, the pain and tenderness in the affected area may intensify. Other symptoms include:

- tiredness,
- bad breath (halitosis),
- pressure in the ears,
- loss of taste and smell, and
- a feeling of being generally unwell.

3   Due to the presence of a number of the above symptoms you believe Mr JC has acute sinusitis. What are the predisposing factors for sinusitis?

The predisposing factors are:

- allergic rhinitis,
- asthma,
- cystic fibrosis,
- irritants that cause a blocked or runny nose, such as chemical pollutants like exhaust fumes,
- a weakened immune system that is caused by an illness such as HIV, or from treatment, such as chemotherapy, and
- certain inflammatory disorders.

Smoking and a blockage in the sinus drainage cavities, such as a nasal polyp, can cause acute sinusitis. Sometimes, an infected tooth can cause the maxillary sinuses to become infected.

4   What are the treatment options?

First-line treatment of acute sinusitis is with oral analgesics; paracetamol, ibuprofen or aspirin. Mr JC should try a full dose of paracetamol (i.e. 1 g q.d.s.). Due to his history of asthma, aspirin and ibuprofen are not the drugs of choice (if the patient has never taken them in the past). He should be told that the symptoms are usually self-limiting and should not persist for longer than 7 days. The use of a topical decongestant may relieve nasal symptoms. They are thought to promote mucociliary clearance and sinus drainage but should not be used for more than 7 days as rebound congestion will occur.

5   Should the patient be given beclometasone nasal spray?

Intranasal corticosteroids are not routinely recommended for acute sinusitis. Any beneficial effect is likely to take at least a week to develop. However, they may have a role in chronic sinusitis.

6   A week later Mr JC returns to the pharmacy with a slight improvement of his symptoms until yesterday when he developed fever and dizziness and slight hearing loss and ear pain. What would you now recommend?

It is likely that the patient's sinusitis has an infective element and therefore a referral to the GP for antibiotic treatment is the next step.

7   The new junior GP calls you and asks your advice on which antibiotic to prescribe.

Amoxicillin is the first-line treatment as it treats most pathogens involved in sinusitis. However, Mr JC is allergic to penicillin and therefore alternative antibiotics are indicated; doxycycline or a macrolide antibiotic would be a suitable alternative in this patient.

8   Mr JC returns to the pharmacy with a prescription for doxycycline 100mg 2 stat then 1 daily for 7 days. How would you counsel this patient?

Your advice should include the following:

- Take with a full glass of water while sitting or standing to avoid oesophageal irritation.
- Do not take with iron or indigestion remedies or milk as absorption is compromised.
- Avoid exposure to sunlight or sunlamps (causes photosensitivity).
- Complete the course.

Case study level Mb – Glaucoma – see page 280

1   What is glaucoma, define different types and why is it important to be treated when diagnosed?

Glaucoma is a condition in which an increase in production of, or decrease in drainage of aqueous humour in the eyes leads to increased pressure in the anterior cavity of the eyeball. The increased pressure in the eye compresses the blood vessels that supply the retina and ultimately damages the cells responsible for seeing, the optic nerve and the nerve fibres running towards it from the retina. The damaged parts of the nerve and seeing cells in the retina lead to permanent patches of vision loss. Untreated glaucoma is one of the world's leading causes of blindness, but blindness can be prevented if glaucoma is diagnosed and treated early enough.

There are two types of glaucoma:

- Primary open-angle glaucoma is a very common form (also known as chronic simple or wide-angle glaucoma). It results from obstruction in the trabecular meshwork which acts as the drainage system for the aqueous humour.
- Primary angle closure glaucoma (also known as acute close-angle or narrow-angle glaucoma) results from blockage of aqueous humour flow into the anterior chamber. The condition develops very quickly with a sudden increase in eye pressure. The eyes become very painful and red.

2   What are the risk factors for developing glaucoma? Identify the possible causes of worsening of his glaucoma condition.

The risk factors for developing glaucoma include:

- age,
- long-term steroid therapy, and
- drug/disease interactions, including long-term treatments with drugs that precipitate glaucoma (e.g. antimuscarinics).

Two possible explanations for worsening of symptoms include:

- gradual deterioration in his condition, especially since he stopped using latanoprost treatment, and
- adverse drug reactions from his current medications.

Tolterodine is an antimuscarinic (anticholinergic) drug used extensively to treat urinary incontinence. The anticholinergics can cause acute angle-closure glaucoma (narrow-angle glaucoma) by decreasing aqueous inflow and outflow by possibly partially antagonising alpha-adrenergic receptors in the eye and hence increase intraocular pressure.

A small number of cases of acute angle-closure glaucoma have been reported in patients treated with a combination of nebulised salbutamol and ipratropium bromide, caused possibly by local absorption of mist containing both products. A combination of nebulised salbutamol with nebulised anticholinergics should therefore be used cautiously. Patients should receive adequate instruction in correct administration and be warned not to let the solution or mist enter the eyes. Use of a mouthpiece rather than a mask for administration would reduce the risk associated with this.

3   Why are some drugs contraindicated in certain diseases even if they are given as eye drops?

With some drugs that are delivered via eye drops, some systemic absorption can occur which in turn can cause systemic side-effects. For example, timolol (a beta-blocker) can worsen or precipitate bronchospasm in asthmatic and COPD patients.

4   How does latanoprost work in the treatment of glaucoma? Discuss the range of drugs and route of administration that can be used to treat this patient's glaucoma.

Topical beta-blockers can precipitate asthma and therefore must not be used to treat this patient's glaucoma. Topical prostaglandin analogues (e.g. latanoprost drops) are used as first-line treatment of glaucoma together with a sympathomimetic agent, brimonidine, as an alternative to beta-blockers in asthmatic and COPD patients.

Latanoprost increases the uveosceleral outflow, thereby lowering the intra-ocular pressure.

It may be necessary to combine these or add another agent such as oral acetazolamide and/or dorzolamide eye drops, which are both carbonic anhydrase inhibitors that reduce aqueous humour production.

5   What other treatment options are available for treating this patient's incontinence?

Tolterodine can only affect the narrow-angle glaucoma (primary closed-angle glaucoma) and is contraindicated in uncontrolled cases of this type of glaucoma. It is therefore necessary to establish if the deterioration in the patient's vision is due to tolterodine use. In order to prevent optical nerve dam-age, an earlier appointment with the consultant is possibly warranted and there-fore the patient should be advised to contact the consultant for further advice.

Flavoxate has inhibitory action on the smooth muscle of the bladder and has no antimuscarinic properties. It may be considered, therefore, as an alter-native therapy to tolterodine.

There are mixed outcomes for flavoxate when compared with antimus-carinic medication; one study showed equal efficacy to oxybutynin, while other studies failed to demonstrate any beneficial effects.

In cases where tolterodine cannot be used, non-pharmacological interven-tions, such as use of urinary sheaths or catheterisation, may be considered.

12

Skin case studies

Tracy Garnier and Gary Moss

Case study level 1 – Cold sores

Learning outcomes

Level 1 case study: You will be able to:

- describe the risk factors
- describe the disease
- describe the pharmacology of the drug
- outline the formulation, including drug molecule, excipients, etc. for the medicines
- summarise basic social pharmacy issues (e.g. opening containers, large labels).

Scenario

A 25-year-old man, Mr MB, presents at your pharmacy complaining about his cold sores. He would like advice on how to treat them and how to stop them coming back time after time.

Questions

1a What are cold sores?
1b What causes cold sores, and what are the risk factors?
2a What type of drugs are used to treat cold sores?
2b What type of formulations are used to deliver cold sore medications?
2c What is the mechanism of action of this class of drugs?
2d What are the common side-effects of these drugs?
3a How are cold sores treated?

3b   What formulations of aciclovir are available for the treatment of cold sores?
3c   How are these formulations administered?
4a   How would you counsel the patient in the use of his prescription?
4b   What other advice would you give the patient to help with this treatment?

General references

Blenkinsopp A, Paxton P and Blenkinsopp J (2005) *Symptoms in the Pharmacy*, 5th edn. Oxford: Wiley Blackwell.

Edwards C and Stillman P (2006) *Minor Illness or Major Disease?*, 4th edn. London: Pharmaceutical Press.

Joint Formulary Committee (2008) *British National Formulary 55*. London: British Medical Association and Royal Pharmaceutical Society of Great Britain, March.

NHS Direct (2008) Herpes simplex virus. Available at http://www.nhsdirect.nhs.uk/articles/article.aspx?articleId=194&sectionId=1 [Accessed 02 July 2008].

Case study level 2 – Severe acne

Learning outcomes

Level 2 case study: You will be able to:

- interpret relevant lab and clinical data
- identify monitoring and referral criteria
- explain treatment choices
- describe goals of therapy including monitoring and the role of the pharmacist/clinician
- describe issues – counselling points, adverse drug reactions, drug interactions, complementary/alternative therapies and lifestyle advice.

Scenario

A 17-year-old girl, Miss EV, presents in your pharmacy with her regular prescription for Microgynon 30. Three months ago she had complained of problems of acne so you recommended that she try an over-the-counter topical benzoyl peroxide formulation. Her acne does not appear to have improved from the treatment so you recommend that she makes an appointment to see her GP. The following week she presents a new prescription for oxytetracycline tablets (500 mg b.d.).

Questions

1   What is acne?

2a   Explain the type of topical formulations of benzoyl peroxide which are available and discuss the differences between them?

2b   Why would an aqueous gel be recommended instead of an alcoholic gel? Give an example of each.

2c   How would you counsel a patient to use a topical formulation of benzoyl peroxide?

3a   What group of drugs does oxytetracycline belong to?

3b   What is the mechanism of action for the tetracyclines?

3c   How would you counsel Miss EV to take her oxytetracycline tablets? Should any particular precautions be taken by Miss EV?

3d   What are the common side-effects of oxytetracycline? Give five examples.

4   Miss EV is concerned about the problem of resistance developing. What do you advise? She also asks you when she should expect to see an improvement in her acne and usually how long the treatment should last.

5   What are the alternative treatment options instead of tetracyclines for severe acne?

General references

Clinical Knowledge Summaries (2006) Acne vulgaris. Available at http://cks.library.nhs. uk/acne_vulgaris [Accessed 1 July 2008].

Cunliffe B (2001) Diseases of the skin and their treatment: acne. *The Pharmaceutical Journal* 267: 749–752.

Delgado JN and Remers WA (1998) *Wilson and Gisvold's Textbook of Organic Medicinal and Pharmaceutical Chemistry*, 10th edn. London: Lippincott-Raven Publishers.

Joint Formulary Committee (2008) *British National Formulary 55*. London: British Medical Association and Royal Pharmaceutical Society of Great Britain, March.

Summary of Product Characteristics (2006) Oxytetracycline tablets BP 250mg. Available at http://www.emc.medicines.org.uk [Accessed 25 October 2006].

Case Study Level 3 – Acute cellulitis

Learning outcomes

Level 3 case study: You will be able to:

- interpret clinical signs and symptoms
- evaluate laboratory data
- evaluate treatment options
- state goals of therapy
- describe a pharmaceutical care plan to include advice to a clinician
- describe the prognosis and long-term complications
- describe the social pharmacy issues which could include supply (e.g. complex treatments at home, concordance and compliance) and lifestyle issues.

Scenario

Mrs PG, mother of 10-year-old Tanya, came into the pharmacy a few days ago with a prescription for her daughter. The prescription requested penicillin V oral solution 250 mg/5 mL, 250 mg four times a day and flucloxacillin syrup 125 mg/5 mL, 125 mg four times a day, at least 30 minutes before food. Her mother requests information on her daughter's condition, cellulitis. You notice from your patient medication records that Tanya had recently been treated for athlete's foot.

A few days later, Mrs PG returns to your pharmacy asking for your advice. Her daughter has developed a red rash on her back.

Questions

1a What is cellulitis?
1b What are the risk factors for developing cellulitis?
1c Does Tanya have any of the risk factors for developing cellulitis?
2a Both penicillin V and flucloxacillin are penicillins, which belong to the beta-lactams. What other antibiotics belong to the beta-lactams?
2b Why do both of these antibiotics require reconstitution before use? What are the specific storage conditions following reconstitution?
2c What is the difference in antibiotic activity between penicillin V and flucloxacillin – explain your answer using structural diagrams for both drugs.
2d Why should penicillin V and flucloxacillin be taken on an empty stomach?

2e   What are the common side-effects of penicillins? Give three examples.
3   What is the mechanism of action for the beta-lactam pencillins?
4   Co-amoxiclav is an alternative treatment to penicillin V and flucloxacillin. What does this consist of and what formulations are available?
5a   Parenteral benzylpenicillin (Crystapen) and flucloxacillin is an alternative treatment option instead of oral antibiotics for severe cellulitis. Why is benzylpenicillin only available as a parenteral formulation?
5b   What pH is this formulation buffered to and why?
6   Penicillins should be used with caution in renal impairment – why?
7   Resistance is a problem with antibiotics. Explain the mechanisms of resistance for the beta-lactam antibiotics?
8a   Tanya may be suffering from a side-effect due to her medication. What do you think might be causing this?
8b   How common are allergic reactions to penicillins?
8c   What alternative treatment might a GP prescribe?

General references

Clinical Knowledge Summaries (2008) Cellulitis. Available at http://cks.library.nhs.uk/ cellulitis [Accessed 1 July 2008].
Delgado JN and Remers WA (1998) *Wilson and Gisvold's Textbook of Organic Medicinal and Pharmaceutical Chemistry*, 10the edn. London: Lippincott-Raven.
Joint Formulary Committee (2008) *British National Formulary 55*. London: British Medical Association and Royal Pharmaceutical Society of Great Britain, March.
Summary of Product Characteristics (2006) Floxapen. Available at http://www.emc. medicines.org.uk [Accessed 25 October 2006].

Case study level Ma – Atopic eczema

Learning outcomes

Level M case study: You will be able to:

- interpret clinical signs and symptoms
- evaluate laboratory data
- critically appraise treatment options
- state goals of therapy
- describe a pharmaceutical care plan to include advice to a clinician
- describe the prognosis and long-term complications
- describe the social pharmacy issues which could include supply (e.g. complex treatments at home, concordance and compliance) and lifestyle issues
- describe the monitoring of therapy.

Mr DP, 35 years, has been taking asthma medication for 12 years and occasionally also suffers from eczema. His regular prescription is for salbutamol inhaler (100 micrograms/metered inhalation); 1–2 puffs as required and Clenil-Modulite (100 micrograms/dose); 2 puffs twice daily. Today he presents in your pharmacy with a new prescription for Betnovate scalp application.

A week later, Mr DP returns to your pharmacy complaining of worsening symptoms. Upon examination, you notice redness on an area of his scalp and the skin has a crusted appearance. You explain to Mr DP that the worsening of his symptoms may be due to a bacterial infection and that he must make an appointment to see the GP.

1   What is atopic eczema?

2   State the main causes of atopic eczema?

3a What are the main therapies available for treating atopic eczema?

3b Coal tar has been used to manage a variety of dry-skin conditions. Is this appropriate for treatment of atopic eczema?

4a What family of drugs does betamethasone belong to? Explain the general mechanism of action for this family.

4b Explain the terms 'glucocorticoid' and 'mineralocorticoid' activity. Give an example of one drug associated with each activity.

5a How should the Betnovate scalp application be applied?

5b List the excipients that are contained within Betnovate scalp application. Explain the possible role for each excipient.

5c The Summary of Product Characteristics for Betnovate scalp application states that it contains betamethasone valerate BP 0.122% w/w. Calculate the total amount in grams (to three decimal places) of betamethasone in 100 g of the formulation. The formula and molecular weight for betamethsone valerate are $C_{27}H_{37}FO_6$ and 476.577 g/mol respectively. The formula and molecular weight for betamethasone are $C_{22}H_{29}FO_5$ and 392.461 g/mol respectively.

5d Clenil-Modulite contains beclometasone (as dipropionate). Betnovate scalp application contains betamethasone (as valerate). Explain, using the chemical formulas shown in Figure Q12.1 overleaf, the difference in log P values between beclometasone and their respective salts.

6a Beclometasone (as dipropionate) is a pro-drug. Define the term 'pro-drug' and explain the pharmacodynamics involved.

6b How is beclometasone (as dipropionate) metabolised? State the metabolites involved.

6c State the main excipients in Clenil-Modulite and briefly describe why they are used in this formulation.

7   Discuss both the systemic and local adverse effects associated with using corticosteroids, giving examples of each. What factors increase the risk of adverse effects and why?

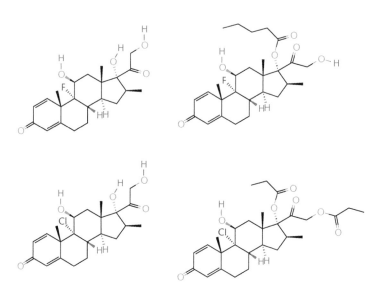

Figure Q12.1 Betamethasone (top left), betamethasone (as valerate) (top right), beclometasone (bottom left) and beclometasone dipropionate (bottom right).

8a   Mr DP's worsening symptoms are probably due to a bacterial infection. What is the most common cause of bacterial infected eczema?

8b   What is the recommended first-line treatment for bacterial infected eczema?

General references

Clinical Knowledge Summaries (2006) Atopic eczema. Available at http://cks.library.nhs.uk/eczema_atopic [Accessed 1 July 2008].

Delgado JN and Remers WA (1998) *Wilson and Gisvold's Textbook of Organic Medicinal and Pharmaceutical Chemistry*, 10th edn. London: Lippincott-Raven.

Hoare C, Li Wan Po A and Williams H (2000) Systematic review of treatments for atopic eczema. *Health Technology Assessment* 4: 1–191.

Joint Formulary Committee (2008) *British National Formulary 55*. London: British Medical Association and Royal Pharmaceutical Society of Great Britain, March.

Lund W (ed.) (1994) *The Pharmaceutical Codex (Principles and Practice of Pharmaceutics)*, 12th edn. London : Pharmaceutical Press.

National Prescribing Centre (2003) Atopic eczema in primary care. *MeRec Bulletin* 14(1). Available at http://www.npc.co.uk/MeReC_Bulletins/2003Volumes/V0114n01.pdf [Accessed 1 July 2008].

Rowe R, Sheskey P and Owen S (2005) *Handbook of Pharmaceutical Excipients: Chlorofluorocarbons* (CFC). London: Pharmaceutical Press. Available at: http://www.medicinescomplete.com/ [Accessed 4 July 2008].

Simonsen L, Hoy G, Didriksen E *et al.* (2004) Development of a new formulation combining calcipotriol and betamethasone dipropionate in an ointment vehicle. *Drug Development and Industrial Pharmacy* 30: 1095–1102.

Summary of Product Characteristics (2008) Betnovate Scalp Application. http://www. emc.medicines.org.uk [Accessed 1 July 2008].

Case study level Mb – Psoriasis

Learning outcomes

Level M case study: You will be able to:

- interpret clinical signs and symptoms
- evaluate laboratory data
- critically appraise treatment options
- state goals of therapy
- describe a pharmaceutical care plan to include advice to a clinician
- describe the prognosis and long-term complications
- describe the social pharmacy issues which could include supply (e.g. complex treatments at home, concordance and compliance) and lifestyle issues
- describe the monitoring of therapy.

Scenario

This case study relates to a 47-year-old male patient, Mr GM, with severe psoriasis. The patient has been suffering with psoriasis on and off for 2 years, mostly in the form of widespread irritation. However, over the last few months the occurrence of the dry, scaly, shiny red lesions has become more regular and has spread across his body, after being initially confined to his elbows, knees and lower back.

Previous treatment has focused on the use of topical products. Initially, these were over-the-counter products which provided relief but which also caused irritation at times. The patient took paracetamol and ibuprofen to help manage irritation, pain and swelling associated with psoriasis and the topical products.

After a consultation approximately a year ago, the patient's GP recommended the use of prescription topical products (corticosteroids). These were used regularly but with variable results. The patient commented that he was sick of waiting for the products to do something, and usually after two or three weeks he stopped or lessened their use, exasperated at their failure to work.

He was then moved to PUVA (psoralen and UVA) treatment and this had limited success. Currently, the patient is taking acitretin.

Questions

1a   What is psoriasis? What are the different types of psoriasis? (In your answer focus on topical psoriasis.)

1b   What causes psoriasis, and what are the risk factors?

1c   Given the description of Mr GM, which type(s) of psoriasis do you think he has?

1d   Is Mr GM at risk of developing any further types of psoriasis, or any related illnesses?

2a   What type of medicaments are used to treat psoriasis at each of the stages of therapy, i.e. (i) topical therapies, (ii) phototherapies, (iii) combination therapies, (iv) systemic drug therapies (i.e. oral and i.v.)?

2b   Mr GM is currently being treated with acitretin, and the topical application of emollients. How would you counsel him on their side-effects and use?

2c   How may side-effects affect the compliance of the patient in this case? In particular, focus on the patient's analgesic use, and review how this may affect the proposed systemic drug therapy.

3a   Review the stages of treatment, including formulations and their administration, available for psoriasis. Evaluate the treatment provided to the patient and suggest any issues in the previous treatment regimen.

3b   Discuss a suitable long-term care plan for Mr GM. Clearly addressing the goals of therapy, discuss how this plan will be monitored and how compliance will be assured. Address long-term care issues and discuss possible alternative treatments available to Mr GM.

3c   Are there any other treatments available to Mr GM?

General references

Abel EA, DiCicco LM, Orenberg EK *et al.* (1986) Drugs in exacerbation of psoriasis. *Journal of the American Academy of Dermatology* 15: 1007–1022.

Clinical Knowledge Summaries (2008) Patient information leaflet psoriasis. Available at http://cks.library.nhs.uk/patient_information_leaflet/psoriasis [Accessed 1 July 2008].

Gudjonsson JE, Karason A, Antonsdottir AA *et al.* (2002) HLA-Cw6-positive and HLA-Cw6-negative patients with psoriasis vulgaris have distinct clinical features. *Journal of Investigative Dermatology* 118: 362–365.

Joint Formulary Committee (2008) *British National Formulary 55*. London: British Medical Association and Royal Pharmaceutical Society of Great Britain, March.

Lebwohl M, Yoles A, Lombardi K and Lou W (1998) Calcipotriene ointment and halobetasol ointment in the long-term treatment of psoriasis: Effects on the duration of improvement. *Journal of the American Academy of Dermatology* 39: 447–450.

Mallon E, Newson R and Bunker CB (1999) HLA-Cw6 and the genetic predisposition to psoriasis: a meta-analysis of published serologic studies. *Journal of Investigative Dermatology* 113: 693–695.

Michaëlsson G, Gerdén B, Hagforsen E *et al.* (2000) Psoriasis patients with antibodies to gliadin can be improved by a gluten-free diet. *British Journal of Dermatology* 142: 44.

Parish J (1981) Phototherapy and photochemotherapy of skin diseases. *Journal of Investigative Dermatology* 77: 167–171.

Syed TA, Ahm AS, Holt AH *et al.* (1996) Management of psoriasis with Aloe vera extract in a hydrophilic cream: a placebo-controlled, double-blind study. *Tropical Medicine and International Health* 1: 505–509.

Van Dooren-Greebe RJ, Kuijpers ALA, Mulder J *et al.* (1994) Methotrexate revisited: effects of long-term treatment in psoriasis. *British Journal of Dermatology* 130: 204–210.

Answers

Case study level 1 – Cold sores – see page 294

1a   What are cold sores?

Cold sores are caused by the herpes simplex virus. They are characterised by groups of closely packed fluid-filled blisters, which usually appear on the skin or mucous membranes. They are most usually associated with the mouth and lips as the skin in these areas may not be as resistant as in other parts of the body, although infection of the eye and mucous membranes are also common. Infection of other skin areas is common in immunodeficient patients. The blisters can be tender and painful. They will normally heal without scarring. Cold sore infections can last for 1–3 weeks and are characterised by tingling and/or itching 24 hours prior to the appearance of lesions. Cold sores can recur.

1b   What causes cold sores, and what are the risk factors?

Cold sores are caused by the herpes simplex virus serotype 1 (HSV-1). A person may become infected by transmission from another individual who has a cold sore, for example, by kissing. The virus passes through the skin and travels up the nerve, where it usually lies dormant until triggered. Common risk factors include emotional stresses, fatigue, colds and viruses that may weaken the body's immune system, menstruation and environmental factors such as cold weather and strong winds.

2a   What type of drugs are used to treat cold sores?

Cold sores are treated by the administration of antiviral drugs such as aciclovir or famciclovir.

2b   What type of formulations are used to deliver cold sore medications?

The most common form of treatment is by the application of topical creams (e.g. Zovirax). More severe cases may be treated by, progressively, oral (normally tablets) or i.v. preparations.

2c   What is the mechanism of action of this class of drugs?

Drugs used to treat HSV-1, such as aciclovir, act as nucleoside analogues. Viral thymidine kinase converts the drugs into the monophosphate form. This is then converted to the active triphosphate form, aciclo-GTP, which inhibits viral DNA polymerase, resulting in chain termination (highly selective for infected cells). These drugs are inactive against latent viruses in the nerve ganglia. Therefore, they will treat cold sores when they arise but they will not eradicate the virus from the body.

2d   What are the common side-effects of these drugs?

Nausea, vomiting, abdominal pain, diarrhoea and headache. Side-effects may depend upon the way that the drug is administered (i.e. topical, tablet).

3a   How are cold sores treated?

Initial treatment of cold sores is usually by the application of topically applied creams, such as Zovirax. More severe cases are treated with oral products, such as conventional or dispersible tablets. In very severe cases treatment may be via intravenous infusion.

3b   What formulations of aciclovir are available for the treatment of cold sores?

Formulations available include:

- topical products, including those for ophthalmic use,
- tablets, including conventional and dispersible tablets, and
- products for intravenous infusion.

3c   How are these formulations administered?

Topical products are applied directly to the cold sore. Tablets are taken orally with water (five times a day at regular intervals, for 5 days, or longer if new lesions appear), and parenteral products are administered under supervision from healthcare professionals in a clinical setting.

4a   How would you counsel the patient in the use of his prescription?

The medicine should be used exactly as advised by the patient's doctor. The patient should be asked about other medications or current health issues and lifestyle and advised on how to help reduce infections (see below).

4b   What other advice would you give the patient to help with this treatment?

Other products may help to soothe the itching associated with cold sores. These include balm mint extract or tea tree oil. Over-the-counter medicines such as paracetamol may be taken to relieve the pain and itching associated with cold sores. Witch hazel may also be applied to the sore to reduce pain. The patient should wash his hands frequently and avoid sharing towels, etc.

Mr MB should be advised to avoid picking at or touching the cold sore as it may spread the virus to other parts of the body, and it may also make the cold sore become infected. He should avoid kissing (i.e. newborn babies or those with weak immune systems) and eating salty, spicy or acidic foods which may irritate the sore. In severe cases eating 'soft' foods, such as soup, may be less painful, as less chewing and movement of the mouth is required. The patient should also be advised to maintain a good level of hydration.

Persistent and severe cold sores may be exacerbated by a range of underlying issues, such as fatigue, emotional or stress-related problems, a cold (or other viruses which may weaken the body's defences), and menstrual periods (which is not directly applicable to this patient). Particular weather conditions, such as strong sunlight (the use of sun-block may be an issue) or wind, may make the cold sore worse. Triggers are different for each person, and any underlying issues should be referred to the patient's doctor.

For recurrent problems, start treatment as soon as a 'tingling' sensation is felt around the lips.

Case study level 2 – Severe acne – see page 295

1   What is acne?

Acne is an inflammatory disease of the sebaceous glands and hair follicles of the skin. It is characterised by the eruption of pimples or pustules, especially on the face.

2a   Explain the type of topical formulations of benzoyl peroxide which are available and discuss the differences between them?

Benzoyl peroxide is available as Brevoxyl cream, PanOxyl aquagel/cream/gel and wash. Compound preparations with antimicrobials are also available as Benzamycin gel, Duac Once Daily gel and Quinoderm cream.

2b   Why would an aqueous gel be recommended instead of an alcoholic gel? Give an example of each.

Alcoholic formulations (e.g. PanOxyl gel) are not recommended for people with sensitive skin or asthmatics. An aqueous gel such as PanOxyl aquagel would be more suitable.

2c   How would you counsel a patient to use a topical formulation of benzoyl peroxide?

Apply once or twice daily, preferably after washing with soap and water. Treatment should be started with lower strength formulations. Adverse effects can include local skin irritation, such as scaling and redness, particularly on commencement of therapy. If this occurs advise the patient to reduce the frequency of application. Benzoyl peroxide formulations can also cause bleaching of clothes.

3a   What group of drugs does oxytetracycline belong to?

Oxytetracycline is a tetracycline antibiotic. It is a broad-spectrum antibiotic.

3b   What is the mechanism of action for the tetracyclines?

Tetracyclines inhibit protein biosynthesis by acting on the 70S and 80S ribosomes.

3c   How would you counsel Miss EV to take her oxytetracycline tablets? Should any particular precautions be taken by Miss EV?

Oxytetracycline is licensed to be taken four times a day, but can be taken twice a day for the treatment of acne (two 250 mg tablets twice a day). These oxytetracycline tablets should be taken 1 hour before or 2 hours after meals, followed by a glass of water. They should NOT be taken at the same time as milk, food or antacids, as they can make the medicine less effective. Tablets should be swallowed when either sitting or standing and they should not be taken immediately before going to bed. The complete course of prescribed tablets should be completed.

Miss EV is taking the combined oral contraceptive (COC) pill and should be advised to use additional contraception (with a barrier contraceptive) for three weeks when starting the course of oral oxytetracyclines. She should also be advised to start the next pack of COCs without taking a 7-day break. After three weeks, additional precautions are not necessary as the bacterial flora (responsible for recycling ethinylestradiol from the large bowel) develop resistance.

3d   What are the common side-effects of oxytetracycline? Give five examples.

Side-effects may include vomiting, nausea, diarrhoea, dysphagia and oesophageal irritation.

4   Miss EV is concerned about the problem of resistance developing. What do you advise? She also asks you when she should expect to see an improvement in her acne and usually how long the treatment should last.

Resistance of *Propionibacterium acnes* to topical and systemic antibiotics is increasing. Therefore you should recommend that Miss EV complete the full course of the prescribed treatment. You should also advise that she should only use antibiotics when absolutely necessary.

In general, six months should be adequate for oral antibiotics (two months for topical antibiotics). Maximum improvement generally occurs after 4–6 months.

5   What are the alternative treatment options instead of tetracyclines for severe acne?

Tetracyclines are recommended as first-line treatment. When tetracyclines are not tolerated or contraindicated, erythromycin is an alternative. However erythromycin has problems with resistance and gastrointestinal adverse effects. If compliance is a problem, either doxycycline or lymecycline may be prescribed (can be taken once daily with food). Minocycline is second-line treatment (e.g. if oral antibiotic has failed).

Case study level 3 – Acute cellulitis – see page 297

1a   What is cellulitis?

Cellulitis is a skin infection of the dermis and subcutaneous tissues. It is characterised by redness, swelling, pain and inflammation. A common symptom is fever. Cellulitis is caused by bacterial infection, most commonly *Streptococcus* (group A) and *Staphylococcus*.

1b   What are the risk factors for developing cellulitis?

Risk factors include athlete's foot, swollen legs or obesity, a previous episode of cellulitis, poor immune status or poorly controlled diabetes.

1c   Does Tanya have any of the risk factors for developing cellulitis?

Athlete's foot is fungal skin infection that may result in cracked skin between the toes. Through these breaks in the skin, bacteria can enter and multiply under the skin surface, resulting in cellulitis.

2a   Both penicillin V and flucloxacillin are penicillins, which belong to the beta-lactams. What other antibiotics belong to the beta-lactams?

The beta-lactams include the penicillins, aminocillins, cephalosporins, carbapenems, and monobactams.

2b   Why do both of these antibiotics require reconstitution before use? What are the specific storage conditions following reconstitution?

Penicillins are susceptible to hydrolysis, as the highly reactive beta-lactam has a carbonyl C7 (within the lactam ring) susceptible to both nucleophilic and electrophilic attack. Hydrolysis and degradation is influenced by pH. Therefore, penicillins are formulated as dry powders which require reconstitution just prior to use. Once dispensed, the penicillin solutions should be stored in the fridge and used usually within 14 days.

2c What is the difference in antibiotic activity between penicillin V and flucloxacillin – explain your answer using structural diagrams for both drugs.

The chemical structures of phenoxymethylpenicillin (penicillin V) and flucloxacillin are shown in Figure A12.1.

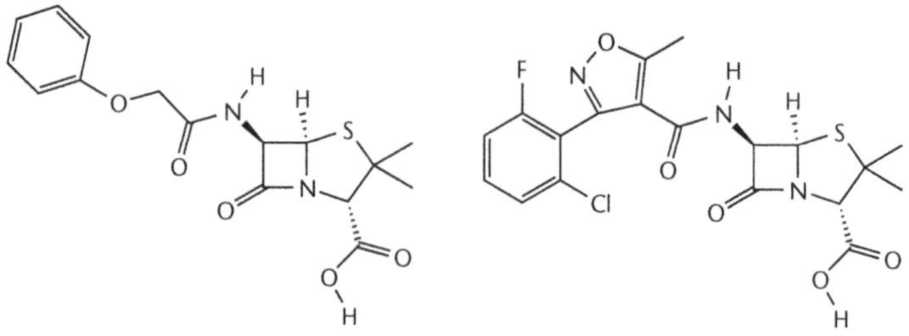

Figure A12.1 Phenoxymethylpenicillin (penicillin V) (left) and flucloxacillin (right).

Penicillin V is a narrow-spectrum penicillin and has similar antibacterial activity to benzylpenicillin. It is active against many streptococcal infections, but it is inactivated by penicillinases. Flucloxacillin is a penicillinase-resistant antibiotic and is effective against infections caused by penicillin-resistant staphylococci. In comparison to penicillin V, attachment of carbocyclic/heterocyclic ring directly to the C6 carbonyl group confers resistance to beta-lactamases due to steric hindrance around the amide group.

2d Why should penicillin V and flucloxacillin be taken on an empty stomach?

Both penicillin V and flucloxacillin should be taken on an empty stomach since they are not absorbed well into the bloodstream. Taking these medicines on an empty stomach helps to improve the absorption profile.

2e What are the common side-effects of penicillins? Give three examples.

Common side-effects (≥1% of patients) associated with use of the penicillins include: gastrointestinal disturbances (diarrhoea, nausea), hypersensitivity (rash, urticaria) and superinfection (e.g. candida infection).

3   What is the mechanism of action for the beta-lactam pencillins?

Beta-lactam penicillins prevent the biosynthesis of a dipeptidoglycan which forms the peptidoglycan cell wall in bacteria. This results in cell death and bactericidal activity. Specifically, they acylate a specific bacterial D-transpeptidase, which inactivates this enzyme and it therefore cannot form peptide crosslinks of two linear peptidoglycan strands for cell wall formation.

4   Co-amoxiclav is an alternative treatment to penicillin V and flucloxacillin. What does this consist of and what formulations are available?

Co-amoxiclav consists of amoxicillin, a broad-spectrum penicillin, and clavulanic acid, a beta-lactamase inhibitor. It is available as tablets, an oral suspension and as an injection formulation.

5a   Parenteral benzylpenicillin (Crystapen) and flucloxacillin is an alternative treatment option instead of oral antibiotics for severe cellulitis. Why is benzylpenicillin only available as a parenteral formulation?

Benzylpenicillin is unstable to acid because it does not contain an electron-withdrawing group on the α-carbon to prevent electronic displacement. Therefore it is not given orally as it would be inactivated by the low pH of the gastric environment.

5b   What pH is this formulation buffered to and why?

Benzylpenicillin is buffered to pH 7 since it is acid unstable and therefore given parenterally.

6   Penicillins should be used with caution in renal impairment – why?

Penicillins are mainly cleared by renal tubular secretion and therefore should be used with caution in renal impairment, as penicillin half-lives may be increased in this condition.

7   Resistance is a problem with antibiotics. Explain the mechanisms of resistance for the beta-lactam antibiotics?

Resistance to beta-lactam antibiotics may occur through a number of mechanisms:

- Bacteria may prevent the antibiotic from binding with and entering the organism (seen in certain resistant *P. aeruginosa*).
- Bacteria may produce an enzyme that inactivates the antibiotic (i.e. beta-lactamase enzymes in the case of resistant *H. influenzae*). This type of resistance can be transmitted to other bacteria through a process known as transference.

■ Change in the internal binding site of the antibiotic may occur (i.e. alterations in the penicillin-binding proteins in the case of penicillin-resistant *S. pneumoniae*).

8a Tanya may be suffering from a side-effect due to her medication. What do you think might be causing this?

This might be caused by hypersensitivity to penicillins.

8b How common are allergic reactions to penicillins?

Allergic reactions to penicillins typically occur in 1–10% of the population.

8c What alternative treatment might a GP prescribe?

Alternative treatment for cellulitis in a patient hypersensitive to penicillins is the macrolide erythromycin.

Case study level Ma – Atopic eczema – see page 298

1 What is atopic eczema?

Atopic eczema is a chronic, relapsing, inflammatory skin condition. Typically it is characterised by an itchy red rash (often associated with the skin flexures). It is associated with a family history of other atopic diseases such as asthma and hay fever. Due to the reduced barrier function of the dry skin, eczematous skin can be particularly sensitive to irritants.

2 State the main causes of atopic eczema?

Atopic eczema occurs in individuals who are genetically predisposed to this condition when exposed to environmental irritants (abrasive fabrics, soaps, detergents, extremes of temperature/humidity) and allergies (dust mites, pollen, moulds, diet). It may be worsened by endogenous factors (e.g. hormones, stress).

3a What are the main therapies available for treating atopic eczema?

Skin dryness is treated with emollients which should be applied liberally and used regularly. Topical corticosteroids are generally used intermittently to control flare-ups. Oral antibiotics may be indicated for moderate to severe infection. Treatment of lichenification may initially be with a potent corticosteroid. Other therapies include ichthammol paste (reduces itching), zinc oxide and potassium permanganate solution (exudating eczema). Newer treatment options include drugs acting on the immune system such as pimecrolimus and tacrolimus.

3b Coal tar has been used to manage a variety of dry-skin conditions. Is this appropriate for treatment of atopic eczema?

There is little evidence to support the use of coal tar in treating atopic eczema and it would therefore be inappropriate. In addition, hypersensitivity reactions may be caused by the use of coal tar.

4a What family of drugs does betamethasone belong to? Explain the general mechanism of action for this family.

Betamethasone is a corticosteroid. Corticosteroids are very lipophilic (due to their hydrocarbon skeleton) and as a result can passively diffuse into target cells. It acts by binding to the intracellular corticosteroid receptor protein, which is found within the cytosol. The resulting complex translocates to the nucleus and induces synthesis of mediator proteins (e.g. metabolic enzymes and lipocortin). The binding of steroid hormones to their receptors causes changes in gene transcription and cell function. Corticosteroids reduce the inflammatory reaction by limiting capillary dilatation and vascular permeability.

4b Explain the terms 'glucocorticoid' and 'mineralocorticoid' activity. Give an example of one drug associated with each activity.

Glucocorticoid activity refers to anti-inflammatory, immunosuppressive and metabolic activities (e.g. diabetes). Dexamethasone shows significant glucocorticoid activity. Mineralocorticoid refers to the effects on both fluid and salt balance (e.g. sodium and water retention, potassium loss). Fludrocortisone (Florinef) shows marked mineralocorticoid activity.

5a How should the Betnovate scalp application be applied?

Initially apply to the affected area of the scalp both morning and evening. After removing the cap, the nozzle of the bottle should be placed on the affected area of the scalp. The bottle should be gently squeezed until the affected area is covered with a thin layer of the liquid, which may be rubbed into the scalp. The scalp will begin to feel cold as the liquid evaporates to leave the active ingredient. Wash hands after use.

5b List the excipients that are contained within Betnovate scalp application. Explain the possible role for each excipient.

Betnovate scalp application is an aqueous suspension and contains carbomer, isopropyl alcohol, sodium hydroxide and purified water. Carbomer is a thickening agent and it is used to increase the stability of suspension/emulsion formulations. Isopropyl alcohol is often used in topical formulations. It may be used as a solvent or as a disinfectant (if >70% concentration). Sodium hydroxide would be used to adjust the pH of the formulation, specifically in this case to neutralise the carbomer polymer and therefore increase viscosity. Purified water is used as a solvent.

5c The Summary of Product Characteristics for Betnovate scalp application states that it contains betamethasone valerate BP 0.122% w/w. Calculate the total amount in grams (to three decimal places) of betamethasone in 100 g of the formulation. The formula and molecular weight for betamethsone valerate are $C_{27}H_{37}FO_6$ and 476.577 g/mol respectively. The formula and molecular weight for betamethasone are $C_{22}H_{29}FO_5$ and 392.461 g/mol respectively.

Betamethasone valerate BP 0.122% w/w means 0.122 g of the salt, betamethasone valerate, in 100 g of the formulation. The weight of betamethasone can be calculated as follows:

0.122 g of betamethasone valerate $\equiv$ 476.577 g/mol
Let x g of betamethasone $\equiv$ 392.461 g/mol
Therefore x g = 0.122 g $\times$ (392.461/476.577) = 0.1004 g

To three decimal places is 0.100 g of betamethasone.

5d Clenil-Modulite contains beclometasone (as dipropionate). Betnovate scalp application contains betamethasone (as valerate). Explain, using the chemical formulas shown in Figure A12.2, the difference in log P values between beclometasone and their respective salts.

Betamethasone valerate and beclometasone dipropionate both mask the polar hydroxyl groups to increase lipophilicity. This increases the topical penetration for topical formulations used in eczema and psoriasis and aerosol formulations used in asthma. The log $P_{\text{octanol/pH7}}$ value of betamethasone is 2.01, whereas the log $P_{\text{octanol/pH7}}$ value for betamethasone (as valerate) is 3.60.

6a Beclometasone (as dipropionate) is a pro-drug. Define the term 'pro-drug' and explain the pharmacodynamics involved.

Beclometasone (as dipropionate) is a pro-drug with weak glucocorticoid receptor-binding activity. It is hydrolysed via esterase enzymes to the active metabolite beclometasone-17-monopropionate (B-17-MP), which has high topical anti-inflammatory activity.

6b How is beclometasone (as dipropionate) metabolised? State the metabolites involved.

Beclometasone (as dipropionate) undergoes extensive first-pass metabolism and is rapidly excreted from the systemic circulation. The main active metabolite is beclometasone-17-monopropionate and the minor inactive metabolites are beclometasone-21-monopropionate and beclometasone.

6c   State the main excipients in Clenil-Modulite and briefly describe why they are used in this formulation.

Clenil-Modulite contains HFA-134a, ethanol and glycerol. The propellant 1,1,1,2-tetrafluoroethane (HFA-134a) is a non-chlorofluorocarbon (CFC). Ethanol is commonly used in pharmaceutical formulations as a solvent and can act as a preservative and skin penetrant. Glycerol acts as a humectant, preservative and increases formulation viscosity.

7   Discuss both the systemic and local adverse effects associated with using corticosteroids, giving examples of each. What factors increase the risk of adverse effects and why?

Adverse effects of corticosteroids may be classified as either systemic or local. Systemic side-effects are due to hypothalamus-pituitary-adrenal (HPA) suppression which may lead to Cushing's syndrome. However systemic side-effects are most likely to occur with very potent corticosteroids used in large quantities for a prolonged period. These adverse effects are more likely to occur in young children (large surface area in relation to body weight) or if an occlusive dressing (increases drug absorption) is used. Other adverse effects may include gastrointestinal disturbance, musculoskeletal effects, neuropsychiatric effects, and ophthalmic effects.

Local side-effects may include skin thinning, skin 'burning' sensation and irritation. Factors that may increase the risk of skin thinning again include using very potent corticosteroids in large quantities for a prolonged period, thin skin and flexural areas and occlusive dressings. Other adverse effects may include striae (stretch marks), blood vessel dilation, bruising and discoloration.

8a   Mr DP's worsening symptoms are probably due to a bacterial infection. What is the most common cause of bacterial infected eczema?

Staphylococcus aureus is the most common cause of bacterial infected eczema as 90% of atopic eczema patches are colonised by this organism.

8b   What is the recommended first-line treatment for bacterial infected eczema?

Flucloxacillin is recommended as first-line oral antibiotics. If the patient is allergic to penicillins, then erythromycin is prescribed.

Case study level Mb – Psoriasis – see page 301

1a   What is psoriasis? What are the different types of psoriasis? (In your answer focus on topical psoriasis.)

Psoriasis is a chronic immune system disease affecting the skin and joints. It is most commonly associated with inflammation of the skin and is characterised by hyperproliferation (thickening) of dermal keratinocytes. The most common form of psoriasis is plaque psoriasis (psoriasis vulgaris), which accounts for approximately 80% of all cases of psoriasis. It is characterised by the presence of raised, inflamed lesions, red in colour and covered in a silvery-white scale. It is normally found on the knees, elbows, lower back and the groin, although it may spread to other parts of the body, particularly the scalp.

Erythrodermic psoriasis results in a widespread erythema that affects most of the body. It is often associated with pustular psoriasis. Oedema, particularly around the ankles, is common, as is excessive exfoliation of the skin and severe itching and/or pain.

Inverse psoriasis is similar to plaque psoriasis, although the reddened skin areas are not associated with a scaly plaque. It is associated with skin folds and in moist areas, including the axillae, beneath the breasts, groin and in skin folds.

Guttate psoriasis is more often associated with children or young adults. It is characterised by small, red spots (not as deep or large as plaque psoriasis) on the skin, usually on the trunk of the body. Its onset can be rapid and has been associated with infections, particularly of the upper respiratory tract, or as a side-effect of certain drugs, including beta-blockers.

Pustular psoriasis manifests itself as a series of white blisters, surrounded by reddened skin, which usually contain white blood cells. It is normally localised to the hands and feet. Normally the skin reddens and this is then followed by the formation of pustules and associated scaling.

It is typical for patients to have only one form of psoriasis at a time, although two or more forms can occur simultaneously.

1b   What causes psoriasis, and what are the risk factors?

The exact causes of psoriasis are unknown, although it is generally believed to be a disorder of the immune system. This manifests itself as psoriasis when T-cells abnormally trigger in the dermis, causing hyperproliferation of skin keratinocytes. This causes the skin to grow more rapidly than normal and, in the case of plaque psoriasis, causes the development of raised plaques on the skin surface. Recent research has indicated that psoriasis may have a genetic basis. Specifically, genes that regulate the human leucocyte antigen system have been implicated in an increased risk of psoriasis. The presence of the *HLA-Cw6* allele in patients is consistent with an increased risk of psoriasis.

Psoriasis is thought to be more likely if there is a history of it in a patient's family. However, there are also a range of other 'triggers' implicated in the development of psoriasis. It is commonly associated with emotional stresses in a patient's life, and often associated with deficiencies in the immune system. Plaque psoriasis has also been associated with injury to the skin, including sunburn (although moderate exposure to the sun has been shown to be beneficial in the treatment of psoriasis), skin infections or excessive scratching of the skin due to irritation or inflammation. Smokers and drinkers of alcohol (particularly middle-aged males) are also at increased risk of developing psoriasis, particularly plaque psoriasis. Hormonal changes, particularly during the menopause or the postpartum period, can also exacerbate the condition. Infections, particularly of the upper respiratory tract, have been associated with particular types of psoriasis (e.g. streptococcal infections and guttate psoriasis). Psoriasis has also been associated as being a side-effect of certain drug therapies, including beta-blockers, antimalarials and antidepressants. The use of NSAIDs is often avoided in patients with psoriasis. HIV infection can worsen the effects of psoriasis.

1c   Given the description of Mr GM, which type(s) of psoriasis do you think he has?

Mr GM is most likely suffering from plaque psoriasis. There is evidence to suggest that he may also have suffered from erythrodermic psoriasis.

1d   Is Mr GM at risk of developing any further types of psoriasis, or any related illnesses?

Mr GM's psoriasis has worsened. It was initially characterised by extensive reddening of the skin (which was possibly erythrodermic psoriasis) but it has progressed to a plaque psoriasis. It has failed to respond effectively to treatment so, while it is unlikely that other types of psoriasis will develop, the plaque psoriasis has, and continues to, spread across his body. However, given the drug therapies and issues of Mr GM's compliance, it is possible that initial plaque psoriasis has deteriorated into more unstable forms of the disease, such as erythrodermic psoriasis.

2a   What type of medicaments are used to treat psoriasis at each of the stages of therapy, i.e. (i) topical therapies, (ii) phototherapies, (iii) combination therapies, (iv) systemic drug therapies (i.e. oral and i.v.)?

Psoriasis has no known cure, so all the therapies listed below are used to control the spread of the disease, or to lessen its extent.

The first line of treatment is usually the application of topical products, ranging from over-the-counter products to topical steroids. Emollients may be used to reduce dryness and scaling, as well as reducing the hyperproliferation associated with plaque psoriasis. The use of vitamin D analogues, tazarotene, dithranol or coal tar preparations aims to lessen or remove the patient's scaly plaques. However, excess use can irritate the skin and their use is not recommended for the more irritant forms of psoriasis. Tar baths and tar shampoos (containing coal tar) may help with managing the condition. Treatment, if non-irritating, should be continued for 4–6 weeks and thereafter assessed. Emollients may also be used in the treatment of erythrodermic or pustular psoriasis. They should be used copiously and frequently. Inflammatory psoriasis should be treated with emollients or mild to moderate corticosteroids. Analogues of vitamin D, such as calcipotriol and tacalcitol, affect cell division and differentiation. They normally irritate less than other vitamin D analogues and are less likely to suffer from problems of cosmetic/social acceptability that affect coal tar products. Dithranol is used for chronic plaque psoriasis. It may be irritating to individual patients so its use needs to be carefully and frequently monitored, starting with low concentrations of the drug, as treatment commences. The strength of treatment can be increased on a daily basis from 0.1% to 3.0%, or to a tolerable level for the patient. It may also stain the skin and clothes, and its application to non-psoriatic skin, particularly on the face or scalp may cause irritation. Tazarotene is also effective, but irritation is common and as such should be used sparingly, if at all appropriate, and its use on normal, healthy skin should be avoided.

Topical corticosteroids are usually given in combination with other topical treatments for the treatment of chronic plaque psoriasis. Sensitive areas, such as the face, should be treated with a mild corticosteroid and other areas, such as the scalp, with moderate to potent corticosteroids. In general, use should be maintained as early improvements in the condition are not maintained if use is halted. Such a pattern of use may worsen the condition, possibly causing a deterioration of the condition to unstable forms, such as erythrodermic or pustular psoriasis. Co-administration of topical medicaments usually involves alternating administration of each product. Scalp psoriasis is normally treated with softening emollients in combination with salicylic acid with coal tar or sulphur.

If topical therapies are unsuccessful, they may be considered in combination with other therapies, including phototherapy or systemic drug therapy.

Phototherapy involves exposing the skin to specific wavelengths of non-ionising electromagnetic (ultraviolet) light with or without the use of exogenous (systemic) photosensitisers to facilitate treatment. Mechanistically, phototoxicity or the photochemical alteration of extracellular metabolites are likely, and result in a reduction of the rate of abnormal cell growth. Superficially, both techniques have many similarities. However, their mechanisms of action are fundamentally different and may affect long-term benefits and risks to patients. Normally, treatment involves UVB phototherapy, where the skin is exposed to artificial UVB light for a set duration. This may be used with or without topical emollients or drugs. Usually, the patient is required to prepare for treatment by bathing for up to 30 minutes prior to treatment. Sensitive skin areas, such as the neck, lips, backs of hands and pigmented areas of the torso, are normally protected during treatment. This treatment normally takes place in a clinic, although home treatment is increasing. Alternatively, psoralen photochemotherapy (PUVA) may be used. It involves the oral or topical administration of the psoralen, which facilitates and enhances the photoactivity of the UVA.

Treatment is usually stopped after the plaques have disappeared. If the plaques reappear, patients are advised to recommence treatment three times a week.

Systemic drug therapy is normally used only where the above treatments have failed to improve the condition of plaque psoriasis, or for unstable forms of psoriasis. Treatments include acitretin or drugs that act on the immune system, such as ciclosporin or methotrexate. Their use is rare in psoriasis treatment due to the possibility of rebound deterioration when the dose is reduced. Acitretin also poses a risk of teratogenicity up to 2 years after ceasing administration, and causes reversible irritation and damage to epithelial cells, manifesting itself in the form of dry and cracked lips, dry skin and mucosa, and thinning hair. Use of acitretin also requires monitoring of liver function.

2b Mr GM is currently being treated with acitretin, and the topical application of emollients. How would you counsel him on their side-effects and use?

Acitretin causes reversible irritation and damage to epithelial cells, manifesting itself in the form of dry and cracked lips, dry skin and mucosa, and thinning hair. Use of acitretin also requires regular monitoring of liver function. Social and cosmetic issues are associated with some emollients, including salicylic acid and in particular coal tar preparations. This can result in reduced compliance and a prolonging or worsening of the condition.

2c How may side-effects affect the compliance of the patient in this case? In particular, focus on the patient's analgesic use, and review how this may affect the proposed systemic drug therapy.

Mr GM took NSAIDs to alleviate the pain and irritation associated with his psoriasis. NSAIDs, such as ibuprofen and indometacin, have been shown to exacerbate psoriasis. Mr GM should be appropriately counselled in his use of pain medication. Further, the patient has failed to give treatment enough time to work in the past, citing associated pain and irritation of his condition. This may be due to the patient's use of ibuprofen, but also to the premature cessation of treatment. The patient should be counselled with regard to the duration of the treatments, and to the possible exacerbation of his condition should he cease treatment too soon. The provision of systemic drugs should be given with caution as, for example, premature cessation of systemic corticosteroid therapy will result in rebound deterioration of the condition.

Notes: Drugs associated with the exacerbation of psoriasis include lithium, beta-adrenergic receptor blocking agents and antimalarials. Withdrawal of corticosteroid therapy may activate pustular psoriasis. NSAIDs, such as ibuprofen or indometacin, have been reported to worsen psoriasis. Drugs used for the treatment of psoriasis will sometimes cause a flare-up due to irritation, phototoxicity or hypersensitivity reactions which usually result in a Koebner phenomenon. Psoriasis is a very complex and unpredictable disease to manage, and as such systematic and meaningful clinical studies on adverse drug effects on psoriasis have been difficult to conduct.

3a   Review the stages of treatment, including formulations and their administration, available for psoriasis. Evaluate the treatment provided to the patient and suggest any issues in the previous treatment regimen.

The main issue with treatment has been the use of NSAIDs and the premature ending of particular treatments by the patient. Compliance therefore is an issue, and may impact upon the choice of treatment. Treatment has progressed as the disease has spread and the seriousness of the therapies administered may be confused due to compliance issues and the side-effects of NSAID use. Review the extent of the latter and counsel on issues related to the former.

3b   Discuss a suitable long-term care plan for Mr GM. Clearly addressing the goals of therapy, discuss how this plan will be monitored and how compliance will be assured. Address long-term care issues and discuss possible alternative treatments available to Mr GM.

The main issues associated with treatment are compliance and management of side-effects. Mr GM has not tolerated previous treatments well, and this, along with the use of particular over-the-counter analgesics, may have reduced the effectiveness of his therapy. His condition has worsened and systemic therapy with or without PUVA treatment is the next step in treatment. There is substantial evidence to suggest that long-term oral/systemic therapy can be tolerated by the vast majority of patients. Mr GM has also been intolerant of completing previous therapies and monitoring of such a care plan should be attempted by his pharmacist.

The goals of therapy are to see an improvement in the condition of his psoriasis using a treatment regimen that is compliant with the patient's social needs.

Monitoring is by regular contact with his pharmacist and possibly a dietician, to review how the treatment is progressing and how compliant the patient is with his treatment. Unfortunately, a lot of the treatments or treatment options are experimental, and may or may not work, so the patient is to be encouraged to persist with a recommended treatment as long as possible and to not finish treatment early.

One possibility is that the original treatment which Mr GM did not complete should be attempted again.

3c   Are there any other treatments available to Mr GM?

'Alternative' treatments for psoriasis are of increasing popularity. In light of possible compliance issues, Mr GM might be able to use such treatments in combination with pharmaceutical intervention and improve his condition.

A number of alternative approaches have been cited as being beneficial in the treatment of psoriasis. These range from the use of Chinese medicine, particularly acupuncture and diet-based approaches, to homeopathy. Little evidence is available to substantiate the claims often made for these approaches to treatment. 'Natural' topical treatments have also been suggested, including the use of capsaicin, tea tree oil (while bathing), evening primrose oil (orally or topically) and aloe vera. The claims for such products are variable and inconsistent, although a randomised, double-blind clinical trial indicated that 0.5% w/w aloe vera extract was significantly better than placebo in treating psoriasis.

Diet has been indicated as a possible trigger for psoriasis, and several diet regimens have been suggested. These include low-protein, high-carbohydrate or starvation diets. The evidence for their success is variable, although it has been demonstrated clinically that patients with antibodies to gliadin can see an improvement in their condition by adopting a gluten-free diet. Although the use of dietary supplements is also suggested to help alleviate the symptoms of psoriasis, their use has not been quantitatively proven. In some cases they can exacerbate the condition, for example in the case of St John's wort, which can influence levels of ciclosporin and cause sensitivity to light. The latter in particular can have a significant impact on UV treatments.

'Physical' alternatives, including massage (specifically for psoriatic arthritis) and sun and water therapies, are increasingly used alongside conventional treatments for psoriasis patients. Again, their efficacy is currently unproven.

13

Immunology case studies

Niall McMullan

Case study level 1 – Tetanus

Learning outcomes

Level 1 case study: You will be able to:

- describe the risk factors
- describe the disease
- describe the pharmacology of the drug
- outline the formulation, including drug molecule, excipients, etc. for the medicines
- summarise basic social pharmacy issues (e.g. opening containers, large labels).

Scenario

Ms AR and her son, a boisterous 5-year-old boy, come into your pharmacy for the first time, seeking advice about a gash junior had sustained on his shoulder a few days earlier. The boy had sustained the wound after falling from a tree in a nearby field. There had been some soil in the wound, and although Ms AR had cleaned the area and applied some antiseptic cream, the skin around the area lacked vitality. You suspected a possible tetanus infection and advised her to see her GP. The family had moved around a lot in junior's short life and it was established that he had never been immunised against tetanus. Some days later, Ms AR informed you that junior had been given an anti-tetanus and was due to start a course of immunisations.

1a What is tetanus?
1b What are the risk factors for developing tetanus?
2   What is human tetanus immunoglobulin (anti-tetanus immunoglobulin)?
3   How does human tetanus immunoglobulin work?
4   What additional advice should be given to Ms AR?

General references

Mimms CA, Playfair J, Roitt IM *et al.* (1998) *Medical Microbiology*, 2nd edn. London: Mosby.

Therapy Areas (2008) Immunoglobulins. Summary of product and patient information leaflet. Available at http://www.bpl.co.uk/public/therapy_areas/immunoglobulins/tetanus.asp [Accessed 2 July 2008].

Case study level 2 – Idiopathic thrombocytopenic purpura

Learning outcomes

Level 2 case study: You will be able to:

- interpret relevant lab and clinical data
- identify monitoring and referral criteria
- explain treatment choices
- describe goals of therapy, including monitoring and the role of the pharmacist/clinician
- describe issues – counselling points, adverse drug reactions, drug interactions, complementary/alternative therapies and lifestyle advice.

You have received a hospital prescription from the paediatric unit for human normal immunoglobulin (HNIG) for i.v. injection. The patient, Master OB, is a 5-year-old boy, height 110 cm and weight 19 kg. He has a history of bruising and started bleeding from his gums following routine dental hygiene. His dentist referred him due to concerns about the bleeding. The clinical history also reveals pinpoint-sized reddish-purple spots on the boy's legs. Haematological tests showed platelet levels of 120×10^9/L, but other blood cell numbers were normal. The doctor has prescribed a single dose (i.v.) of 15 g of HNIG. Master OB is in good form and can be heard singing merrily throughout the corridors.

Questions

1   What is idiopathic thrombocytopenic purpura (ITP)?
2   What are the signs and symptoms of ITP?
3   What laboratory findings confirm a diagnosis of ITP?
4a   How is ITP treated?
4b   What is human normal immunoglobulin?
4c   What other aspects of HNIG administration should be considered?
5   What advice should be given about the use of HNIG?
6   How might ITP affect lifestyle?

General references

British Committee for Standards in Haematology (2003) Guidelines for the investigation and management of idiopathic thrombocytic purpura in adults, children and in pregnancy. *British Journal of Haematology* 120: 574–596.

Joint Formulary Committee (2008) *British National Formulary* 55. London: British Medical Association and Royal Pharmaceutical Society of Great Britain, March.

Wells JV (2001) Haematologic diseases. In: *Medical Immunology*, 10th edn. New York: McGraw-Hill, pp. 434–450.

Case study level 3 – Chronic granulomatous disease

Learning outcomes

Level 3 case study: You will be able to:

- interpret clinical signs and symptoms
- evaluate laboratory data
- evaluate treatment options
- state goals of therapy
- describe a pharmaceutical care plan to include advice to a clinician
- describe the prognosis and long-term complications
- describe the social pharmacy issues which could include supply (e.g. complex treatments at home, concordance and compliance) and lifestyle issues.

You receive a request for interferon gamma for subcutaneous injection, three times weekly. The patient, Master CG is 18 months old, 80 cm tall, weighs 10 kg and has been admitted to the paediatric unit, following referral by his GP. The child has a history of recurrent bacterial infections, complicated with a fungal infection and has been on both prophylactic antibacterial regimens and therapeutic regimens of antibiotics and antifungal drugs. The child is now experiencing a sustained episode of infections, skin lesions are apparent on his face and other parts of his body and he has a tender abdomen.

1   What is chronic granulomatous disease?
2   What are the pathogenetic factors associated with chronic granulomatous disease?
3   What is the laboratory diagnosis of chronic granulomatous disease?
4a   What is the treatment strategy for chronic granulomatous disease?
4b   How should the dose of interferon gamma be calculated for a child such as Master CG?
4c   What is interferon gamma?
5a   What adverse reactions are associated with interferon gamma treatment?
5b   How is the response to interferon gamma treatment monitored?
6a   What additional advice should be given?
6b   What is the prognosis for Master CG?

General references

Assari T (2006) Review. Chronic granulomatous disease; fundamental stages in our understanding of CGD. *Medical Immunology* 5: 4. Available at http://www.medimmunol.com/content/5/1/4 [Accessed 2 July 2008].

Roberts RL and Stiehm ER (2001) Phagocytic dysfunction diseases. In: *Medical Immunology*, 10th edn. New York: McGraw-Hill, pp. 333–340.

Summary of Product Characteristics (2008) Immukin. Available at http://emc.medicines.org.uk/emc/assets/c/html/displaydoc.asp?documentid=312 [Accessed 2 July 2008].

Case study level Ma – Chronic hepatitis B infection

Learning outcomes

Level M case study: You will be able to:

- interpret clinical signs and symptoms
- evaluate laboratory data
- critically appraise treatment options
- state goals of therapy
- describe a pharmaceutical care plan to include advice to a clinician
- describe the prognosis and long-term complications
- describe the social pharmacy issues which could include supply (e.g. complex treatments at home, concordance and compliance) and lifestyle issues
- monitoring of therapy.

Scenario

Mr JJ has a prescription for interferon alfa in pre-filled injection pens, 15 million units per mL available as 1.5-mL cartridges. He is 27-years-old and was an intravenous drug user for 9 years. He is well known to you, having been a frequent visitor to your pharmacy for some years. Mr JJ is of slight build, 180 cm in height, weight 55 kg. He has been 'clean' for several months but has been in hospital recently due to serious health problems. Laboratory tests showed increased levels of serum alanine aminotransferase (ALT), antibodies to hepatitis B_e antigen (HB_eAg) and DNA polymerase activity.

Questions

1a What is hepatitis B infection?
1b What are the risk factors for developing hepatitis B virus (HBV) infection?
2 How is HBV infection diagnosed?
3 How can hepatitis B infection be prevented?
4a What is interferon alfa and how does it work in the management of HBV infection?
4b What formulations of interferon alfa are available?
5 What additional treatments are used for chronic hepatitis B infection and how do they act?
6 How should interferon alfa treatment be monitored?
7 What additional advice should be given?

General references

Mills J (2001) Viral infections. In: Parlow TG, Stites DP, Terr IA and Imboden JB (eds) *Medical Immunology*, 10th edn. New York: McGraw-Hill, pp. 617–635
Mohanty SR, Kupfer SS and Khiani V (2006) Treatment of chronic hepatitis B. *Nature Clinical Practice Gastroenterology and Hepatology* 3: 446–458.
NICE (National Institute for Health and Clinical Excellence) (2006) Guidance on the use of adefovir dipivoxil and pegylated interferon alpha-2b for the treatment of chronic hepatitis B. Available at http://www.nice.org.uk/guidance/TA96 [Accessed 2 July 2008].

Case study level Mb – Rheumatoid arthritis

Learning outcomes

Level M case study: You will be able to:

- interpret clinical signs and symptoms
- evaluate laboratory data
- critically appraise treatment options
- state goals of therapy
- describe a pharmaceutical care plan to include advice to a clinician
- describe the prognosis and long-term complications
- describe the social pharmacy issues which could include supply (e.g. complex treatments at home, concordance and compliance) and lifestyle issues
- describe the monitoring of therapy.

Scenario

Ms RR is 32 years of age and has been visiting your pharmacy for 2 years. She is approximately 150 cm in height and weighs approximately 55 kg. Her fingers appear swollen at the knuckles and her hands appear slightly deformed. In the time you have known her, she had complained of stiffness in her fingers and wrists, especially in the mornings, and now her mobility appears to have diminished. She has been taking ibuprofen for that time. In the last year, Ms RR had been on methotrexate and sulfasalazine. Recent laboratory findings indicate an erythrocyte sedimentation rate (ESR) of 85 mm/hour, the presence of rheumatoid factor (RF) in serum and normochromic, normocytic anaemia. She is now presenting with a prescription for etanercept. The drug is to be administered as a 25-mg dose by subcutaneous injection, twice weekly.

Questions

1 What is rheumatoid arthritis?
2 What are the predisposing factors associated with rheumatoid arthritis?
3 What are the laboratory findings associated with rheumatoid arthritis?
4a How is rheumatoid arthritis treated?
4b What are TNF-α inhibitors?
5 When would etanercept be prescribed and is it appropriate for Ms RR?
6 What type of preparation is etanercept?
7 How should the response to etanercept be monitored?
8 What advice should you give Ms RR?

General references

Arthritis Research Campaign (2008) Physiotherapy and arthritis: an information sheet. Available at http://www.arc.org.uk/about_arth/infosheets/6256/6256.htm [Accessed on 2 July 2008].

Ledingham J and Deighton C (2005) Update on the British Society for Rheumatology guidelines for prescribing TNFa blockers in adults with rheumatoid arthritis (update of previous guideline of April 2001). *Rheumatology* 44: 157–163.

NICE (National Institute for Health and Clinical Excellence) (2007) Adalimumab, etanercept and infliximab for the treatment of rheumatoid arthritis. Available at http://www.nice.org.uk/nicemedia/pdf/TA130guidance.pdf [Accessed 2 July 2008].

Sullivan JT, Ni L, Sheelo C *et al.* 2006) Bioequivalence of liquid and reconstituted lyophilized etanercept subcutaneous injections. *Journal of Clinical Pharmacology* 46: 654.

Answers

Case study level 1 – Tetanus – see page 320

1a   What is tetanus?

Tetanus is a condition characterised by prolonged, involuntary contraction of the skeletal muscles. The condition can be localised or generalised. Tetanus is caused by the bacterium *Clostridium tetani*, an obligate, anaerobic, Gram-positive rod-shaped bacterium. The pathogen produces an exotoxin called tetanospasmin. Tetanospasmin is a potent neurotoxin which blocks neurotransmitter release from inhibitory neurons resulting in muscular contractions. *C. tetani* is not an invasive microbe, rather the spread of the toxin is due to tetanospasmin entering neurons via neuromuscular junctions and travelling to the spinal cord where it blocks the inhibitory neurons. Clinical signs typically present within 7 days post infection. Initially, the upper part of the body is affected first, most notably the facial muscles, resulting in 'lockjaw'. Untreated, tetanus may result in death.

1b   What are the risk factors for developing tetanus?

Infection usually occurs when spores of *C. tetani* are introduced into a wound from contaminated soil, farmyard manure or rusty metals. Burns more than 6 hours old are susceptible to infection. Tissues typically show devitalised areas around the wound site.

2   What is human tetanus immunoglobulin (anti-tetanus immunoglobulin)?

Human tetanus immunoglobulin is a solution of human immunoglobulin G (IgG) containing a high level of anti-tetanus toxin antibodies. It is prepared from the plasma of screened, human donors immunised against tetanus toxin and is administered by intramuscular injection. The product also contains iso-tonic sodium chloride, glycine, as a stabiliser, sodium acetate and a small amount of sodium hydroxide used to maintain pH. The product is generally well-tolerated.

3   How does human tetanus immunoglobulin work?

The anti-tetanus antibodies bind specifically to tetanus toxin and neutralise the toxin by inhibiting its binding to neuromuscular receptors. This product is used in cases where there is a likely risk of tetanus infection or where clinical tetanus is observed. Human tetanus immunoglobulin should be administered as soon as possible after possible infection.

4   What additional advice should be given to Ms AR?

Anti-tetanus immunoglobulin is an example of passive immunisation (refer to 'Immunoglobulins' in *BNF* for other examples). It is designed to give immediate, short-term protection. It does not confer long-term immunity to tetanus and Ms.AR should be advised that her son should be immunised with the tetanus vaccine at an appropriate time. A full course of the tetanus vaccine should ensure protection for several years.

Case study level 2 – Idiopathic thrombocytopenic purpura – see page 321

1   What is idiopathic thrombocytopenic purpura (ITP)?

Idiopathic thrombocytopenic purpura, also referred to as immune thrombocytopenic purpura, is a bleeding disorder characterised by destruction of platelets. Antiplatelet autoantibodies are present, suggesting an autoimmune aetiology. These antibodies label the platelets for destruction by macrophages in the spleen. The condition may be acute or chronic. Acute ITP is the most common form and is found most often in children. Some cases are associated with recent viral infections and immunisations, notably the measles, mumps, rubella (MMR) vaccine. Typically, the disease is transient with no evidence of vaccine-associated recurrence. The peak incidence occurs between the ages of 2 and 6 years. Typically, acute ITP resolves within six months. Chronic ITP persists for longer than six months and is most often associated with adults between 20 and 30 years of age. Cases of chronic ITP may develop in children over the age of 10.

2   What are the signs and symptoms of ITP?

The signs of ITP include: sudden appearance of petechiae (small, pinpoint-sized reddish-purple spots), usually on the lower legs due to bleeding into the skin; easy or excessive bruising; spontaneous gingival or nasal bleeding and bleeding in the gastrointestinal tract (blood appears in stools) or genitourinary tract (blood in urine). Bleeding from small cuts may be prolonged. Excessive bleeding requires emergency treatment. Most patients appear well and do not report any sensation of being unwell.

3   What laboratory findings confirm a diagnosis of ITP?

Laboratory diagnosis is confirmed by persistent, low levels of platelets (thrombocytopenia), typically $<150 \times 10^9$/L (normal reference range $150–450 \times 10^9$/L). A full blood count should be performed and this should not show any other abnormalities. Antiplatelet antibody tests may be performed but the latter may occur in other conditions so are not truly diagnostic. White and red blood cell counts are typically normal. Thrombocytopenia with the associated signs, and the general feeling of well-being, are usually confirmatory. However, thrombocytopenia may be associated with serious bone marrow disorders. Typically these are accompanied by a feeling of illness, but must still be eliminated from the diagnosis. Secondary causes, such as systemic lupus erythematosus, drug-induced thrombocytopenia and anti-HIV antibodies due to HIV infection should be investigated and eliminated.

4a   How is ITP treated?

In children, acute ITP is often self-resolving and observation may be all that is necessary. Corticosteroid treatment, oral prednisolone at 1 mg/kg body weight per day for 2–4 weeks, is the first-line therapeutic approach. Where active treatment is required, due to ongoing clinical episodes, such as prolonged bleeding, i.v. injection of human normal immunoglobulin (HNIG) is the preferred treatment. Normal dose of i.v. Ig is 0.8 g/kg for 1 or 2 days. A 5-day course may be used (0.4 g/kg). Either regimen typically achieves the goal of increasing platelet numbers. In some instances, repeat courses may be necessary. HNIG should NOT be administered by intramuscular or subcutaneous injection in ITP patients because of the risk of bleeding.

4b   What is human normal immunoglobulin?

Human normal immunoglobulin (HNIG) is prepared from screened, human plasma. The antibody fraction is extensively purified and contains immunoglobulins in glycine. Some products may contain sorbitol (refer to product information). HNIG is also used to treat possible infections as it contains antibodies to infectious pathogens against which the donors have been immunised.

4c   What other aspects of HNIG administration should be considered?

HNIG is supplied at various concentrations with recommended volumes given to achieve the required dosage. Depending on the formulation available, the actual volume required may vary. Where large volumes are required, the solution should be left to stand at room temperature prior to injection.

5   What advice should be given about the use of HNIG?

HNIG may interfere with immunisations, either recent or those scheduled in the next few weeks. Before administration of HNIG, patient history should be checked for adverse reactions to other blood products and excipients. Any side-effects should be reported immediately to your doctor. Side-effects include chills, fever, malaise and rarely anaphylaxis.

In the most severe of cases, where HNIG does not achieve normal platelet numbers and corticosteroids are inappropriate or ineffective, a splenectomy may be advised. This is rarely performed in children as the condition normally resolves spontaneously within six months. Where splenectomy is performed, the patient is more susceptible to infection but serious infections are rarely a problem in otherwise healthy individuals.

6   How might ITP affect lifestyle?

Although ITP usually resolves in children, physical activities should be avoided where there is a risk of impact injuries or cuts until the condition has resolved.

Case study level 3 – Chronic granulomatous disease – see page 322

1   What is chronic granulomatous disease?

Chronic granulomatous disease (CGD) is a condition characterised by recurrent, bacterial and fungal infections. CGD is rare, the incidence being 1 in 250 000, with 80% of patients being male children. Clinical presentation is typically first observed between the first 2–5 years of life. The most common presentations include; skin infections, pneumonia, lung abscesses, enteritis and enlarged liver, spleen and lymph nodes. Granulomas are often formed in the skin, gastro-intestinal and genitourinary tracts. These granulomas may be obstructive. Gastrointestinal granulomas may cause abdominal pain, dysphagia and vomiting. Granulomas in the genitourinary tract may cause urine retention. Patients often present with infections caused by opportunistic, normally non-pathogenic, microorganisms. People with CGD are particularly at risk from catalase-positive microbes such as *Staphylococcus aureus*.

2   What are the pathogenetic factors associated with chronic granulomatous disease?

The primary cause of this condition is an inherited defect in phagocytic cells. The disorder is usually inherited as an X-linked disorder although an autosomal recessive inheritance may be the cause in one-third of cases. Genetic screening of family members helps to identify the likely type of inheritance. The defect is in a gene encoding the components of the phagocyte-oxidase system, namely cytochrome b_{588}. As a result, the phagocytes are unable to produce superoxide anions that are central to the killing of microbial pathogens.

3   What is the laboratory diagnosis of chronic granulomatous disease?

The most common laboratory diagnostic is the nitroblue tetrazolium (NBT) test which detects impaired function, inability to produce reactive oxygen species, in isolated leucocytes. Female carriers may be identified by this test.

4a   What is the treatment strategy for chronic granulomatous disease?

CGD patients receive daily prophylaxis of bacterial infections with tri-methoprim–sulfamethoxazole. In patients with active bacterial infections, initial parenteral administration of more aggressive antibiotic therapies are pursued. Fungal infections are treated with antifungal agents, notably itraconazole. Interferon gamma is recommended for treatment during severe infectious episodes. The drug increases leucocyte killing of microbes. Interferon gamma (recombinant) is administered by subcutaneous injection at a dose of 50 micro-grams/m², three times a week in children with a body surface area (BSA) greater than 0.5 m² or at 1.5 micrograms/kg in patients with a body surface of less than 0.5 m² (refer to *BNF*).

4b How should the dose of interferon gamma be calculated for a child such as Master CG?

The BSA for Master CG must be calculated. Various formulas have been proposed. The Haycock formula for calculating BSA in children is: BSA = 0.024265 × weight (kg)$^{0.5378}$ × height (cm)$^{0.3964}$. (The average BSA for a 2-year old child is 0.5 m².)

4c What is interferon gamma?

Interferon gamma belongs to the cytokine family of immunoregulatory molecules. The main cellular sources are T-helper cells and natural killer cells. Interferon gamma is a potent activator of macrophages and is important for the killing of intracellular pathogens, most notably mycobacterial pathogens. The formulation used is a recombinant form of interferon gamma in a preparation containing D-mannitol, disodium succinate hexahydrate, polysorbate 20, suc-cinic acid and water for injection. The product does not contain a preservative.

5a What adverse reactions are associated with interferon gamma treatment?

The most common adverse events include flu-like symptoms and skin rashes. More serious adverse effects are less common and are typically transient. The latter may include CNS toxicity and drug-induced anaemia.

5b How is the response to interferon gamma treatment monitored?

Monitoring typically involves observing the response of the infection by moni-toring symptoms and by microbiological laboratory assessment. As with all cytokine-based therapies, the patient should be monitored for blood cell counts, kidney and liver status.

6a What additional advice should be given?

Interferon gamma is usually given by a trained, healthcare professional. However, the treatment may be given at home. The preparation should be stored in a refrigerator and checked for cloudiness prior to injection. If the solu-tion is discoloured or cloudy, it should not be used. Do not shake the solution prior to use. The thighs or upper arms are the usual sites for injection and the site of injection should be varied to avoid tissue damage or irritation. The dosage instructions recommended by the doctor must be followed. Refer to patient information leaflet for additional information.

6b   What is the prognosis for Master CG?

Prognosis is variable depending on the type of CGD. The X-linked form is usually most severe and life expectancy may be 25–30 years. In other forms of the disease, normal life expectancy may not be reduced.

Case study level Ma – Chronic hepatitis B infection – see page 324

1a   What is hepatitis B infection?

Hepatitis B infection is caused by the viral pathogen, hepatitis B virus (HBV). HBV is a non-enveloped, double-stranded DNA virus belonging to the family, *hepadnaviridae*, class 7 (International Committee for the Taxonomy of Viruses). These viruses are unique in that they replicate via an RNA intermediate. The genomic DNA of progeny viruses is synthesised by reverse transcription of the RNA intermediate. HBV is a major cause of acute and chronic hepatitis and is also a major cause of hepatocellular carcinoma. Following infection, the virus replicates in hepatocytes. Liver damage occurs secondary to antiviral cellular immune responses. HBV is not cytopathic. The liver damage associated with infection is due to the immune response, in particular the action of specific cytotoxic T lymphocytes (CTLs). Acute infection may be self-limiting in the presence of anti-HBV antibodies directed towards the HBV surface protein (HBsAg). These antibodies label the viral particles for removal from the blood. HBV encodes a protein, pX, implicated in the progression of chronic hepatitis to hepatocellular carcinoma.

1b   What are the risk factors for developing hepatitis B virus (HBV) infection?

HBV transmission is predominantly through sexual contact, contaminated needles used for injection of drugs, contaminated blood products and by perinatal transmission from infected mothers to their newborn.

2   How is HBV infection diagnosed?

HBV infection, acute or chronic, is diagnosed initially by the detection of HBsAg in the blood of infected individuals. The presence of IgM antibodies to the HBV core antigen (anti-HBcAg-IgM) is indicative of acute infection. Chronic

HBV infection is diagnosed by the presence of anti-HBc antibodies, absence of anti-HBsAg antibodies and the presence of HBsAg in serum. HBeAg is indicative of active disease. Liver biopsy will show the presence of HBV DNA and liver damage, as indicated by elevated levels of serum alanine aminotransferases (ALTs).

3   How can hepatitis B infection be prevented?

Infection can be prevented by immunisation. The vaccine is a recombinant form of the HBsAg and induces strong neutralising antibody responses. High serum antibody titres to HBV are protective in the early stages of infection, effectively preventing establishment of disease.

4a   What is interferon alfa and how does it work in the management of HBV infection?

The cytokine interferon-alpha (IFN-α) belongs to the interferon family (includes IFN-β and IFN-γ). IFN-α is produced, *in vivo*, by leucocytes and inhibits viral replication and increases expression of HLA class I molecules, thus aiding presentation of viral peptides to cytotoxic T lymphocytes. IFN-α also activates natural killer (NK) cells, which destroy virally infected cells.

4b   What formulations of interferon alfa are available?

Therapeutic formulations contain a recombinant form of IFN-α (either interferon alfa-2a or interferon alfa-2b). These are available as powders for reconstitution or as prefilled injection pens. The drug is administered by subcutaneous injection (or intravenous for reconstituted powder formulations) and intramuscular injection. The dosage is usually stated as units per millilitre (refer to *BNF* for various preparations and dosages). Powder formulations of interferon alfa-2b also contain glycine, sodium phosphate (mono- and dibasic) and human albumin; prefilled pens contain sodium chloride, edetate disodium, polysorbate 80 and *m*-cresol as a preservative.

Interferon alfa-2a formulations contain excipients sodium chloride, polysorbate, ammonium acetate, and benzyl alcohol as a preservative. Interferon alfa is also approved for use in the treatment of several other disorders.

Peginterferon formulations are also available (polyethyleneglycol-conjugated interferon alfa). These have an extended serum half-life compared with non-conjugated forms.

5   What additional treatments are used for chronic hepatitis B infection and how do they act?

Interferon alfa should typically be used in combination with antiviral agents such as lamivudine or adefovir dipivoxil (refer to *BNF*), the first-line treatment for chronic hepatitis B infection. Lamivudine and adefovir dipivoxil belong to a class of antiviral compounds known as nucleoside analogues. These substances are incorporated into nascent DNA chains and prevent elongation of the viral DNA. In this sense, they are also referred to as 'chain terminators'.

6   How should interferon alfa treatment be monitored?

Mr JJ should be monitored regularly for efficacy. If there is no significant improvement in the condition, as determined by laboratory measurements of liver function (ALT test) and viral DNA load, then treatment with interferon alfa should be discontinued. In addition, white blood cell counts should be monitored, as should cardiovascular function. Fluid replacement may be required to correct hypotension.

7   What additional advice should be given?

The reported side-effects of interferon alfa include: cardiovascular problems such as arrhythmia, tachycardia and hypotension in the absence of history of such conditions, severe myelosuppression, depression and suicidal behaviour, opthalmic disorders, anorexia and 'flu-like' symptoms and hypersensitivity reactions. Mr JJ should be advised of these and of the actions to be taken. The patient should be informed that under no circumstances should he switch treatments as different formulations may contain different dosages. Furthermore, he should be made aware of the proper disposal of used pens/syringes and to take extra care if blood enters the dispensers, as described in the product literature. Hepatitis B support groups are available. Dietary advice may be offered as cytokine-based treatments often cause reduced appetite.

Case study level Mb – Rheumatoid arthritis – see page 325

1   What is rheumatoid arthritis?

Rheumatoid arthritis is a chronic, recurrent systemic inflammatory disorder that primarily affects the joints. The incidence is typically between 1% and 3% of the UK population with a female preponderance of 3:1. Age of onset is typically between the ages of 20 and 40 years. The small joints of the hands and feet are usually affected first and presentation is usually symmetrical. Deformities may arise and the condition may progress to larger joints. In the most severe of cases, extra-articular tissues may be affected, including the lungs, muscle tissues and blood vessels. Additional complications may include Sjögren's syndrome and Felty's syndrome.

2   What are the predisposing factors associated with rheumatoid arthritis?

The pathogenesis of rheumatoid arthritis is unclear, however there is a clear immunopathology in the progression of the disease. Possible initiating factors proposed include infection. Several first presentations occur following infections, although a clear link is difficult to establish. There may be some genetic predisposition, in particular, the HLA-DRB4 allele is more prevalent in the patient population than in the healthy population (relative risk 6.0). The HLA association suggests immunological involvement in the pathogenesis. This is further supported by the finding of rheumatoid factors – antibodies to the Fc region of IgG antibodies – in the synovial fluid of affected individuals. Experimental arthritis (collagen-induced arthritis) can be induced in laboratory animals immunised with certain collagen products. There is a suggestion that autoreactive T cells may respond to peptides derived from collagen. Activated macrophages are present in inflamed synovia along with elevated levels of the proinflammatory cytokines interleukin 1 (IL-1) and tumour necrosis factor-alpha (TNF-α).

3   What are the laboratory findings associated with rheumatoid arthritis?

Typically, serum and synovial fluid from patients contain rheumatoid factors (>80% of patients) although serum rheumatoid factors are found in other autoimmune disorders affecting connective tissues, and in some chronic infections. The presence of small joint involvement along with the presence of rheumatoid factors is usually taken as diagnostic, however other disorders, such as systemic lupus erythematosus, need to be eliminated by clinical presentation and associated laboratory observations.

4a   How is rheumatoid arthritis treated?

Initial treatment may involve exercise, under the observation of a physiotherapist, and the use of anti-inflammatory agents. The latter may include both non-steroidal anti-inflammatory drugs (NSAIDs) and corticosteroids. The latter are administered by intra-articular injection. The goals of such approaches are to maintain mobility (exercise) and pain relief. Most cases respond to the cytotoxic drug methotrexate (methotrexate is also classed alongside disease-modifying antirheumatic drugs – DMARDs). In addition, immunomodulatory drugs are being used increasingly in the treatment of rheumatoid arthritis. Specifically, these drugs are cytokine inhibitors that block the proinflammatory cytokine TNF-α.

4b   What are TNF-α inhibitors?

These drugs fall into two types: soluble TNF-α receptors, such as etanercept, and 'humanised' monoclonal antibodies against TNF-α. Etanercept is a fusion protein containing the extracellular domain of the TNF-α receptor. The drug binds soluble TNF-α *in vivo*, thus reducing or preventing TNF-α binding to endogenous receptors on the patients's cells. Anti-TNF-α antibodies bind free TNF-α and prevent the cytokine binding to the cell receptors.

5   When would etanercept be prescribed and is it appropriate for Ms RR?

Etanercept is prescribed where the physician feels that other treatments are not achieving the goals of giving pain relief and, indirectly, increased mobility. Cytokines typically have wide-ranging effects and inhibitors of such biomolecules must be treated with caution. Patients who obtain only partial relief on other treatments, or where the disease is not responding, may be recommended for treatment with TNF-α inhibitors. There is little evidence to suggest that switching from one type of TNF-α inhibitor (e.g. etanercept) to another (e.g. infliximab) brings any different outcome or additional benefit.

6   What type of preparation is etanercept?

Etanercept is available as a preservative-free powder for reconstitution or as a solution in prefilled syringes. The powder should be reconstituted in bacteriostatic water, containing 0.9% benzyl alcohol, to a final concentration of etanercept of 25 mg/mL. The prefilled syringes contain 25 mg or 50 mg etanercept in a 1% sucrose solution containing sodium phosphate, sodium chloride and L-arginine. Both preparations are administered by subcutaneous injection.

7   How should the response to etanercept be monitored?

Ms RR should be monitored for symptomatic relief, particularly joint mobility and pain. Laboratory monitoring should include erythrocyte-sedimentation rate (ESR) determination, a decrease in ESR approaching normal reference range (<20 mm/hour) indicates a positive response. Note: ESR values are variable and fluctuate in various disease states. They are not diagnostic for rheumatoid arthritis *per se*, but levels often correlate with disease severity.

8   What advice should you give Ms RR?

Ms RR should be familiar with the injection procedure and advised on how to store the drug and maintain sterility. There are several side-effects associated with the drug and the patient should be advised to read the patient information leaflet. Adverse effects, although uncommon, include itching, bleeding, nausea, fever, rash, chills and difficulty in breathing and swallowing. The most serious adverse effects include serious infections and some fatalities have been reported. Cases of tuberculosis (TB) have been reported and patients must be closely monitored for emergence of TB symptoms. There is a slight risk of cancer associated with TNF-α inhibitors.

The patient may benefit from physiotherapy and she should enquire at her local surgery or hospital. The Arthritis Research Campaign also publishes support information.

Note: Ms RR should be registered on the British Society for Rheumatology Biologics Register (BSRBR).

14

Liver disease case studies

Caron Weeks and Mark Tomlin

In this chapter Case studies levels 1–3 explore the management of a patient with alcoholic liver disease. The patient has alcoholic liver cirrhosis and first presents with alcohol withdrawal (Case study level 1), then the patient's risk of bleeding and treatment for the maintenance of alcohol abstinence are considered (Case study level 2). The patient then goes on to develop encephalopathy (Case study level 3). Case studies levels Ma and Mb consider two patients: one presents with TB and the other liver failure.

Case study level 1 – Alcoholic cirrhosis; alcohol withdrawal

Learning outcomes

Level 1 case study: You will be able to:

- describe the risk factors
- describe the disease
- describe the pharmacology of the drug
- outline the formulation, including drug molecule, excipients, etc. for the medicines
- summarise basic social pharmacy issues (e.g. opening containers, large labels).

Scenario

Mrs MW, 59 years old, is divorced and unemployed. She was admitted to an acute medical ward at the hospital presenting with general malaise, a grossly distended abdomen, swollen ankles and jaundice. It was also noted that she smelt of alcohol and was showing signs of alcohol withdrawal.

1   What is cirrhosis of the liver?
2   List possible causes of cirrhosis.
3   What other clinical signs and symptoms may Mrs MW present with?
4   What drug treatment, including dose, would you recommend for Mrs MW's alcohol withdrawal? What recommendations would you make if the patient was unable to take the medication orally?

General references

Schuppan D and Afdhal NH (2008) Liver cirrhosis. *Lancet* 371: 838–851.
Heidelbaugh JJ and Sherbondy M (2006) Cirrhosis and chronic liver failure: Part II. Complications and treatment. *American Family Physician* 74: 767–776.
Joint Formulary Committee (2008) *British National Formulary 55*. London: British Medical Association and Royal Pharmaceutical Society of Great Britain, March.
Vincent WR, Smith KM, Winstead PS and Lewis DA (2007) Review of alcohol withdrawal in the hospitalized patient: management. *Orthopedics* 30: 446–449.

Case study level 2 – Alcoholic cirrhosis; management of bleeding risk and treatment for the maintenance of alcohol abstinence

Learning outcomes

Level 2 case study: You will be able to:

- interpret relevant lab and clinical data
- identify monitoring and referral criteria
- explain treatment choices
- describe goals of therapy, including monitoring and the role of the pharmacist/clinician
- describe issues – counselling points, adverse drug reactions, drug interactions, complementary/alternative therapies and lifestyle advice.

Mrs MW, 59 years old, is divorced and unemployed. She was admitted to an acute medical ward at the hospital presenting with general malaise, a grossly distended abdomen, swollen ankles and jaundice. It was also noted that she smelt of alcohol and was showing signs of alcohol withdrawal.

Mrs MW weighs 61 kg (with the ascites) and her laboratory data are as follows:

Total protein	49 g/L (63–80 g/L)
Albumin	20 g/L (32–50 g/L)
Total bilirubin	114 micromol/L (<17 micromol/L)
ALP	382 IU/L (100–300 IU/L)
ALT	88 IU/L (5–42 IU/L)
INR	1.6
GGT	306 IU/L (<50 IU/L)

Diagnosis of alcoholic cirrhosis of the liver was made based on Mrs MW's clinical features, liver function tests, abdominal ultrasound, CT scan and liver biopsy.

Questions

1   Describe how Mrs MW's laboratory results relate to her diagnosis.
2   What treatment would you recommend to reduce her risk of bleeding?
3   What medications would you advise Mrs MW to avoid in view of her bleeding risk?
4   What treatment options are available to help Mrs MW abstain from alcohol in the future?

General references

Joint Formulary Committee (2008) *British National Formulary* 55. London: British Medical Association and Royal Pharmaceutical Society of Great Britain, March.

Mason P (2004) Blood tests used to investigate liver, thyroid or kidney function and disease. *The Pharmaceutical Journal* 272: 446–448.

Shea CW (2008) From the neurobiologic basis of alcohol dependency to pharmacologic treatment strategies: bridging the knowledge gap. *Southern Medical Journal* 101: 179–185.

Case study level 3 – Hepatic encephalopathy and ascites

Learning outcomes

Level 3 case study: You will be able to:

- interpret clinical signs and symptoms
- evaluate laboratory data
- evaluate treatment options
- state goals of therapy
- describe a pharmaceutical care plan to include advice to a clinician
- describe the prognosis and long-term complications
- describe the social pharmacy issues which could include supply (e.g. complex treatments at home, concordance and compliance) and lifestyle issues.

Scenario

Mrs MW, 59 years old, is divorced and unemployed. She was admitted to an acute medical ward at the hospital presenting with general malaise, a grossly distended abdomen, swollen ankles and jaundice. It was also noted that she smelt of alcohol and was showing signs of alcohol withdrawal.

On examination, Mrs MW was found to be encephalopathic. The doctors decided to treat her encephalopathy and ascites.

Questions

1   What is hepatic encephalopathy? What are the clinical signs and symptoms?
2   What factors may precipitate hepatic encephalopathy?
3   List two treatment options for the management of Mrs MW's hepatic encephalopathy. Describe the mechanism of action for one of these.
4   What factors are likely to have contributed to the development of ascites in Mrs MW?
5   Name two treatment options for the management of Mrs MW's ascites. Describe the pharmacology of these therapies, including any potential side-effects. What would you monitor in order to determine whether the therapy was effective?

General references

Heidelbaugh JJ and Sherbondy M (2006) Cirrhosis and chronic liver failure: Part II. Complications and treatment. *American Family Physician* 74: 767–776.

Joint Formulary Committee (2008) *British National Formulary* 55. London: British Medical Association and Royal Pharmaceutical Society of Great Britain, March.

Moore KP and Aithal GP (2006) Guidelines on the management of ascites in cirrhosis. *Gut* 55: vi1–vi12.

Case study level Ma – Pulmonary tuberculosis

Learning outcomes

Level M case study: You will be able to:

- interpret clinical signs and symptoms
- evaluate laboratory data
- critically appraise treatment options
- state goals of therapy
- describe a pharmaceutical care plan to include advice to a clinician
- describe the prognosis and long-term complications
- describe social pharmacy issues which could include supply (e.g. complex treatments at home, concordance and compliance) and lifestyle issues
- describe the monitoring of therapy.

Scenario

JS, a 46-year-old male patient, returned from India with cough, malaise, weight loss and night sweats. Sputum culture showed acid-fast bacilli and 3 days later *Mycobacterium tuberculosis* was isolated.

Questions

1   What is TB, what causes it and what is the most common source of infection?
2   How does it present in the UK?
3   What drugs could be used to treat it, what makes resistance likely?

This patient was commenced on triple therapy with rifampicin 600 mg daily, isoniazid 300 mg daily and streptomycin 750 mg daily. All three agents are bactericidal against fast growing extracellular bacilli so they produce rapid sterilisation of sputum to decrease spread. Rifampicin is also active against dormant intracellular organisms that undergo phases of rapid growth. The patient was already taking carbamazepine 200 mg b.d. throughout admission for epilepsy.

4   Are there any problems with this, and how might they be managed?
5   JS received only 750 mg daily of streptomycin. Why was this reduced and how should it be monitored?

Three weeks later he was admitted to hospital complaining of increasing malaise, muscular aches, nausea, decreased appetite, shortness of breath, cough and fever. He was jaundiced with hepatomegaly, blood pressure 120/70 mmHg, pulse 76 beats per minute, regular. Chest X-ray showed a right plural effusion and biochemistry showed increased bilirubin, ALP, ALT and AST; albumin was low.

6   What is likely to be causing these signs and symptoms?

JS was diagnosed as having drug-induced hepatitis and all anti-TB medication was stopped.

7   What can be done to reduce drug-related toxicity?
8   With reference to the biochemistry results: (a) What is the significance of the raised INR on day 19 of admission? (b) What is the significance of the raised ESR on day 23? (c) Why is the white count stable at 4.7–7.3? (d) Compare the profile of bilirubin, GGT, ALT and ALP?

A week after stopping the anti-TB drugs his liver function tests had settled and isoniazid was re-introduced at 150 mg dose, after 3 days increased to 300 mg daily. Rifampicin was then started initially at 300 mg then increased to 600 mg daily. Three weeks into the admission streptomycin was recommenced and 4 days after commencing streptomycin levels were checked and found to be trough: <1 mg/L, peak: 23 mg/L (target peak: <40 mg/L, trough: <3 mg/L). Note rifampicin can increase risk of streptomycin-induced renal dysfunction.

A week later he went home on full anti-tuberculosis drugs with stable liver function tests and carbamazepine and the addition of pyridoxine. The white count does not suggest resistance has emerged during this treatment gap but should be monitored over the full treatment course. Any acute liver insult on top of this treatment would be very difficult to resolve. Compliance with the pyridoxine is very important to prevent any toxicity.

General references

Ashley C and Morlidge C (eds) (2008) Introduction to Renal Therapeutics. London: Pharmaceutical press.

Bircher J, Benhamou J, McIntyre N *et al.* (eds) (1999) Oxford Textbook of Clinical Hepatology, 2nd edn. Oxford: Oxford Medical Publications.

Farrell GC (1994) Drug-induced Liver Disease. London: Churchill Livingstone.

South African Medicines Formulary. http://web.uct.ac.za/depts/mmi/jmoodie/lhea html.html

Stricker BHCH (1992) Drug-induced Hepatic Injury, 2nd edn. Amsterdam: Elsevier Science.

Zimmerman HJ (ed) (1999) Hepatotoxicity: The adverse effects of drugs and other chemicals on the liver. Philadelphia: Lippincott Williams & Wilkins.

Case study level Mb – Liver failure

Learning outcomes

Level M case study: You will be able to:

- interpret clinical signs and symptoms
- evaluate laboratory data
- critically appraise treatment options
- state goals of therapy
- describe a pharmaceutical care plan to include advice to a clinician
- describe the prognosis and long-term complications
- describe the social pharmacy issues which could include supply (e.g. complex treatments at home, concordance and compliance) and lifestyle issues
- describe the monitoring of therapy.

Scenario

A 43-year-old woman was admitted to hospital in December feeling unwell with a two-week history of urinary symptoms. She had decompensated cirrhosis of her liver on ultrasound and was taking pentoxifylline (oxpentifylline, Trental), co-amoxiclav, omeprazole and thiamine. She was jaundiced and confused with respiratory failure limiting speech to partial sentences. There was a marked deterioration in liver function overnight and she went into acute renal failure.

The hepatic team managed her care for 5 days because she was known to consume 1 L vodka per day. Cultures from urine grew *Escherichia coli* and sepsis from this was presumed.

On the medical ward she was self-ventilating with oxygen saturations of 90% on 4 L/min oxygen, her respiration rate was 25 per minute and she was unable to speak. Her blood pressure was 98/60 mmHg, pulse 120 beats per minute.

She was admitted to intensive care with type 1 respiratory failure (low oxygen). She had rising lactate, chest sepsis and worsening liver function tests and raised INR.

Her laboratory results are:

WCC	11×10^9/L	$(4–11 \times 10^9$/L)
INR	1.6	(0.8–1.2)
APTR	0.9	(0.8–1.2)
Na$^+$	125 mmol/L	(135–145 mmol/L)
K$^+$	2.8 mmol/L	(3.5–5 mmol/L)
Urea	18 mmol/L	(3–6.5 mmol/L)
Creatinine	174 micromol/L	(60–125 micromol/L)
Amylase	315 iu/L	(36–126 iu/L)
Bilirubin	113 micromol	(<20 micromol/L)
ALP (alkaline phosphatose)	131 iu/L	(100–300 iu/L)
ALT (alanine phosphatose)	53 iu/L	(5–42 iu/L)

She had good cardiac output with a raised heart rate (109) and central venous pressure of 18 mmHg with bilateral wheeze and fluid overload. The family were told she had a 50–50 chance of survival.

She was given vancomycin infusion, Tazocin and terlipressin.

The raised amylase suggests acute alcohol-induced pancreatitis.

The patient was developing hepatorenal syndrome with hypernatraemia, a coagulopathy and was agitated. The lactate continued to rise to 8, urea 89, creatinine 158 and urine output fell to <30 mL/h.

The next day the patient had decreased respiratory rate, became tired with falling blood sugar and acidosis. She had acute renal failure with urine output <30 mL/h and was in fluid overload. The doctors started her on terlipressin 2 mg q.d.s. and HAS (Human Albumin Solution) 20% to maintain central venous pressure 8–12 mmHg and prevent hepatorenal syndrome. Terlipressin is a pro-drug for vasopressin.

Questions

1 Just before intensive care unit admission this patient has a low blood pressure and a high heart rate. What is the most likely cause of this?
2 How can you link sepsis and liver failure with a high lactate?
3 What is the usual cause of raised serum sodium?
4 Why does sodium rise and potassium fall in liver failure. The reverse happens in hepatorenal syndrome, why?
5 What is hepatorenal syndrome and how does liver failure worsen renal function?
6 Why does hepatic dysfunction make infection more likely?
7 The respiratory failure may be due to pulmonary oedema. Why does liver failure produce oedema?
8 Terlipressin is a prodrug for vasopressin. What does it do?

References

Ashley C and Morlidge C (eds) (2008) Introduction to Renal Therapeutics. London: Pharmaceutical Press.

Bircher J, Benhamou J, McIntyre N et al. (eds) (1999) Oxford Textbook of Clinical Hepatology, 2nd edn. Oxford: Oxford Medical Publications.

Farrell GC (1994) Drug-induced Liver Disease. London: Churchill Livingstone.

South African Medicines Formulary. http://web.uct.ac.za/depts/mmi/jmoodie/lhea html.html

Stricker BHCH (1992) Drug-induced Hepatic Injury, 2nd edn. Amsterdam: Elsevier Science.

Zimmerman HJ (ed) (1999) Hepatotoxicity: The adverse effects of drugs and other chemicals on the liver. Philadelphia: Lippincott Williams & Wilkins.

Answers

Case study level 1 – Alcoholic cirrhosis; alcohol withdrawal see page 338

1   What is cirrhosis of the liver?

Cirrhosis is defined as the histological development of regenerative nodules surrounded by fibrous bands in response to chronic liver injury. It is an advanced stage of liver fibrosis that is accompanied by distortion of the hepatic vasculature.

2   List possible causes of cirrhosis

Causes of cirrhosis can usually be identified by the patient's history combined with serological and histological investigation. Alcoholic liver disease and hepatitis C and B are the most common causes of cirrhosis. The association of excessive alcohol consumption with liver disease has been recognised for centuries. After the identification of the hepatitis C virus and of non-alcoholic steatohepatitis in obese patients with diabetes, the diagnosis of cirrhosis without an apparent cause (cryptogenic cirrhosis) is rarely made. Genetic causes of cirrhosis include haemochromatosis and Wilson's disease.

Epidemiological studies have identified a number of factors that contribute to the risk of developing cirrhosis. Regular (moderate) alcohol consumption, age older than 50 years, and male gender are examples that increase cirrhosis risk in chronic hepatitis C infection, and older age, obesity, insulin resistance or type 2 diabetes, hypertension and hyperlipidaemia in non-alcoholic steatohepatitis.

3   What other clinical signs and symptoms may Mrs MW present with?

Cirrhosis is often asymptomatic until complications of liver disease are present. Mrs MW may present with itching, jaundice, dark urine, pale fatty stools, abdominal pain, nausea, fatigue, bleeding – such as nose bleeds, hepatic encephalopathy, hepatomegaly, ascites, distended abdominal veins, spider angiomata, palmar erythema and asterixis. She may also present with the signs and symptoms of alcohol withdrawal, which include irritability, anxiety, tachycardia, tremor, sweating, confusion and hallucinations.

4   What drug treatment, including dose, would you recommend for Mrs MW's alcohol withdrawal? What recommendations would you make if the patient was unable to take the medication orally?

Long-acting benzodiazepines (e.g. diazepam and chlordiazepoxide) are used to attenuate alcohol withdrawal symptoms but they also have a dependence potential. To minimise the risk of dependence, administration should be for a limited period only (e.g. chlordiazepoxide 20 mg 4 times daily, gradually reducing to zero over 7–14 days). Mild alcohol withdrawal symptoms may be treated with a lower starting dose, such as 15 mg four times a day. In all cases, the patient should be counselled about the proposed length of the treatment course. Benzodiazepines should not be prescribed if the patient is likely to continue drinking alcohol.

In patients unable to take medication by the oral route, diazepam may be administered by intramuscular or slow intravenous injection (into a large vein, at a rate of not more than 5 mg/min), at a dose of 10 mg, repeated if necessary after not less than 4 hours. Alternatively, diazepam may be administered via the rectal route as a rectal solution or suppository. The intramuscular route should only be used when both the oral and intravenous routes are not possible.

Case study level 2 – Alcoholic cirrhosis; management of bleeding risk and treatment for the maintenance of alcohol abstinence – see page 339

1   Describe how Mrs MW's laboratory results relate to her diagnosis.

Albumin is synthesised in the liver and has a long half-life of around 20 days. Mrs MW's low serum albumin is indicative of chronic liver disease. Albumin synthesis is also depressed in states of poor nutrition.

Bilirubin is carried within the plasma by albumin to the liver, where it is conjugated by glucuronidation. Subsequently, low circulating albumin levels and/or damage to the liver cells result in reduced conjugation of the bilirubin. Blockage of the biliary tract (e.g. cholestasis) will result in increased levels of conjugated bilirubin. Bilirubin levels of more than 35 micromol/L can result in visual signs of jaundice. The concentration of both the unconjugated and conjugated bilirubin are likely to be raised in Mrs MW. However, only total bilirubin was measured in this case.

Alkaline phosphatase (ALP) is present in high concentrations in the cells lining the biliary tract and an ALP level exceeding 300 IU/L, together with a raised bilirubin as in the case of Mrs MW, is indicative of cholestasis. Jaundice becomes progressively more severe in unrelieved cholestasis.

Alanine aminotransferase (ALT) is present in high concentrations in the liver and the enzyme is released during hepatocellular damage and a modestly raised level like Mrs MW's is indicative of chronic liver disease.

The increased susceptibility to bleeding observed in patients with liver failure (raised INR) results from depressed fibrinogen levels and the reduced synthesis of clotting factors by the cirrhotic liver. In addition, the absorption of fat-soluble vitamin K is impaired in cholestasis and subsequently the synthesis of vitamin K-dependent clotting factors is reduced.

Gamma-glutamyl transferase (GGT) is found in the liver, but this test is relatively non-specific. It is released following tissue damage and is raised in cholestasis in parallel with ALP. GGT release is stimulated by alcohol and some drugs (such as phenytoin and carbamazepine), and therefore the GGT level can be used to assess abstinence in alcoholics, like Mrs MW.

2   What treatment would you recommend to reduce her risk of bleeding?

Mrs MW has a raised INR value of 1.6 and is therefore at increased risk of bleeding. Vitamin K can be given to correct the vitamin deficiency, either as an intravenous injection or orally. Konakion MM is phytomenadione (10 mg/mL) in a mixed micelles vehicle. Konakion MM may be administered by slow intravenous injection or by infusion in glucose 5%.

For oral administration, the water-soluble preparation menadiol sodium phosphate, is used in patients with hepatic disease, especially biliary obstruction. The usual dose is 10 mg daily. Alternatively, phytomenadione tablets may be used in those patients who do not have impaired fat absorption.

If vitamin K is ineffective in controlling the clotting times (monitored via the INR result) then fresh frozen plasma may be required.

3   What medications would you advise Mrs MW to avoid in view of her bleeding risk?

Medications known to increase the risk of bleeding in cirrhotic patients include aspirin, clopidogrel, dipyridamole, corticosteroids, NSAIDs, heparin and warfarin. Mrs MW would need to be counselled about the risks associated with these medications and advised to always check with the pharmacist before buying any medications over the counter.

4   What treatment options are available to help Mrs MW abstain from alcohol in the future?

Disulfiram is an aversive therapy that works by inhibiting acetaldehyde dehydrogenase. Interactions between disulfiram and alcohol can result in potentially severe reactions, such as myocardial infarction, congestive heart failure, respiratory depression and death. Patients taking disulfiram should be warned of the possible presence of alcohol in liquid medicines, tonics, foods and even in toiletries and mouthwashes. Patient adherence to disulfiram is poor and there is a lack of strong evidence for its effectiveness, thus it is not routinely recommended.

Acamprosate is indicated for the maintenance of abstinence in alcohol-dependent adults. It appears to decrease brain hyperexcitability during alcohol withdrawal, which may reduce alcohol consumption. Treatment should be initiated as soon as possible after the alcohol-withdrawal period is complete. The recommended period of treatment with acamprosate is one year and treatment should be combined with counselling. The GGT level can be monitored as a marker of abstinence from alcohol.

Case study level 3 – Encephalopathy – see page 341

1   What is hepatic encephalopathy? What are the clinical signs and symptoms?

Hepatic encephalopathy is a neuropsychiatric syndrome which may complicate almost all types of liver disease. It may occur intermittently and be reversible or may occur acutely, with rapid progression to coma and death. Mrs MW presented with signs of hepatic encephalopathy including flapping tremor of the hands, intellectual deterioration, slurred speech, confusion, drowsiness and irritability.

2   What factors may precipitate hepatic encephalopathy?

Factors that may precipitate hepatic encephalopathy include:

- hypokalaemia and/or profound diuresis caused by a brisk response to a potent diuretic,
- diarrhoea and vomiting, because of the resulting fluid and electrolyte imbalance,
- constipation,
- a large protein meal or gastrointestinal haemorrhage,
- infection, especially peritonitis, and
- CNS depressant drugs, such as opioids or benzodiazepines.

3   List two treatment options for the management of Mrs MW's hepatic
encephalopathy. Describe the mechanism of action for one of these.

Treatment goals for hepatic encephalopathy include provision of supportive
care, identification and removal of precipitating factors, reduction in the
nitrogenous load from the gut and optimisation of long-term therapy.

Therapy should be directed toward improving mental status via bowel
cleansing with lactulose or with enemas. The dose of lactulose should be titrated
to give two soft stools per day without diarrhoea. Lactulose is metabolised in the
colon to lactic, acetic and formic acids, causing the pH of the colon to drop from
7 to 5. Colonic acidification with lactulose alters the bacterial population and
favours the growth of weak ammonia-producing bacteria rather than proteolytic
ammonia producers such as *E. coli*. In addition, the drop in colon pH leads to
ionisation of nitrogenous products with a subsequent reduction in their absorption from the gastrointestinal tract into the blood. Third, the osmotic laxative
effect speeds the intestinal transit, thereby decreasing the time available for the
absorption of potentially toxic nitrogen compounds. It is imperative to monitor
Mrs MW's bowel frequency while treating with lactulose since fluid and electrolyte imbalances secondary to diarrhoea may precipitate hepatic encephalopathy.
Mrs MW's mental test score should also be repeated to assess benefit.

Neomycin (4 g daily in divided doses) is a non-absorbable antibiotic
which may be used to reduce the number of bacteria in the bowel that normally
break down protein. Neomycin therapy is usually limited to one week's therapy because some absorption may occur with a risk of nephrotoxicity and
ototoxicity.

4   What factors are likely to have contributed to the development of ascites in Mrs
MW?

Mrs MW presented with a swollen abdomen, swollen ankles, pitting oedema
and breathlessness. There are two key factors involved in the pathogenesis of
ascites formation, namely, sodium and water retention and portal hypertension.

The development of renal vasoconstriction in cirrhosis is partly a homeostatic response involving increased renal sympathetic activity and activation of
the renin–angiotensin system to maintain blood pressure during systemic
vasodilatation. Decreased renal blood flow decreases glomerular filtration rate
and thus the delivery and fractional excretion of sodium. Cirrhosis is associated
with enhanced reabsorption of sodium both at the proximal tubule and at the
distal tubule. Increased reabsorption of sodium in the distal tubule is due to
the increased circulating concentrations of aldosterone, occurring secondary
to the reduced hepatic metabolism of aldosterone. However, some patients with
ascites have normal plasma concentrations of aldosterone, leading to the suggestion that sodium reabsorption in the distal tubule may be related to
enhanced renal sensitivity to aldosterone.

In compensated cirrhosis, sodium retention can occur in the absence of vasodilatation and effective hypovolaemia. Sinusoidal portal hypertension can reduce renal blood flow even in the absence of haemodynamic changes in the systemic circulation, suggesting the existence of a hepatorenal reflex. Portal hypertension increases the hydrostatic pressure within the hepatic sinusoids and favours transudation of fluid into the peritoneal cavity.

Systemic vasodilatation, the severity of liver disease and portal pressure contribute to the abnormalities of sodium handling in cirrhosis.

5   Name two treatment options for the management of Mrs MW's ascites. Describe the pharmacology of these therapies, including any potential side-effects. What would you monitor in order to determine whether the therapy was effective?

Management of ascites aims to mobilise ascitic fluid, relieve abdominal discomfort and breathlessness and to exclude infection. Diuretics have been the mainstay of treatment of ascites since the 1940s when they first became available.

Spironolactone, an aldosterone antagonist, is the drug of choice since secondary hyperaldosteronism often coexists in patients with hepatic ascites. Aldosterone is usually metabolised by the liver and is highly protein bound, therefore the free aldosterone levels are raised in cirrhosis. Spironolactone competes with aldosterone for receptor sites in the distal tubule, resulting in potassium retention and sodium and water loss. The initial dose of spironolactone is 100–200 mg and can be slowly increased according to response. There is a lag of 3–5 days between the beginning of spironolactone treatment and the onset of the natriuretic effect.

The aim is to remove the fluid gradually with a maximum weight loss of 0.5 kg/day in the absence of peripheral oedema, or 1.0 kg/day if peripheral oedema is present. Too rapid a diuresis will result in intravascular fluid loss rather than the peripheral oedema. The diuretic should be stopped if the serum sodium falls below 120 mmol/L or if there is a rising serum creatinine. Urinary electrolytes should be monitored to ensure that the spironolactone therapy is effective. The aim is to reverse the sodium/potassium ratio in the urine so that more sodium than potassium is excreted. Most frequent side-effects of spironolactone are those related to its anti-androgenic activity, such as decreased libido, impotence and gynaecomastia in men and menstrual irregularities in women. Other side-effects include hyperkalaemia, uraemia, hyponatraemia and nausea.

In addition to spironolactone, ascites can be managed by paracentesis. That is the removal ('tapping') of ascitic fluid from the peritoneal cavity under aseptic conditions. A colloid (human albumin solution (20%)) is infused (40 mL (8 g of albumin) per litre of ascites drained) intravenously during paracentesis, in order to prevent intravascular volume depletion and the onset of renal failure. Following paracentesis, ascites recurs in the majority (93%) if diuretic therapy is not reinstituted, but recurs in only 18% of patients treated with spironolactone. Cirrhotic ascites can become infected and if peritonitis occurs survival depends on early, vigorous antibiotic therapy. The patient should be monitored for signs of infection.

Case study level Ma – Pulmonary tuberculosis– see page 342

1   What is TB, what causes it and what is the most common source of infection?

Tuberculosis (TB) is an infection with mycobacterium causing the presence of tubercles. The most common single source of infection is the lungs. If the tubercles are within the blood and more than two tissues sites (e.g. lungs and liver) then it is called miliary tuberculosis. Tuberculosis is caused by *Mycobacterium tuberculosis* or more rarely *Mycobacterium bovis*. Infection spreads by inhalation of infected droplets.

2   How does it present in the UK?

The most common presentation is in people returning from holiday in Asia or Africa. It is also seen in immunocompromised patients (oncology, HIV patients, and i.v. drug abusers) and those living on the streets or in cramped accommodation. Steroids can reactivate dormant tubercles so it may present after a course of corticosteroids.

3   What drugs could be used to treat it and what makes resistance likely?

The drugs used to treat TB include capreomycin, cycloserine, ethambutol, isoniazid, pyrazinamide, rifabutin, rifampicin and streptomycin. Resistance is most likely with long courses of treatment of antimicrobial agents and treatment courses are six (or even nine) months long.

4   Are there any problems with this, and how might they be managed?

Isoniazid can cause convulsions and therefore should be prescribed with caution in patients with epilepsy. Isoniazid is an enzyme inhibitor and may increase carbamazepine levels. Rifampicin is an enzyme inducer and may decrease carbamazepine levels.

5   JS received only 750 mg daily of streptomycin. Why was this reduced and how should it be monitored?

This dose is used in patients over 40 years of age if they have subclinical renal failure. Streptomycin is an aminoglycoside so is associated with oto- and nephrotoxicity. Monitoring is by blood levels with peak 1 hour post dose below 40 mg/L and trough below 3 mg/L.

6   What is likely to be causing these signs and symptoms?

Rifampicin can cause renal failure, transient disturbances of liver function tests, hyperbilirubinaemia or severe hepatotoxicity and other side-effects. Strepto-mycin can cause renal and ototoxicity. The combination of rifampicin and streptomycin increases the risk of streptomycin-induced renal failure.

Isoniazid-induced hepatitis has an incidence estimated at 0.1%, but is higher in fast acetylators.

Rifampicin is an enzyme inducer and can increase the incidence and sever-ity of isoniazid-induced hepatitis. Carbamazepine is an enzyme induction agent and interacts with isoniazid, increasing its hepatotoxicity. Isoniazid toxicity is associated with fast acetylator genotype. Although his phenotype was unknown, the interaction with carbamazepine increases risk of this toxicity.

Isoniazid is an enzyme inhibitor and may increase carbamazepine levels so this was checked. Carbamazepine levels were checked and normal at 16 micro-mol/L (17–50 micromol/L).

7   What can be done to reduce drug-related toxicity?

- Various detoxifying products have been tried with variable success.
- If severe, the medication should be stopped. This stops the input of substrate, reduces the drive to speed up (increase quantity) of metabolic enzymes and reduces the generation of toxic metabolites.
- Thiamine is given for alcohol-induced liver toxicity (to prevent Wernicke's encephalopathy).
- Pyridoxine was commenced to prevent any isoniazid-induced peripheral neuropathy, particularly as the patient was a vegetarian of Asian ethnicity and prone to this vitamin deficiency.
- Vitamin C and E are given to provide antioxidants and reduce oxygen-free radicals.
- Acetylcysteine is given as a glutathione precursor in paracetamol overdose and in many other liver failures, including septic shock.

8   With reference to the biochemistry results: (a) What is the significance of the raised INR on day 19 of admission? (b) What is the significance of the raised ESR on day 23? (c) Why is the white count stable at 4.7–7.3? (d) Compare the profile of bilirubin, gamma-GT, ALT and ALP?

- An abnormal INR is the fastest indicator of altered liver function. Clotting relies on both the synthesis of clotting factors and then their activation as required. A raised INR shows that liver synthetic function may have slowed or stopped.
- A raised ESR indicates an inflammatory process in progress. Immuno-globulins stick to the red blood cells, causing then to settle out of solution at a faster rate.
- The infection appears to be being treated, hence white blood cells are only required to finish off and clear the wounded bacteria. In a viral infection a

huge white blood cell response may be required with cytokines to kill the viral particles.

- GGT shows the most significant change, with peaks 5.5 times baseline, but it is not a routine test.
- Bilirubin is triggered in line with INR and rapidly shows that red blood cells are being destroyed, its peak-to-baseline ratio is similar to that of GGT, it starts to fall relatively quickly and it is a routine test.
- ALT gives an early signal of hepatocellular damage but with a peak-to-baseline ratio of less than 4, it falls slower than bilirubin.
- ALP rises relatively early and settles very late but the peak-to-baseline ratio is less than 2. This is because it shows sludging of the bile duct as a secondary event to the hepatocellular damage.

Case study level Mb – Liver failure – see page 344

1   Just before intensive care unit admission this patient has a low blood pressure and a high heart rate. What is the most likely cause of this?

Peripheral vasodilatation or a loss of blood volume will reduce systemic blood pressure. The heart tries to compensate and maintain cardiac output by increasing the heart rate. Sepsis causes vasodilatation and reflex tachycardia.

2   How can you link sepsis and liver failure with a high lactate?

Lactate is a by-product of carbohydrate metabolism. It is burnt in the Krebs cycle normally but when there is an insufficiency of oxygen the normal production of carbon dioxide from glucose is not possible. Vasodilatation is a consequence of sepsis and produces abnormal blood flows, especially to the liver. So the liver does not metabolise glucose properly and lactate and acid are produced. Sepsis causes hypoxia and abnormal liver blood flow. The liver normally clears lactate.

3   What is the usual cause of raised serum sodium?

Serum sodium usually rises due to excess salt intake or dehydration.

4   Why does sodium rise and potassium fall in liver failure. The reverse happens in hepatorenal syndrome, why?

Aldosterone retains sodium in exchange for secreting potassium into the renal tubular fluid, serum potassium therefore falls. In liver failure aldosterone is not metabolised so it accumulates. Therefore in liver failure serum sodium will rise and potassium fall.

5   What is hepatorenal syndrome and how does liver failure worsen renal function?

The liver metabolises nutrients and toxins. The waste products overall are vasodilators and they are usually converted by the liver into water-soluble compounds that can be excreted by the kidneys. In the failing liver the metabolites are not eliminated and a net vasodilatation occurs. The major capillary beds are in the lungs and legs and skin, thus the metabolites divert blood away from the kidneys.

6   Why does hepatic dysfunction make infection more likely?

The spleen stores white blood cells and the liver produces the antibodies for infection. A lack of albumin causes tissue oedema. When the gut becomes oedematous bacteria can translocate from the gut lumen into the bloodstream.

7   The respiratory failure may be due to pulmonary oedema. Why does liver failure produce oedema?

The liver does not synthesise enough albumin and does not metabolise aldosterone. A lack of albumin in the vascular space reduces colloid oncotic pressure and water flows out of the blood vessels to form tissue oedema or ascites (oedema in the peritoneal cavity). Water oozing from the pulmonary arteries causes pulmonary oedema.

8   Terlipressin is a prodrug for vasopressin. What does it do?

Terlipressin is the lysine ester of vasopressin. Vasopressin is a vascular constrictor particularly in the portal vein. It prevents oesophageal varices from enlarging by decreasing portal vein blood flow. It also counteracts peripheral vasodilatation and generally diverts blood flow back to the kidneys.

15

Renal disease case studies

Caroline Ashley

Case study level 1 – Acute pyelonephritis

Learning outcomes

Level 1 case study: You will be able to:

- describe the risk factors
- describe the disease
- describe the pharmacology of the drug
- outline the formulation, including drug molecule, excipients, etc. for the medicines
- summarise basic social pharmacy issues (e.g. opening containers, large labels).

Scenario

Miss WS is a 26-year old woman, previously fit and well, admitted with a 2-day history of shaking chills, accompanied by a high fever and pain in the joints and muscles including flank pain, which is made worse on movement. She also complains of nausea, loss of appetite and headache. On examination:

- temperature = 38.5°C
- urinalysis – signs of frank haematuria, and unpleasant odour
- serum creatinine = 136 micromol/L (normal range 65–115 micromol/L)
- serum urea = 8.4 mmol/L (normal range 3.0–6.5 mmol/L).

The doctor ordered a full set of blood tests, including U&E, full blood count, blood cultures, urine sample for urinalysis and culture, and a renal ultrasound.

A diagnosis of acute bacterial pyelonephritis was made, which was later confirmed when urine culture grew *Escherichia coli*.

1   Where in the body are the kidneys located?
2   How do the kidneys work?
3   What are the functions of the kidneys?
4   How would you monitor renal function?
5   How may renal function be calculated?
6   What is acute pyelonephritis and what are the risk factors associated with developing the condition?

Miss WS is prescribed ciprofloxacin, initially 400 mg twice daily by intravenous infusion, converting after 48 hours to a dose of 500 mg twice a day orally for a total of 14 days' treatment.

7   How would you counsel Miss WS on her medication, and what would you monitor to assess its effectiveness?

General references

Ashley C (2008) What are the functions of the kidney? In: Ashley C, Morlidge C (eds) *Introduction to Renal Therapeutics*. London: Pharmaceutical Press, 1-7.

Cockcroft DW and Gault MH (1976) Prediction of creatinine clearance from serum creatinine. *Nephron* 16: 31–41.

Lamerton E (2008) Laboratory tests and investigations. In: Ashley C, Morlidge C (eds) *Introduction to Renal Therapeutics*. London: Pharmaceutical Press, 9-19.

Levey AS, Bosch JP, Lewis JB *et al.* (1999) A more accurate method to estimate glomerular filtration rate from serum creatinine: a new prediction equation. Modification of Diet in Renal Disease Study Group. *Annals of Internal Medicine* 130: 461–470.

Case study level 2 – NSAIDs and ACE inhibitors

Learning outcomes

Level 2 case study: You will be able to:

- interpret relevant lab and clinical data
- identify monitoring and referral criteria
- explain treatment choices
- describe goals of therapy including monitoring and the role of the pharmacist/clinician
- describe issues – counselling points, adverse drug reactions, drug interactions, complementary/alternative therapies and lifestyle advice.

Scenario

Mr VC is a 65-year-old man (68 kg, 175 cm) who presents to the accident and emergency department feeling increasingly unwell. He is on a short holiday with his wife, and unable to return home to see his GP. Two weeks ago he presented to his GP with a painful right metatarsal pharyngeal joint (due to gout), for which his GP prescribed:

- indometacin 50 mg three times a day and
- ranitidine 150 mg twice daily.

The gout pain is now resolving.

On admission Mr VC was pale, lethargic and breathless. His past medical history includes hypertension for 1 year and type 2 diabetes for 5 years. His routine medication comprises:

- bendroflumethiazide 5 mg o.m. (for the last six months – increased from 2.5 mg)
- ramipril 2.5 mg o.m. (started six months ago)
- gliclazide 40 mg b.d.

Mr VC's biochemistry results are as follows:

Na$^+$	137 mmol/L (135–150 mmol/L)
K$^+$	6.9 mmol/L (3.5–5.2 mmol/L)
Urea	28.5 mmol/L (3.2–6.6 mmol/L)
Creatinine	268 micromoll/L (60–110 micromol/L)
Bicarbonate	18 mmol/L (22–31 mmol/L)
Phosphate	1.7 mmol/L (0.9–1.5 mmol/L)
Corr. calcium	2.6 mmol/L (2.2–2.5 mmol/L)
pH	7.26 (7.36–7.44)
Glucose	10.8 mmol/L
24-hour urine output	600 mL

Mr VC is admitted to hospital under the diabetic team.

Questions

1. Calculate Mr VC's renal function using both Cockcroft–Gault and the Modification of Diet in Renal Disease (MDRD) equations.
2. What patient and pharmaceutical factors may have precipitated acute renal failure in this patient?
3. By what mechanism can non-steroidal anti-inflammatory drugs (NSAIDs) cause renal impairment?
4. By what mechanism can ACE inhibitors cause renal impairment?

5 What are the main medical/pharmaceutical problems now? Relate these to the patient's test results.

6 How might these problems be managed?

General references

Ashley C (2008) Acute renal failure. In: Ashley C, Morlidge C (eds) *Introduction to Renal Therapeutics*. London: Pharmaceutical Press, 3-34.

Pearson J (2008) Drug-induced kidney disease. In: Ashley C, Morlidge C (eds) *Introduction to Renal Therapeutics*. London: Pharmaceutical Press, 139-144.

Slack A, Ho S, Forni LG (2007) The management of acute renal failure. *Medicine* 35: 434–437.

Stevens P (2007). Assessment of patients presenting with acute renal failure (acute kidney injury). *Medicine* 35: 429-433

Case study level 3 – Pre-dialysis patient with anaemia

Learning outcomes

Level 3 case study: You will be able to:

- interpret clinical signs and symptoms
- evaluate laboratory data
- evaluate treatment options
- state goals of therapy
- describe a pharmaceutical care plan to include advice to a clinician
- describe the prognosis and long-term complications
- describe the social pharmacy issues which could include supply (e.g. complex treatments at home, concordance and compliance) and lifestyle issues.

Scenario

Mrs HK is a 75-year-old woman who presents to her GP with a six-week history of lethargy and weakness. She has a 10-year history of type 2 diabetes mellitus and 15-year history of hypertension.

The patient has evidence of end-organ damage as a result of her diabetes and has previously received photocoagulation therapy for her retinopathy.

On examination Mrs HK is pale and lethargic. She has mild effort dyspnoea and the following blood results:

Serum creatinine   266 µmol/L (eGFR = 16 mL/min/1.73 m²)
Blood pressure   160/88 mmHg
Hb   7.9 g/dL.

Her stools were negative for occult blood.

The patient's medication comprises:

- glibenclamide 10 mg twice daily
- ramipril 10 mg once daily
- amlodipine 100 mg once daily
- diltiazem 240 mg daily
- doxazosin XL 4 mg once daily
- furosemide 40 mg once daily
- domperidone 10 mg three times a day
- pravastatin 10 mg at night
- insulin human Mixtard 30 22 units am, 20 units pm.

Questions

1   Comment on Mrs HK's results.
2   What therapy would you recommend?
3   Describe the differences between erythropoietin and darbepoetin alfa.
4   What dosing schedule would you recommend?
5   What haemoglobin level would you aim for?
6   What concomitant therapy might Mrs HK require to treat her renal anaemia?
7   What would you do if Mrs HK failed to respond to her epoetin therapy?

General references

Sexton J (2008) Renal Anaemia. In: Ashley C, Morlidge C (eds) *Introduction to Renal Therapeutics*. London: Pharmaceutical Press, 45-56.

NICE (National Institute for Health and Clinical Excellence) (2006) Anaemia management in chronic kidney disease. Available at http://www.nice.org.uk/nicemedia/pdf/ AMCKD_NICE_guideline_v8.1.pdf [Accessed 4 July 2008].

Case study level Ma – Diabetes and renal impairment

Learning outcomes

Level M case study: You will be able to:

- interpret clinical signs and symptoms
- evaluate laboratory data
- critically appraise treatment options
- state goals of therapy
- describe a pharmaceutical care plan to include advice to a clinician
- describe the prognosis and long-term complications
- describe the social pharmacy issues which could include supply (e.g. complex treatments at home, concordance and compliance) and lifestyle issues
- describe the monitoring of therapy.

Scenario

CM is a 27-year-old white woman with type 1 diabetes diagnosed at age 14 when she presented with diabetic ketoacidosis. Her initial insulin treatment was complicated by poor glycaemic control, frequent hypoglycaemia and weight gain.

Two years ago she developed hypertension, which was treated with bendroflumethiazide, 5mg daily. At that time, her blood urea level was 8.2 mmol/L, serum creatinine was 80 µmol/L, and dipstick urinalysis was negative for protein. She was also noted to have non-proliferative diabetic retinopathy, and given a course of laser treatment.

She has now been admitted via A&E complaining of nausea and vomiting. On examination, she was dehydrated and her breath smelled of ketones. She was conscious and alert. Her finger-prick blood glucose was 25.4 mmol/L and the urine dipstick was strongly positive for glucose, ketones and protein. She was diagnosed as being in diabetic ketoacidosis and was transferred to the intensive care unit for further management.

On admission to the intensive care unit her laboratory results were as follows:

Na^+	127 mmol/L	(135–150 mmol/L)
K^+	4.5 mmol/L	(3.5–5.2 mmol/L)
Blood pH	7.15	(7.36–7.44)
Base excess	−20.9 mmol/L	
Bicarbonate	5.8 mmol/L	(22–31 mmol/L)
Urea	18.3 mmol/L	(3.5–5.2 mmol/L)

Creatinine	546 micromol/L	(60–110 micromol/L)
Glucose	40.1 mmol/L	
HbA1c	(3.9–6.1%)	

Her weight is 54 kg, and she is 160 cm tall.

Questions

1   What is diabetic ketoacidosis?

CM was started on intravenous insulin, fluids, and electrolyte replenishment. Her nausea and vomiting resolved and, although initially, she required 60–70 units of insulin intravenously per day to attain glycaemic control, her blood glucose dropped to 7.4 mmol/L after 4 days of intensive care. However, despite treatment of her diabetic ketoacidosis, including significant rehydration therapy, CM was still found to have an elevated but stable serum creatinine of 246 micromol/L, and so she was transferred from the intensive care unit to the renal unit for further management.

2   Calculate CM's renal function using both the MDRD equation and the Cockcroft–Gault formula.
3   What is the likely cause of CM's renal impairment?
4   What pharmacological and other interventions could be employed to reduce the risk of problems?

As a result of the urethral catheter she had inserted in the intensive care unit, CM develops a urinary tract infection, with an *E. coli* that is resistant to trimethoprim and amoxicillin, but is sensitive to gentamicin. She is prescribed a dose of gentamicin, 7 mg/kg intravenously once daily for 5 days.

5   Comment on this dose of gentamicin.
6   What dose would you recommend?

General references

Ashley C and Currie A (2008) Renal Drug Handbook, 3rd edn. Oxford: Radcliffe Medical Press.

Patel, M (2008) Diabetes management in kidney disease. In: Ashley C, Morlidge C (eds) *Introduction to Renal Therapeutics*. London: Pharmaceutical Press, 205-216.

Strippoli GFM, Craig M, Deeks JJ et al. (2004) Effects of angiotensin converting enzyme inhibitors and angiotensin II receptor antagonists on mortality and renal outcomes in diabetic nephropathy: systematic review. *British Medical Journal* 329: 1–12.

Case study level Mb – Hypertension-associated kidney disease

Learning outcomes

Level M case study: You will be able to:

- interpret clinical signs and symptoms
- evaluate laboratory data
- critically appraise treatment options
- state goals of therapy
- describe a pharmaceutical care plan to include advice to a clinician
- describe the prognosis and long-term complications
- describe the social pharmacy issues which could include supply (e.g. complex treatments at home, concordance and compliance) and lifestyle issues
- describe the monitoring of therapy.

Scenario

Mr WD, 42-year-old Afro-Caribbean man, presents to his GP with six-week history of headaches and lethargy. On examination the following is noted:

- dipstick – proteinuria +++
- Blood pressure 180/105 mmHg (120/80 mmHg)
- Serum creatinine 365 micromol/L (60–110 micromol/L)
- Serum urea 15.8 mmol/L (3.2–6.6 mmol/L)
- Weight 98 kg
- Height 180 cm.

Questions

1 Comment on Mr WD's laboratory results.
2 Calculate Mr WD's renal function using the MDRD equation and the Cockcroft–Gault formula.
3 What do you think may have caused Mr WD's renal impairment?
4 How should Mr WD's hypertension be managed?
5 What therapy would you recommend for the treatment of Mr WD's hypertension?

Mr WD was prescribed nifedipine LA 30 mg once daily and enalapril 10 mg twice daily to treat his hypertension. After one week's treatment, his blood pressure was still only 150/85 mmHg, but the patient was complaining of very swollen ankles. He also mentions that he has developed a persistent cough.

6   What could be the cause of Mr WD's new symptoms?
7   What treatment would you suggest now for Mr WD's hypertension?

References

Braunwald E, Domanski MJ, Fowler SE *et al.* PEACE Trial Investigators (2004) Angiotensin-converting-enzyme inhibition in stable coronary artery disease. *New England Journal of Medicine* 351(20): 2058-68.

Dahlof B, Sever PS, Poulter NR *et al.* for the ASCOT investigators (2005) Prevention of cardiovascular events with an antihypertensive regimen, in the Anglo-Scandinavian Cardiac Outcomes Trial (ASCOT). *Lancet* 366: 895–906.

Douglas J, Greene TH, Toto RD *et al.* (2002) The African-American Study of Kidney Disease and Hypertension (AASK Trial). *Journal of the American Society of Nephrology* 13:131P.

Klag MJ, Whelton PK, Randall BL *et al.* (1996) Blood pressure and end-stage renal disease in men. *New England Journal of Medicine* 334: 13–18.

Lewis EJ, Hunsicker LG, Clarke WR *et al.* (2001) Renoprotective effect of the angiotensin-receptor antagonist irbesartan in patients with nephropathy due to Type 2 diabetes. *New England Journal of Medicine* 345: 851-860.

Morlidge C (2008) Hypertension and hyperlipidaemia. In: Ashley C, Morlidge C (eds) *Introduction to Renal Therapeutics*. London: Pharmaceutical Press, 77-84.

NICE (National Institute for Health and Clinical Excellence) (2006) Hypertension: management of hypertension in adults in primary care. Clinical Guideline CG34. Available at http://www.nice.org.uk/nicemedia/pdf/CG034NICEguideline.pdf [Accessed 4 July 2008].

Ruilope LM and Rodicio JL (1995) Microalbuminuria in clinical practice. *Kidney* 4: 211–216.

Taal MW, Tomson C (2007) Clinical Practice Guidelines: Module 1: Chronic Kidney Disease. 12-13. UK Renal Association. www.renal.org/guidelines [accessed 4 August 2008].

Williams B, Poulter NR, Brown MJ *et al.* The BHS Guidelines Working Party (2004) British Hypertension Society guidelines for hypertension management, 2004 – BHS IV. Summary. *British Medical Journal* 328: 634–640.

General references

Howie AJ (1996) 'Benign' essential hypertension and kidney damage: a histopathologist's view. *Journal of Human Hypertension* 10: 691–694.

Mogensen C (1984) Microalbuminuria predicts clinical proteinuria and early mortality in maturity onset diabetes. *New England Journal of Medicine* 310: 356–360.

Case study level 1 – Acute pyelonephritis – see page 356

1   Where in the body are the kidneys located?

In humans, the kidneys are located in the posterior part of the abdomen. There is one on each side of the spine; the right kidney sits just below the liver, the left below the diaphragm and adjacent to the spleen. Above each kidney is an adrenal gland (also called the suprarenal gland). The asymmetry within the abdominal cavity caused by the liver results in the right kidney being slightly lower than the left one.

The kidneys are retroperitoneal, which means they lie behind the peritoneum, the lining of the abdominal cavity. They are approximately at the vertebral level T12 to L3. The upper parts of the kidneys are partially protected by the 11th and 12th ribs, and each whole kidney is surrounded by two layers of fat (the perirenal and pararenal fat) which help to cushion it.

2   How do the kidneys work?

Each kidney receives its blood supply from a renal artery, two of which branch from the abdominal aorta. Upon entering the hilum of the kidney, the renal artery divides into smaller arteries which in turn give off still smaller branches. Branching off these are the afferent arterioles supplying the glomerular capillaries, which drain into efferent arterioles. Efferent arterioles divide into peritubular capillaries that provide an extensive blood supply to the renal cortex. Blood from these capillaries collects in renal venules and leaves the kidney via the renal vein. Blood supply is intimately linked to blood pressure.

The basic functional unit of the kidney is the nephron, of which there are more than a million within the cortex and medulla of each normal adult human kidney. Nephrons regulate water and soluble matter (especially electrolytes) in the body by first filtering the blood under pressure, and then reabsorbing some necessary fluid and molecules back into the blood while secreting other, unneeded molecules. Reabsorption and secretion are accomplished with both cotransport and countertransport mechanisms established in the nephrons and associated collecting ducts.

The fluid flows from the nephron into the collecting duct system. This segment of the nephron is crucial to the process of water conservation. In the presence of antidiuretic hormone (ADH; also called vasopressin), these ducts become permeable to water and facilitate its reabsorption, thus concentrating the urine and reducing its volume. Conversely, when the organism must eliminate excess water, such as after excess fluid drinking, the production of ADH is decreased and the collecting tubule becomes less permeable to water, rendering urine dilute and abundant.

After being processed along the collecting tubules and ducts, the fluid, now called urine, is drained into the bladder via the ureter, to be finally excreted.

3   What are the functions of the kidneys?

Excretion of waste products

The kidneys excrete a variety of waste products produced by metabolism, including the nitrogenous wastes: urea (from protein catabolism) and uric acid (from nucleic acid metabolism). The kidneys also excrete many drugs or their metabolites, in particular those that are hydrophilic, have a small volume of distribution and a low degree of protein binding.

Homeostasis

The kidney is one of the major organs involved in whole-body homeostasis. Among its homeostatic functions are acid–base balance, regulation of electrolyte concentrations, control of blood volume and regulation of blood pressure. The kidneys accomplish these homeostatic functions independently and through coordination with other organs, particularly those of the endocrine system. The kidney communicates with these organs through hormones secreted into the bloodstream.

Acid–base balance

The processes of metabolism generate hydrogen ions. Approximately 15 000 mmol/24 h acid is produced as a result of carbon dioxide (CO_2) release from oxidative (aerobic) metabolism.

Although CO_2 does not contain hydrogen ions it rapidly reacts with water to form carbonic acid (H_2CO_3), which further dissociates into hydrogen and bicarbonate ions (HCO_3^-). This reaction is shown below:

$$CO_2 + H_2O \rightleftharpoons H_2CO_3^- \rightleftharpoons HCO_3^- + H^+$$

This reaction occurs throughout the body and in certain circumstances is speeded up by the enzyme carbonic anhydrase. Carbonic acid is a weak acid and with bicarbonate, its conjugate base, forms the most important buffering system in the body.

With hydrogen ion concentration being so critical to enzyme function, the body has sophisticated mechanisms for ensuring pH remains in the normal range. Three systems are involved: blood and tissue buffering, excretion of CO_2 by the lungs and the renal excretion of H^+ and regeneration of HCO_3^-.

Buffers
Buffers are able to limit changes in hydrogen ion concentration. This prevents the large quantities of hydrogen ions produced by metabolism resulting in dangerous changes in blood or tissue pH.

Bicarbonate
This is the most important buffer system in the body. Although bicarbonate is not an efficient buffer at physiological pH its efficiency is improved because CO_2 is removed by the lungs and bicarbonate regenerated by the kidney.

Proteins
Many proteins, and notably albumin, contain weak acidic and basic groups within their structure. Therefore, plasma and other proteins form important buffering systems. Intracellular proteins limit pH changes within cells, whilst the protein matrix of bone can buffer large amounts of hydrogen ions in patients with chronic acidosis.

The kidneys not only secrete hydrogen ions but they also regenerate bicarbonate ions. The renal handling of electrolytes also influences acid-base balance.

Regeneration of bicarbonate
Bicarbonate ions are freely filtered by the glomerulus. The concentration of bicarbonate in the tubular fluid is equivalent to that of plasma. If bicarbonate were not reabsorbed the buffering capacity of the blood would rapidly be depleted.

Filtered bicarbonate combines with secreted hydrogen ions forming carbonic acid. Carbonic acid then dissociates to form CO_2 and water. This reaction is catalysed by carbonic anhydrase, which is present in the brush border of the renal tubular cells. This CO_2 readily crosses into the tubular cell down a concentration gradient.

Inside the cell the CO_2 recombines with water, again under the influence of carbonic anhydrase, to form carbonic acid. The carbonic acid further dissociates to bicarbonate and hydrogen ions. The bicarbonate passes back into the blood stream whilst the H^+ passes back into the tubular fluid in exchange for sodium. In this way, virtually all the filtered bicarbonate is reabsorbed in the healthy individual.

Excretion of hydrogen ions

Hydrogen ions are actively secreted in the proximal and distal tubules, but the maximum urinary [H^+] is around 0.025 mmol/L (pH 4.6). Therefore, in order to excrete the 30–40 mmol of H^+ required per day, a urine volume of 1200 litres would have to be produced. However, buffering of hydrogen ions also occurs in the urine. This allows the excretion of these large quantities of H^+ without requiring such huge urine volumes. Hydrogen ion secretion occurs against a steep concentration gradient, 40 nmol/L in plasma against up to 25 000 nmol/L (25×10^3 nmol/L) in urine. Therefore, hydrogen ion secretion is an active process and requires energy in the form of ATP.

The predominant buffers in the urine are phosphate (HPO_4^{2-}) and ammonia (NH_3). Phosphate is freely filtered by the glomerulus and passes down the tubule where it combines with H^+ to form $H_2PO_4^-$. Hydrogen ions are secreted in exchange for sodium ions; the energy for this exchange comes from the sodium-potassium ATPase that maintains the concentration gradient for sodium.

Ammonia is produced in renal tubular cells by the action of the enzyme glutaminase on the amino acid glutamine. This enzyme functions optimally at a lower (more acidic) than normal pH. Therefore, more ammonia is produced during acidosis improving the buffering capacity of the urine. Ammonia is unionised and so rapidly crosses into the renal tubule down its concentration gradient. The ammonia combines with H^+ to form the ammonium ion, which being ionised does not pass back into the tubular cell. The ammonium ion is therefore lost in the urine, along with the hydrogen ion it contains.

Blood pressure

Sodium ions are controlled in a homeostatic process involving aldosterone which increases sodium ion absorption in the distal convoluted tubules.

When blood pressure becomes low, a proteolytic enzyme called renin is secreted by cells of the juxtaglomerular apparatus (part of the distal convoluted tubule) which are sensitive to pressure. Renin acts on a blood protein, angiotensinogen, converting it to angiotensin I (10 amino acids). Angiotensin I is then converted by the angiotensin-converting enzyme (ACE) in the lung capillaries to angiotensin II (8 amino acids), which stimulates the secretion of aldosterone by the adrenal cortex, which then affects the kidney tubules.

Aldosterone stimulates an increase in the reabsorption of sodium ions from the kidney tubules which causes an increase in the volume of water that is reabsorbed from the tubule. This increase in water reabsorption increases the volume of blood, which ultimately raises the blood pressure.

Plasma volume

Any significant rise or drop in plasma osmolality is detected by the hypothalamus, which communicates directly with the posterior pituitary gland. A rise in osmolality causes the gland to secrete antidiuretic hormone, resulting in water reabsorption by the kidney and an increase in urine concentration. The two factors work together to return the plasma osmolality to its normal levels.

Hormone secretion

The kidneys secrete a variety of hormones, including erythropoietin, urodilatin, renin and vitamin D.

4   How would you monitor renal function?

Most doctors use the plasma concentrations of creatinine, urea and electrolytes to determine renal function. These measures are adequate to determine whether a patient is suffering from kidney disease. Protein and amino acid catabolism results in the production of ammonia, which in turn is converted via the urea cycle into urea, which is then excreted via the kidneys. Creatinine is a breakdown product of creatine phosphate in muscle, and is usually produced at a fairly constant rate by the body (depending on muscle mass). Creatinine is mainly filtered by the kidney, though a small amount is actively secreted. There is little to no tubular reabsorption of creatinine. If the filtering of the kidney is deficient, blood levels rise.

Unfortunately, urea and creatinine will not be outside the normal range until 60% of total kidney function is lost. Hence, creatinine clearance is a more accurate measure and is used whenever renal disease is suspected or careful dosing of nephrotoxic drugs is required.

In renal patients, the glomerular filtration rate (GFR) is used. This is calculated by comparing urine creatinine levels with the blood test results. It gives a more precise indication of the state of the kidneys. The GFR is expressed in millilitres per minute. For most patients, a GFR over 60 mL/min is adequate. But, if the GFR has significantly declined from a previous test result, this can be an early indicator of kidney disease requiring medical intervention. The sooner kidney dysfunction is diagnosed and treated, the greater the odds of preserving remaining nephrons, and preventing the need for dialysis.

Very often, the GFR is expressed as mL/min/1.73 m^2. This is an indication that the GFR needs to be corrected for the actual body surface of the patient.

5   How may renal function be calculated?

Cockcroft–Gault formula

A commonly used surrogate marker for actual creatinine clearance is the Cockcroft–Gault formula, which employs creatinine measurements and a patient's age and weight to predict the clearance. It is named after the scientists who first published the formula. The equation is popular because it is easy to calculate.

The formula, slightly modified from that originally published to take account of UK units, is:

$$\text{Creatinine clearance} = \frac{\text{Constant} \times (140 - \text{age}) \times \text{weight}}{\text{Serum creatinine}}$$

This formula expects the patient's weight to be measured in kilograms and creatinine to be measured in micromols per litre. The constant is 1.23 for men and 1.04 for women. This formula is useful because the calculations are relatively simple and can often be performed without the aid of a calculator.

MDRD formula

The most recently advocated formula for calculating the GFR is the one that was developed as a result of the Modification of Diet in Renal Disease (MDRD) study (Levey *et al.*, 1999).

For creatinine in mg/dL (USA units):

Creatinine clearance = $186 \times \text{creatinine}^{-1.154} \times \text{age}^{-0.203} \times \text{constant}$

For creatinine in µmol/L (UK units):

Creatinine clearance = $32\,788 \times \text{creatinine}^{-1.154} \times \text{age}^{-0.203} \times \text{constant}$

The constant is 1 for a white male, and is multiplied with 0.742 for females and multiplied with 1.21 for Afro-Caribbeans.

Creatinine levels in mg/dL can be converted to µmol/L by multiplying them by 88.4. The 32 788 number above is equal to $186 \times 88.4^{1.154}$.
This is a complicated equation to use manually, and the easiest way to calculate an estimated GFR (eGFR) is to use an on-line calculator, for example at http://www.renal.org/eGFR/

6   What is acute pyelonephritis and what are the risk factors associated with developing the condition?

Pyelonephritis is an infection of the kidneys and ureters, usually from bacteria that spread upwards from the bladder. If not properly treated, it can lead to permanent scarring of the kidneys, with resultant kidney damage and loss of kidney function.

The risk factors for developing pyelonephritis include: urinary tract infection, bladder infection, indwelling urinary catheter, urinary tract surgery, pregnancy, prostate enlargement, kidney stones, tumours of the urinary tract, immunocompromised patients, patients on immunosuppressant drugs and steroid therapy. These risk factors are not always a direct cause of the disease, but seem to be associated in some way. Having a risk factor for pyelonephritis makes the chances of developing the condition higher but does not always lead to pyelonephritis. Conversely, the absence of any risk factors does not necessarily mean a person will not develop pyelonephritis.

7   How would you counsel Miss WS on her medication, and what would you monitor to assess its effectiveness?

Miss WS has been prescribed ciprofloxacin 500 mg twice daily for 12 days (she already had 48 hours of intravenous antibiotics). She should be advised:

- to take them at regular intervals (ideally 12 hours apart),
- to complete the prescribed course unless otherwise directed,
- not to take milk, indigestion remedies or medicines containing iron or zinc at the same time of day as the ciprofloxacin,
- to swallow the tablets whole and not chew them,
- to be aware that this medicine may cause drowsiness and may affect her ability to drive motor vehicles, and
- to report any adverse affects to her GP.

To assess the effectiveness of the antibiotics, points to be monitored include:

- patient's temperature,
- patient's pain score,
- urinalysis – should show no blood or protein,
- urine culture – should be negative (i.e. no bacteria should be grown), and
- renal function tests – should return to the normal range.

Case study level 2 – NSAIDs and ACE inhibitors – see page 357

1   Calculate Mr VC's renal function using both Cockcroft–Gault and the Modification of Diet in Renal Disease (MDRD) equations.

Cockcroft–Gault

$$\text{Creatinine clearance} = \frac{1.23\ (140 - \text{age}) \times \text{weight}}{\text{Serum creatinine}} = \frac{1.23\ (140\text{–}65) \times 68}{268} = 23.4\ \text{mL/min}$$

MDRD

Creatinine clearance = 22 mL/min

2   What patient and pharmaceutical factors may have precipitated acute renal failure in this patient?

■   The patient is elderly.
■   He has previously been prescribed bendroflumethiazide on an escalating dose. This in turn precipitated an episode of gout. At this point the thiazide should have been stopped, since thiazide diuretics are contraindicated in gout. This did not happen.

The GP then added in indometacin, which compromised renal perfusion. The combination therapy of an NSAID, an ACE inhibitor and a diuretic in an elderly patient who because of his age already has reduced renal function, induced a state of acute renal failure.

■   A previous medical history of non-insulin dependent diabetes mellitus and hypertension are added risk factors for developing acute renal failure, as they will predispose the patient to having a degree of chronically impaired renal function.
■   Acute gout could cause urate uropathy, whereby uric acid crystals are deposited within the renal tubules, causing intrinsic renal damage.

3   By what mechanism can non-steroidal anti-inflammatory drugs (NSAIDs) cause renal impairment?

Non-steroidal anti-inflammatory drugs are associated with renal damage, and even a short course of an NSAID (such as diclofenac) has been associated with acute renal failure, especially in older patients. The main cause of NSAID-induced renal damage is inhibition of prostaglandin synthesis in the kidney, particularly prostaglandins E_2, D_2 and I_2 (prostacyclin). These prostaglandins are all potent vasodilators and consequently produce an increase in blood flow to the glomerulus and the medulla. The maintenance of blood pressure in a variety of clinical conditions, such as volume depletion, biventricular cardiac failure, or hepatic cirrhosis with ascites, may rely on the release of vasoconstrictor substances such as angiotensin II. In these states, inhibition of prostaglandin synthesis may cause unopposed renal arteriolar vasoconstriction, which again leads to renal hypoperfusion. NSAIDs impair the ability of the renovasculature to adapt to a fall in perfusion pressure or to an increase in vasoconstrictor balance.

4   By what mechanism can ACE inhibitors cause renal impairment?

Angiotensin-converting enzyme (ACE) inhibitors may also produce a reduction in renal function by preventing the angiotensin-II-mediated vasoconstriction of the efferent glomerular arteriole, which contributes to the high pressure gradient across the glomerulus. This problem is important only in patients with renal vascular disease, particularly those with bilateral renal artery stenoses, causing renal perfusion to fall. In order to maintain the pressure gradient across the glomerulus, the efferent arteriolar resistance must rise. This is predominantly accomplished by angiotensin-induced efferent vasoconstriction. If ACE inhibitors are administered, this system is rendered inoperable and there is no longer any way of maintaining an effective filtration pressure. This leads to a fall in GFR and acute renal failure.

5 What are the main medical/pharmaceutical problems now? Relate these to the patient's test results.

The main pharmaceutical problems are:

- acute renal failure (grossly elevated serum creatinine and urea, and 24-hour urine output only 600 mL),
- hyperkalaemia (raised serum potassium level),
- metabolic acidosis (low serum bicarbonate level, and blood pH below the normal range), and
- hyperglycaemia (fasting blood glucose level high).

6 How might these problems be managed?

Treatment of acute renal failure

There is no actual treatment *per se* for acute renal failure. Just provide supportive measures, for example, renal replacement therapy (dialysis), treat the symptoms, and if possible, the underlying cause, and wait to see if renal function is recovered.

Many texts suggest using high-dose loop diuretics such as furosemide to try and force the kidneys to work. Furosemide should only be given if the patient is euvolaemic or fluid overloaded, and if the drug fails to induce a diuresis, then it should be discontinued, as further use merely increases renal damage. Mannitol has been used, as theoretically it induces an osmotic diuresis, while low-dose dopamine was advocated for many years, as it was said to dilate the renal vascular bed, increase renal perfusion, and thereby improve renal function. However, there is no evidence that either mannitol or dopamine are of any benefit, and their use in acute renal failure is by and large now historic.

Review all oral medications to assess their potential toxicity given the patient's current state. Suggest stopping the indometacin, ramipril and gliclazide, with a view to restarting the latter two when the patient is more stable. Continue the ranitidine, as the patient is at risk of developing stress ulceration.

Treatment of hyperkalaemia

The hyperkalaemia is the most life-threatening symptom at present. Initially, the patient could be given salbutamol nebulisers, since salbutamol acts via beta-receptors to drive potassium back into cells (one of its side effects is hypokalaemia). This could be followed by intravenous insulin (e.g. 15 units of a soluble, short-acting insulin) plus glucose (typically 50 mL of glucose 50% given intravenously). Intravenous calcium gluconate may also be given to stabilise the myocardium against the effects of the high serum potassium, and thereby reduce the risk of cardiac arrhythmias. Insulin allows glucose to enter cells where it is utilised during cell metabolism. As glucose enters cells, potassium enters with it; hence a sudden dose of insulin will have the effect of acutely lowering the serum potassium level. The 50% glucose is given intravenously to counteract the effects of the insulin on the blood glucose level, and prevent the patient going into a hypoglycaemic coma. Finally, if necessary, an ion-exchange resin such as Calcium Resonium may be given. This swaps calcium ions for potassium ions across the intestinal wall, and thus lowers serum potassium. It may be given either orally or rectally, but should always be given with an osmotic laxative such as lactulose to prevent constipation.

Treatment of metabolic acidosis

Metabolic acidosis involves a build-up of hydrogen ions in the blood, thus lowering blood pH. Under normal physiological conditions, the kidneys excrete excess hydrogen ions, and release more bicarbonate ions into the bloodstream to buffer the excess acid. However, in renal failure, or in diabetic ketoacidosis, this mechanism either fails, or is unable to compensate to an adequate extent. Hence, metabolic acidosis is usually treated with sodium bicarbonate, either intravenously (1.26% or 8.4% i.v. solution) or orally (typically 1 g three times a day). Sodium bicarbonate 1.26% intravenous solution is isotonic with plasma (and with sodium chloride 0.9%), so may be given in large volumes (1–2 L) by peripheral venous catheter to correct metabolic acidosis and provide fluid replacement at the same time. Sodium bicarbonate 8.4% may only be given by central venous catheter.

Treatment of hyperglycaemia

The hyperglycaemia will respond to the insulin and glucose used to treat the hyperkalaemia. The patient is unstable, and it is evident his usual oral diabetic medication is insufficient to control his diabetes at present. Therefore he should be put on a sliding scale insulin infusion until such time that his glycaemic control has improved and he is considered stable enough to re-introduce the oral gliclazide therapy. Blood glucose levels should be monitored very closely.

Case study level 3 – Pre-dialysis patient with anaemia – see page 359

1   Comment on Mrs HK's results.

From Mrs HK's results it would appear that she has severe renal impairment (an eGFR of 16 mL/min/1.73 m^2 means she has grade 4/5 chronic kidney disease (CKD)). She is not hypertensive, but is symptomatically anaemic, with a haemoglobin of 7.9 g/dL, and she is pale, lethargic and breathless on effort.

2   What therapy would you recommend?

Renal anaemia is generally treated with erythropoiesis-stimulating agents (ESAs), of which three are currently in general use: the erythropoietins, namely epoetin alfa (Eprex), epoetin beta (NeoRecormon) and darbepoetin alfa (Aranesp).

3   Describe the differences between erythropoietin and darbepoetin alfa.

Erythropoietin is a glycoprotein hormone with a molecular mass of approximately 30 000 Da. It has a 165-amino-acid chain, three *N*-linked oligosaccharide side-chains, and is a cytokine for erythrocyte precursors in bone marrow. It may be given by subcutaneous or intravenous injection, although the subcutaneous route is more efficient, and requires lower doses (the intravenous dose is approximately 25% higher). The dosing interval may be anywhere between daily to once a week, although the most popular dosing regimen is three times a week.

Darbepoetin alfa is a second-generation ESA. It is a 165-amino-acid protein, with five *N*-linked oligosaccharide chains resulting from five amino acid substitutions in the erythropoietin peptide backbone. As a result of this, it has a longer half-life than erythropoietin, and so is given either once a week or in some patients, every two weeks. In addition, due to its longer duration of action, the intravenous and subcutaneous doses of darbepoetin alfa are the same.

4   What dosing schedule would you recommend?

Treatment for renal anaemia is divided into two stages – correction and maintenance phase – and the dosage regimens vary according to the preparation used.

Darbepoetin alfa

Correction phase: Initial dose is 0.45 micrograms/kg by subcutaneous or intravenous injection, once weekly. Alternatively, in pre-dialysis patients, an initial dose of 0.75 micrograms/kg may be administered subcutaneously once every two weeks.

If the increase in haemoglobin is inadequate (less than 1 g/dL in four weeks) increase the dose by approximately 25%. Dose increases must not be made more frequently than once every four weeks.

If the rise in haemoglobin is greater than 2 g/dL in four weeks, reduce the dose by 25%, depending on the rate of increase. If the haemoglobin exceeds 12 g/dL a dose reduction should be considered. If the haemoglobin continues to increase, the dose should be reduced by approximately 25%. If, after a dose reduction haemoglobin continues to rise, the dose should be temporarily with-held until the haemoglobin starts to fall, at which point therapy should be re-initiated at approximately 25% lower than the previous dose. The haemoglobin should be measured every one or two weeks until it is stable. Thereafter the haemoglobin can be measured periodically.

Maintenance phase: Darbepoetin alfa may continue to be administered once weekly or once every two weeks.

Epoetin beta

Correction phase: Initial dosage is 20 IU/kg body weight three times per week. The dosage may be increased every four weeks by 20 IU/kg three times a week, if the increase of packed cell volume is not adequate (<0.5% per week).

Maintenance phase: To maintain a packed cell volume of between 30% and 35%, the dosage is initially reduced to half of the previously administered amount.

In the case of subcutaneous administration, the weekly dose can be given as one injection per week or in divided doses three or seven times per week. Patients who are stable on a once weekly dosing regimen may be switched to once every two weeks administration. In this case dose increases may be necessary.

Epoetin alfa

Correction phase: Starting dose of 50 IU/kg, three times per week, followed if necessary by a dosage increase with 25 IU/kg increments (three times per week) until the desired goal is achieved (this should be done in steps of at least four weeks).

Maintenance phase: Dosage adjustment in order to maintain haemoglobin values at the desired level: Hb between 10 and 12 g/dL, dose between 17 and 33 IU/kg, three times per week.

The maximum dosage should not exceed 200 IU/kg, three times per week.

5   What haemoglobin level would you aim for?

In people with anaemia of CKD, treatment should maintain stable haemoglobin levels between 10.5 and 12.5 g/dL for adults and children aged over 2 years, and between 10 and 12 g/dL in children aged under 2 years, reflecting the lower normal range in that age group. This should be achieved by:

- considering adjustments to treatment, typically when Hb rises above 12.0 or falls below 11.0 g/dL,
- taking patient preferences, symptoms and co-morbidity into account and revising the aspirational range and action thresholds accordingly.

6   What concomitant therapy might Mrs HK require to treat her renal anaemia?

Iron status should be evaluated prior to and during treatment and iron supplementation administered if necessary. Patients receiving ESA maintenance therapy should be given iron supplements to keep their serum ferritin between 200 and 500 micrograms/L in both haemodialysis patients and non-haemodialysis patients, and *either* the transferrin saturation level above 20% (unless ferritin >800 micrograms /L) *or* percentage hypochromic red cells (%HRC) less than 6% (unless ferritin >800 micrograms/L). In practice it is likely this will require intravenous iron.

A suggested iron dosage schedule is given in Table A15.1.

Table A15.1 Iron dosage schedule

Haemodialysis patients		Non-haemodialysis patients
Induction phase	Maintenance phase	
Either iron sucrose 200 mg/week for 5 weeks or low molecular weight iron dextran 1 g	Iron sucrose 50 mg/week or 100 mg/fortnight	Either iron sucrose 200 mg/week for 3 doses or low molecular weight iron dextran 1 g

7   What would you do if Mrs HK failed to respond to her epoetin therapy?

Non-response to epoetin alfa therapy should prompt a search for causative factors. These include: iron, folate, or vitamin B12 deficiency; aluminium intoxication; intercurrent infections; inflammatory or traumatic episodes; occult blood loss; haemolysis; and bone marrow fibrosis of any origin.

Case study level Ma – Diabetes and renal impairment – see page 361

1   What is diabetic ketoacidosis?

Diabetic ketoacidosis (DKA) is one consequence of untreated diabetes mellitus and is linked to an impaired glucose cycle. In a diabetic patient, DKA begins with deficiency in insulin. This is most commonly due to undiagnosed diabetes mellitus or, in patients who have been diagnosed with diabetes, failure to take prescribed insulin. DKA has a 100% mortality rate if left untreated.

A key component of DKA is that there is no or very little circulating insulin so it occurs mainly (but not exclusively) in type 1 diabetes (because type 1 diabetes is characterised by a lack of insulin production in the pancreas). It is much less common in type 2 diabetes which is closely related to cell insensitivity to insulin, rather than shortage or absence of insulin.

One of the effects of insulin is to stimulate the formation of glycogen from glucose and inhibition of glycogenolysis; stimulation of fatty acid (FA) production from stored lipids and inhibition of FA release into the blood; stimulation of FA uptake and storage; inhibition of protein catabolism and of gluconeogenesis, in which glucose is synthesised (mostly from some amino acid types, released by protein catabolism). A lack of insulin therefore has significant effects, all of which contribute to increasing blood glucose levels, to increased fat metabolism and protein degradation. Fat metabolism is one of the underlying causes of DKA.

Despite high circulating levels of plasma glucose, the liver will act as though the body is starving if insulin levels are low. In starvation situations, the liver produces another form of fuel: ketone bodies. Ketogenesis, that is fat metabolic processing (beginning with lipolysis), makes ketone bodies as intermediate products in the metabolic sequence as fatty acids (formerly attached to a glycerol backbone in triglycerides) are processed. The ketone bodies beta-hydroxybutyrate and acetoacetate enter the bloodstream and are usable as fuel for some organs such as the brain, though the brain still requires a substantial proportion of glucose to function. If large quantities of ketone bodies are produced, the metabolic imbalance known as ketosis may develop, though this condition is not necessarily harmful. The positive charge of ketone bodies causes decreased blood pH. An extreme excess of ketones can cause ketoacidosis.

Normally, ketone bodies are produced in minuscule quantities, feeding only part of the energy needs of the heart and brain. In DKA, the body enters a starving state. Eventually, neurons (and so the brain) switches from using glucose as a primary fuel source to using ketone bodies. As a result, the bloodstream is filled with an increasing amount of glucose that it cannot use (as the liver continues gluconeogenesis and exporting the glucose it makes). At the same time, massive amounts of ketone bodies are produced, which are acidic. As a result, the pH of the blood begins to move downward towards an acidotic state. The normal pH of human blood is 7.35–7.45; in acidosis the pH dips below 7.35. Very severe acidosis may be as low as 6.9–7.1. The acidic shift in the blood is significant because the proteins (i.e. body tissues, enzymes, etc.) in the body will be permanently denatured by a pH that is either too high or too low, thereby leading to widespread tissue damage, organ failure and eventually death.

Glucose begins to spill into the urine as the proteins responsible for reclaiming it from urine reach maximum capacity. As glucose is excreted in the urine, it takes a great deal of body water with it, resulting in dehydration. Dehydration further concentrates the blood and worsens the increased osmolality of the blood. Severe dehydration forces water out of cells and into the bloodstream to keep vital organs perfused. This shift of intracellular water into the bloodstream occurs at a cost, as the cells themselves need the water to complete chemical reactions that allow the cells to function.

2   Calculate CM's renal function using both the MDRD equation and the Cockcroft–Gault formula.

The standard equations used to calculate renal function may be applied here, as although the serum creatinine is elevated, it is stable. Were it still changing rapidly, the calculations would not be accurate.

MDRD

eGFR = 22 mL/min/1.73 m^2

Cockcroft and Gault

Ideal body weight = 45.5 + (2.3 × 3) = 52.4 kg. Since CM's actual body weight is not more than 15% greater than her IBW, use CM's actual body weight:

$$\text{GFR} = \frac{1.04 \times (140 - \text{Age}) \times \text{Weight}}{\text{Serum creatinine}}$$

$$= \frac{1.04 \times 113 \times 54}{246}$$

$$= \quad 25.8 \text{ mL/min}$$

3   What is the likely cause of CM's renal impairment?

CM appears to have developed diabetic nephropathy, although a renal biopsy would be required to establish the definitive diagnosis. Approximately 40% of people with longstanding type 1 diabetes develop diabetic nephropathy.

Essentially all patients with diabetic nephropathy also have diabetic retinopathy detectable by dilated retinal examination.

In type 1 diabetes, diabetic nephropathy follows a predictable course from onset of diabetes to the onset of microalbuminuria to frank nephropathy to end-stage renal disease or death. Microalbuminuria (a tiny amount of protein in the urine) develops 10–14 years after onset of diabetes. Without treatment, clinical nephropathy follows within 5 years, and severe renal impairment leading to end-stage renal failure develops approximately 5 years later. Hypertension develops in association with microalbuminuria and progresses with diabetic nephropathy, further damaging the kidneys. Once 'end-stage renal disease' (ESRD) is reached, the toxins in the body can no longer be cleared by the kidneys and, unless treated by dialysis, can build up to fatal levels.

The overall risk of developing diabetic nephropathy varies between about 10% of people with type 2 diabetes (diabetes of late onset) to about 30% of people with type 1 diabetes (diabetes of early onset). There are many factors, some known and others not, that affect the individual risk of developing diabetic nephropathy. Some of the factors that are known to increase the likelihood of getting diabetic nephropathy include:

- poor blood sugar control
- high blood pressure
- smoking
- relatives with kidney disease or hypertension
- onset of diabetes in teen years
- male
- Indo-Asian or Afro-Caribbean background.

4   What pharmacological and other interventions could be employed to reduce the risk of problems?

Once the process of diabetic nephropathy has begun, nothing can be done to stop it, and in most cases, eventually the patient will progress to end-stage renal failure. However, a number of clinical management points have been shown to slow the rate of progression of diabetic nephropathy, helping the patient to maintain their residual renal function for longer, and delaying the need to instigate dialysis (Table A15.2).

Good blood glucose control

Good blood glucose control can prevent the development and slow the progression of diabetic nephropathy, as well as preventing the other complications of diabetes, even if kidney failure has developed. This cannot be achieved by insulin alone, but requires a good diet too. Ideally HbA1c levels (a measure of average blood sugar control over three months) should be less than 7%.

Table A15.2 Management of diabetic nephropathy

Stage	Assessment	Treatment
No proteinuria	Monitor blood pressure Monitor blood glucose Screen for microalbuminuria if type 1 diabetes for >5 years or type 2 diabetes	Aim for <130/80 mmHg Aim for <120/70 mmHg if type 1 diabetes Aim for HbA1c <7% Dietary advice for sugar and fat STOP SMOKING
Microalbuminuria	Close monitoring of blood pressure, blood glucose and blood lipid levels Monitor urinary protein	Aim for BP <125/75 mmHg Add further antihypertensive drugs if necessary Add ACE I/ARB if possible Aim for total cholesterol <3.5 mmol/L
Proteinuria	Close monitoring of blood pressure, blood glucose and blood lipid levels Monitor urinary protein	As for microalbuminuria
Declining kidney function		Prepare for dialysis and/or transplantation

Blood pressure control

The recommended target blood pressure is 125/75 mmHg in diabetic patients; however, the lower the blood pressure the lower the risk of problems developing. This rigorous control of blood pressure usually requires more than one type of antihypertensive agent to achieve this desired result, and it is not uncommon to see renal patients on combinations of a beta-blocker, a calcium channel blocker, an alpha-blocker, an ACE inhibitor, an angiotensin II receptor blocker (ARB) and a loop diuretic. If the patient is overweight, losing weight will help too.

Using ACE inhibitors and angiotensin II receptor blockers

Two classes of drug used to control blood pressure deserve special mention. These are the angiotensin-converting enzyme (ACE) inhibitors and angiotensin II receptor blockers (ARBs). These drugs not only reduce blood pressure in the large blood vessels, but also directly in the kidneys' filtering system (the glomeruli). Many studies have documented the beneficial effects of these agents beyond simply blood pressure control to reducing kidney protein leak. Although these drugs are useful, they need to be monitored as they may have a detrimental effect, in particular, in those patients with bilateral renal artery stenosis.

Diet

Diet above and beyond the diabetic diet, not adding any salt and reducing alcohol intake, will have beneficial effects on blood pressure. Other aspects of diet (including energy, calcium and phosphate) are important in renal failure and the assistance of a renal dietitian is normally required if the degree of renal impairment is severe (e.g. CKD stage 4–5).

Controlling blood lipids and cholesterol

Controlling blood triglyceride and cholesterol levels helps prevent heart disease and possibly strokes, and may slow the progression of diabetic kidney disease. The current data point towards a target total cholesterol of <3.5 mmol/L if the patient has microalbuminuria, and statins are very widely prescribed in diabetic patients with renal impairment.

Smoking

Patients really should not smoke, not only for the sake of their kidneys, but also for the sake of their heart and cerebral blood vessels. Smokers die earlier than non-smokers, but diabetic smokers die much earlier and often develop serious circulation problems at a young age.

5   Comment on this dose of gentamicin.

Gentamicin is a drug with a narrow therapeutic index, which is highly nephrotoxic and ototoxic. In order to minimise this toxicity, it is necessary to monitor plasma levels of the drug. Since gentamicin is cleared almost exclusively via the kidneys, there is a risk that in situations where a patient has renal impairment, the drug cannot be excreted at the usual rate and so will accumulate, causing greater toxicity. Hence the usual practice is to reduce the dose in patients with renal impairment and monitor levels very carefully.

6   What dose would you recommend?

Depending on the equation used, CM's GFR has been calculated as being between 22 and 26 mL/min. Given this level of renal function, it would be prudent to recommend giving a dose of 4 mg/kg body weight, and then monitoring plasma levels until a suitable trough level of less than 1.5–2.0 mg/L has been reached. Depending on how well the patient clears the drug, daily dosing may be required, or she may only need a dose every 48 hours.

In addition, it should be remembered that gentamicin is nephrotoxic, so that patient's renal function should be constantly monitored. If it deteriorates (i.e. the serum creatinine rises), then the patient's renal function needs to be recalculated and the dose of gentamicin amended accordingly.

Case study level Mb – Hypertension-associated kidney disease – see page 363

1   Comment on Mr WD's laboratory results.

Mr WD has severe hypertension with a blood pressure of 180/105 mmHg. The proteinuria on dipstick is also indicative of renal damage. His serum creatinine is well above the normal range of 65–115 micromol/L, and his serum urea is also elevated (normal range 3.0–6.5 mmol/L), indicating that he has moderate to severe renal impairment.

2   Calculate Mr WD's renal function using the MDRD equation and the Cockcroft–Gault formula.

MDRD

$$eGFR = 21 \text{ ml/min/1.73 m}^2$$

Cockcroft and Gault

Ideal body weight = 50 + (2.3 x 11) = 75.3 kg.

$$GFR = \frac{1.23 \times (140 - \text{Age}) \times \text{Weight}}{\text{Serum creatinine}}$$

$$= \frac{1.23 \times 98 \times 75.3}{365}$$

$$= \quad 24.8 \text{ mL/min}$$

3   What do you think may have caused Mr WD's renal impairment?

Hypertension can be a consequence as well as a frequent cause of renal dysfunction.

Renal haemodynamic alterations are detectable prior to the diagnosis of hypertension and, along with the elevation of blood pressure, are associated with structural changes in small renal arteries and arterioles. By disturbing the normal pressure–natriuresis relationship, both changes impair sodium and water excretion and thereby are instrumental in raising blood pressure. For unknown reasons, in some hypertensive individuals, related structural changes become progressive and give rise to gross signs of renal dysfunction, including proteinuria and eventually renal failure.

Although the connection between malignant hypertension and end-stage renal disease (ESRD) has been recognised since the nineteenth century, some have proposed that ESRD developing in patients with non-malignant hypertension is secondary to underlying primary renal disease and that hypertension only aggravates progression of the primary disease. Among 332 544 men screened for the Multiple Risk Factor Intervention Trial (MRFIT), there was a graded relationship between levels of both systolic and diastolic blood pressure at baseline and risk of subsequent ESRD, even after considering other predictors of ESRD risk (i.e. age, race, smoking, cholesterol, diabetes, myocardial infarction and income) (Klag et al., 1996). Almost half of the incident cases of ESRD (49%) were attributable to hypertension.

The findings in this study provide the most compelling evidence of a causal relationship between elevated blood pressure and ESRD in people with no other primary renal disease (Klag et al., 1996) . The likelihood of ESRD is greater among minority populations, particularly among Mexican Americans and African Americans. Different rates of ESRD among racial/ethnic groups after adjustment for known risk factors have been attributed to differences in genetic predisposition; however, the particular genetic factors that contribute to differences in risk of ESRD between and within racial/ethnic groups remain unknown.

Until late in the course of hypertensive nephropathy, renal damage is asymptomatic and laboratory findings are subtle. The first objective sign of renal involvement is a small increase in the amount of albumin in the urine.

Increasing evidence suggests that microalbuminuria, reported in 10–40% of non-diabetics with hypertension (Ruilope and Rodicio, 1995), may serve as an early indicator of risk to develop subsequent proteinuria and progressive renal impairment. In both insulin- and non-insulin-dependent diabetes mellitus, these predictive relationships are well established. In non-diabetics with hypertension, microalbuminuria correlates with established predictors of ESRD and/or cardiovascular disease morbidity and mortality including black race, male gender, age, body mass index, blood pressure level and hypertension, plasma cholesterol, triglycerides, glucose, insulin and fibrinogen concentrations, and smoking.

4   How should Mr WD's hypertension be managed?

As a general rule, the treatment of hypertension in patients with renal impairment follows the British Hypertension Society and NICE guidelines, as detailed below.

The drugs commonly used in the treatment of hypertension are:

- thiazide diuretics
- beta-blockers
- alpha-adrenoceptor blockers
- calcium channel blockers
- angiotensin-converting enzyme (ACE) inhibitors
- angiotensin II receptor blockers
- centrally acting drugs
- direct acting vasodilators.

Tight blood pressure control, especially in renal patients, can be difficult to obtain, and may result in patients being on maximum doses of many antihypertensive drugs. In renal patients, the general rule is to start drug therapy at the lowest dose and then increase the dose cautiously according to the patient's response. Beta-blockers, calcium channel blockers and ACE inhibitors have all been shown to improve left ventricular hypertrophy in the general population and are safe in chronic renal failure. In order to maximise 24-hour blood pressure control, long-acting agents are generally preferred. In addition, it does not matter whether a particular drug is excreted via the kidneys or the liver, since the dose will be titrated to an end-point, namely, the adequate control of blood pressure.

The British Hypertension Society recommendations are shown in Figure A15.1 overleaf.

The ASCOT trial (Dahlof *et al.*, 2005) recommends using ACE inhibitors first line for younger patients and calcium channel blockers for older patients. The National Institute for Health and Clinical Excellence (NICE, 2006) recommends:

- For patients over 55 years old or black – a calcium channel blocker or thiazide diuretic first line, ACE inhibitor second line, and a calcium channel blocker or thiazide third line whichever was not used first.
- For patients under 55 years old, an ACE inhibitor first line, a calcium channel blocker or thiazide second line, and a calcium channel blocker or thiazide third line.
- For all patients an alpha-blocker, further diuretic or beta-blocker may be added as a fourth drug, with referral to a specialist.

NICE (2006) also recommends that beta-blockers are not used as an initial therapy for hypertension since they have been shown to be less effective at reducing the risk of a major cardiovascular system event, in particular stroke.

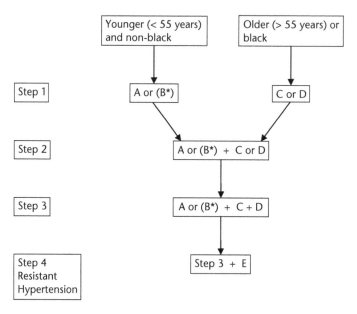

A = Angiotensin-converting enzyme (ACE) inhibitor or angiotensin II receptor blocker
B = Beta-blocker
C = Calcium channel blocker
D = Thiazide diuretic
E = Add either alpha-blocker or spironolactone or other diuretic.
* Combination therapy involving B + D may induce more new-onset diabetes compared
with other combination therapies. (Williams *et al.*, 2004.)

Figure A15.1 British Hypertension Society Recommendations.

Beta-blockers are an alternative to an ACE inhibitor when an ACE inhibitor is contraindicated or not tolerated (for example, in women of childbearing age or those with an increased sympathetic drive).

In patients with renal disease, hypertension can increase the rate of progression to ESRD and therefore the use of antihypertensive drugs can be important in delaying the progression to ESRD. This is the same for all causes of renal impairment. In some cases, initiation of dialysis is needed to control hypertension. In diabetes and some other renal diseases (e.g. glomerulonephritis), controlling the blood pressure with an ACE inhibitor or angiotensin II blocker slows the damage to the kidney and therefore delays the time to onset of ESRD. However, ACE inhibitors should be used with caution in patients with severe renal disease since they can reduce the perfusion of the kidney, thereby reducing kidney function even further, and hence reduce the time until dialysis is required. In all patients, when starting an ACE inhibitor or ARB, renal function should be measured prior to starting therapy and regularly thereafter to detect whether the drug is affecting the patient's renal function.

In patients with renal artery stenosis (RAS), the main blood vessel running to the kidney becomes blocked – partially or fully – due to atherosclerosis. It usually affects both kidneys. It is a common cause of renal failure in older people, especially those who have suffered an MI or stroke (i.e. they are at increased risk of atherosclerosis). In patients with RAS, ACE inhibitors and angiotensin II blockers are generally avoided since they can dramatically reduce the remaining level of renal function, accelerating the progression to ESRD. Occasionally, if the benefits outweigh the risks these drugs may be used under the close supervision of a nephrologist.

Thiazide diuretics are ineffective once the GFR becomes less than 25 mL/min, and loop diuretics are often used at high doses (e.g. furosemide 500 mg to 1 g daily) to gain an effect. Metolazone is effective when combined with a loop diuretic. Potassium-sparing diuretics such as amiloride are not recommended. Spironolactone is not generally used, but is beneficial in low dose for the treatment of heart failure even in patients on dialysis. Beta-blockers and calcium channel blockers are generally well tolerated. Any ankle swelling with calcium channel blockers must not be confused with fluid overload.

It should be remembered that hypertension in patients with renal dysfunction can be particularly difficult to treat, and many patients require more than one antihypertensive agent in order to control their blood pressure. There is some guidance provided by the Renal Association in their Clinical Guidelines document as to choice of therapeutic agent:

> The treatment of hypertension affords the dual benefit of slowing the rate of progression of CKD and reducing cardiovascular risk in patients with CKD. Whereas the evidence that lowering blood pressure confers renal and cardiovascular protection is clear, the optimal level of blood pressure control is less well established. Two large prospective randomised studies have investigated the effect of lower target blood pressures on CKD progression but have failed to provide clear answers. Nevertheless, the MDRD study (1999) did show that the level of proteinuria at baseline significantly modulated the effect of blood pressure lowering such that a lower blood pressure target (125/75 vs. 140/90mmHg) was associated with a slower rate of decline in GFR among patients with >1g/day of proteinuria. Furthermore, secondary analysis revealed significant correlations between rate of GFR decline and achieved blood pressure prompting the authors to suggest blood pressure targets of <130/80mmHg for patients with <1g/day of proteinuria and <125/75mmHg for those with >1g/day of proteinuria. Long-term follow-up of 840 patients from the MDRD study (1999) showed adjusted hazard ratios of 0.68 (0.57–0.82) and 0.77 (0.65–0.91) for ESRD and a composite end-point of ESRD and all-cause mortality, respectively for patients originally randomised to the low blood pressure target. Similarly, a meta-analysis of data from 1860 non-diabetic patients with CKD reported the lowest risk of CKD progression in patients with systolic blood pressure 110–129mmHg but a higher risk of progression associated with SBP<110mmHg.
>
> A similar note of caution has been sounded by a secondary analysis of data from

the Irbesartan Diabetic Nephropathy Trial. Whereas the analysis showed improved renal and patient survival associated with lower achieved systolic blood pressure, there was a significant increase in all-cause mortality among patients with achieved systolic blood pressure <120mmHg.

There is a strong consensus among national and international renal, hypertension and diabetes organisations to recommend a target blood pressure of <130/80mmHg for all patients with CKD. Whereas there is some evidence to support a lower target of <125/75mmHg in patients with >1g/day of proteinuria there is concern that lower blood pressures may be associated with adverse outcomes in some patients.

Several large prospective randomised controlled trials among different groups of patients with CKD provide evidence that ACEI or ARB treatment affords significant renal protection in addition to that attributable to blood pressure lowering. Specifically, ACEI treatment has been shown to slow CKD progression among patients with type 1 diabetes mellitus and established nephropathy as well as patients with non-diabetic CKD and proteinuria >1g/day. Furthermore a recent randomised study has shown that ACEI treatment may afford significant renal protection (43% reduction in risk of doubling serum creatinine, ESRD or death) in non-diabetic patients with advanced renal disease (serum creatinine 264–440mmol/l). A meta-analysis of data from 11 randomized controlled trails that compared ACEI with other antihypertensives among patients with predominantly non-diabetic CKD showed a significantly lower risk of ESRD incidence (relative risk 0.69; 95%CI 0.51–0.94) associated with ACEI treatment after adjustment for differences in level of blood pressure control. The analysis also found greater renal protective benefit associated with ACEI treatment in patients with higher levels of baseline proteinuria and no benefit could be shown for those with proteinuria <0.5g/day. This analysis did not however include data from the AASK study, which reported a lower incidence of the combined end-point of >50% GFR reduction, ESRD or death among African American patients with mild baseline proteinuria (mean 0.6g/day among males and 0.4g/day among females) randomised to ACEI treatment versus a calcium channel blocker or a β-blocker. We have selected a proteinuria threshold of >1g/day to recommend ACEI or ARB treatment because this has the most robust evidence to support it. It should be recognised, however, that some patients with lesser degrees of proteinuria may benefit from ACEI or ARB treatment.

ARB treatment has been shown to afford significant renal protection (risk reduction 16% and 20 or 23% for primary outcome of doubling of serum creatinine, ESRD or death) in two large randomised studies of patients with type 2 diabetes and established nephropathy.

Two large prospective randomised controlled studies have reported significant reductions in cardiovascular morbidity and mortality associated with ACEI treatment among patients with a high risk for future cardiovascular events. On the other hand the primary analysis of one study found no such benefit among patients with stable coronary heart disease and low risk of cardiovascular events. Interestingly a secondary analysis of the PEACE Trial data found a higher risk of death among patients with an estimated GFR of <60ml/min/1.73m^2 at baseline and a significant reduction in all cause mortality associated with ACEI treatment in this subgroup. Whereas none of the above studies specifically included patients with CKD and all excluded patients with moderate or severe renal impairment, these data do provide support for the notion that ACEI treatment reduces cardiovascular risk in high-risk patients. As cardiovascular disease remains the most important cause of death among CKD patients it seems reasonable to recommend ACEI or ARB treatment for reduction of cardiovascular risk as well as slowing of CKD progression.(Taal and Tonsen, 2007)

For a full version of these guidelines, refer to the Renal Association website, http://www.renal.org/pages

5   What therapy would you recommend for the treatment of Mr WD's hypertension?

Following the guidelines of the British Hypertension Society, Mr WD should be prescribed a thiazide diuretic and a calcium channel blocker, so a good combination might be nifedipine LA 20 mg or 30 mg once daily or amlodipine 5 mg once daily, plus bendroflumethiazide 2.5 mg once daily. However, we know that his renal function is poor, with a calculated GFR of approximately 25 mL/min, so he is borderline for thiazides to be clinically effective. In this instance, it might be prudent to prescribe an ACE inhibitor instead, for example, enalapril 5–10 mg twice daily.

6   What could be the cause of Mr WD's new symptoms?

Calcium channel blockers are well known to cause peripheral oedema, in particular ankle oedema. This occurs as the vasodilatation induced by the drug tends to make the blood vessel walls 'leaky', and so fluid escapes to, and accumulates in the surrounding tissues. Unfortunately, this condition is unresponsive to diuretic therapy, and so the only way to reverse it is to discontinue the drug.

ACE inhibitors are known to cause a cough. It is a class-wide effect, and is thought to be due to the fact that apart from converting angiotensin I to angiotensin II, the angiotensin-converting enzyme is also responsible for assisting in the breakdown of bradykinins and other inflammatory mediators within the body. The prescribing of an ACE inhibitor not only inhibits the production of angiotensin II (thereby having an antihypertensive effect), but also means that there will be higher circulating levels of bradykinins since they are not being metabolised. These bradykinins manifest their higher blood levels by inducing a coughing reaction. This may vary from a light tickly cough that does not cause too much inconvenience, to a severe hacking cough that necessitates discontinuation of the drug.

7   What treatment would you suggest now for Mr WD's hypertension?

In view of his cardiovascular status and proteinuria, WD should be on 'anti-ACE' therapy of some kind. If he is unable to tolerate an ACE inhibitor, an alternative might be to try an ARB. This has the advantage of blocking the renin–angiotensin system, thereby achieving the required therapeutic effect, but since ACE itself is not affected, the patient should not develop a cough.

If the patient is finding the ankle oedema caused by the calcium channel blocker distressing, then the drug should be discontinued. Some patients find the symptoms may be reduced by switching to a longer-acting drug within the class, for example, amlodipine. Failing this the drug needs to be discontinued, and an alternative class of drug used, for example, a beta-blocker or an alpha-receptor blocker.

16

Paediatrics case studies

Stephen Tomlin

Case study level 1 – Croup

Learning outcomes

Level 1 case study: You will be able to:

- describe the risk factors
- describe the disease
- describe the pharmacology of the drug
- outline the formulation including drug molecule, excipients, etc. for the medicines
- summarise basic social pharmacy issues (e.g. opening containers, large labels).

Scenario

A mother comes into the pharmacy with a young girl who is seven months old. She tells you that her daughter has a harsh cough which sounds more like a bark than anything else. Although she is not too bad during the day she is terrible at night and really struggles to get to sleep. The mother tells you that she is keen not to have any medicines, but has heard that substances can be inhaled in steam and is keen to try something like that. You decide that the child must have croup.

Questions

1   What is croup?
2   Should steam therapy be recommended by the community pharmacist?
3   What is the first-line treatment of mild to moderate croup?

4   Are there side-effects related to the use of glucocorticoids?
5a   What other treatment has been shown to be effective in severe croup?
5b   How does this treatment work?

General references

Anon (1999) Cough medications in children. *Drugs and Therapeutics Bulletin* 37: 19–21.

Bjornson GC, Klassen TP, Williamson J *et al.* (2004) Paediatric Emergency Research Canada Network. A randomised trial of a single dose of oral dexamethasone for mild croup. *New England Journal of Medicine* 351: 1306–1313.

Johnson D, Williamson J, Craig W *et al.* (2004) Management of croup: practise variation among 21 Alberta hospitals. *Paediatric Research* 55: 113A.

Joint Formulary Committee (2008) *BNF for Children*. London: British Medical Association and Royal Pharmaceutical Society of Great Britain.

Lissauer T and Clayden G (2001) *Illustrated Textbook of Paediatrics*, 2nd edn. St. Louis: Mosby, pp. 217–220.

Case study level 2 – Fever

Learning outcomes

Level 2 case study: You will be able to:

- interpret relevant lab and clinical data
- identify monitoring and referral criteria
- explain treatment choices
- describe goals of therapy, including monitoring and the role of the pharmacist/clinician
- describe issues – counselling points, adverse drug reactions, drug interactions, complementary/alternative therapies and lifestyle advice.

Scenario

A 2-year-old boy is brought into your pharmacy by his parents. He is well wrapped up for the cold weather but they say he has a temperature. He has a cough which he picked up at nursery. The parents want to know if they can have something to prevent febrile convulsions. They are particularly worried as they have an older child with epilepsy. On questioning the parents say that they took his temperature this morning and it was 38°C, but his head still feels very hot.

1   What is a normal temperature and how should it be recorded?
2   What physiological process causes a fever?
3   What basic (non-drug) advice would you give to the family?
4a What medication could be offered to reduce the fever? Discuss available products and issues of use.
4b Should medication be used individually or in combination?
4c Will the medication reduce the chance of the child having febrile convulsions?
5a Are the parents right to be concerned about the additional risk of febrile convulsions due to the given family history?
5b Is there any treatment that can be offered as prophylaxis against febrile convulsions?

General references

Anon (2006) Managing infants with pyrexia. *Nursing Times* 26 September–2 October, 102: 42–43. Review.
Kramer MS and Shapiro ED (1997) Management of the young febrile child. *Paediatrics* 100: 128–134.

Case study level 3 – Diabetes

Learning outcomes

Level 3 case study: You will be able to:

- interpret clinical signs and symptoms
- evaluate laboratory data
- evaluate treatment options
- state goals of therapy
- describe a pharmaceutical care plan to include advice to a clinician
- describe the prognosis and long-term complications
- describe the social pharmacy issues which could include supply (e.g. complex treatments at home, concordance and compliance) and lifestyle issues.

Scenario

DP is a 7-year-old girl, who weighs 22 kg and has always been a healthy, active child. The family have had colds and fevers over the last few weeks, but DP was still suffering from flu-like symptoms and a recurrent stomachache, with occasional nausea and vomiting. Her mum thought she had lost weight over the last few weeks. She has thus been taken to the GP.

On questioning, it was found that DP has been drinking large quantities of water and juice over the last couple of months. She had also been wetting the bed on a number of occasions which her mum has put down to her not getting on well at school.

On testing, her random blood glucose was 14 mmol/L (3.5–10 mmol/L) and her urine tested negative for ketones. A diagnosis of mild ketosis was made presenting secondary to newly diagnosed type 1 diabetes.

Questions

1a Describe the presenting symptoms that led to a diagnosis of type 1 diabetes. Explain the mechanism behind each symptom.

1b How do these symptoms compare to a classic presentation of the disease? Could there have been a misdiagnosis? Consider specifically what is happening at her school.

2 What are the aims of treatment for DP?

DP was initiated on a preloaded pen, using an insulin mix (biphasic) for subcutaneous administration. She was started on a twice daily biphasic insulin regimen based on a total dose of 0.5 units/kg/day with 2/3 given in the morning before breakfast and 1/3 given before the evening meal.

3 How should DP be advised and taught to monitor her regimen?

4 How should she and her carers be taught to inject her insulin?

5 What should her carers be told about her first few months of treatment?

6 Discuss the insulin and devise options for treating type 1 diabetes.

Reference

Diabetes Control and Complications Trial Research Group (1994) The effect of intensive diabetes treatment on the development and progression of long-term complications in adolescents with insulin-dependent diabetes mellitus. *Journal of Pediatrics* 125: 177–188.

General references

National Prescribing Centre (2002) When and how should patients with diabetes test blood glucose? *MeReC Bulletin* 13(1). Available at http://www.npc.co.uk/MeReC_Bulletins/2002Volumes/v0113n01.pdf [Accessed 4 July 2008].

NICE (National Institute for Health and Clinical Excellence) (2004) Type 1 diabetes in children, young people and adults: Available at http://www.nice.org.uk/nicemedia/pdf/CG015NICEguideline.pdf [Accessed 4 July 2008].

Thompson R and Hindmarsh P (2002) Management of type 1 diabetes in children. *Prescriber* 19 April: 77–85.

Young YL and Koda Kimble MA (2001) *Applied Therapeutics: The Clinical Use of Drugs.* Philadelphia: Lippincott Williams & Wilkins.

Case study level Ma – Gastro-oesophageal reflux

Learning outcomes

Level M case study: You will be able to:

- interpret clinical signs and symptoms
- evaluate laboratory data
- critically appraise treatment options
- state goals of therapy
- describe a pharmaceutical care plan to include advice to a clinician
- describe the prognosis and long-term complications
- describe the social pharmacy issues which could include supply (e.g. complex treatments at home, concordance and compliance) and lifestyle issues
- describe the monitoring of therapy.

Scenario

Jim is a three-month-old baby born at 35 weeks' gestation. He has been in hospital since birth with a variety of problems. He is now feeding enterally via a bottle, but is not thriving and his weight is falling off the centile chart. He has been on feed thickeners and ranitidine for the last month for gastro-oesophageal reflux, but symptoms still persist.

Questions

1 What is gastro-oesophageal reflux and what are the main symptoms?

2a What is the rationale behind the ranitidine treatment already started?

2b What alternative class of drug may work in the same way as ranitidine, but be more effective?

2c What are the practical problems of using this second class of medicine in an infant?

3a   Name three prokinetic agents which could be added to the regimen at this stage.

3b   What is the rationale of use of these products?

3c   Briefly mention the potential issues surrounding the use of each product.

Jim gets an ear infection and is started on metronidazole suspension. The current reflux regimen continues.

4   What is the problem of using metronidazole suspension when the gastric content is acid suppressed?

5   What is the other potential risk of using metronidazole alongside ranitidine suspension?

General references

Gold BD and Freston JW (2002) Gastroesophageal reflux in children. *Pediatric Drugs* 4: 673–685.

Rudolph CD, Mazur LJ *et al.* (2001) Guidelines for evaluation and treatment of gastroespophageal reflux in infants and children. *Journal of Pediatric Gastroenterology and Nutrition* 32 (Suppl 2): S1–S31.

Sharma VK (1999) Comparison of 24-hour intragastric Ph using four liquid formulations of lansoprazole and omeprazole. *American Journal of Health-System Pharmacy* 56 (23 Suppl): S18–S21.

Case study level Mb – Asthma

Learning outcomes

Level M case study: You will be able to:

- interpret clinical signs and symptoms
- evaluate laboratory data
- critically appraise treatment options
- state goals of therapy
- describe a pharmaceutical care plan to include advice to a clinician
- describe the prognosis and long-term complications
- describe the social pharmacy issues which could include supply (e.g. complex treatments at home, concordance and compliance) and lifestyle issues
- describe the monitoring of therapy.

A 3-year-old boy comes into A&E with a severe asthma attack. This is his third in the last three months. He is started on nebulised salbutamol, intravenous aminophylline and oral prednisolone. The presenting symptoms include:

- tachycardia
- rapid breathing
- peak expiratory flow rate (PEFR) <50% normal
- unable to talk due to breathlessness.

Three days later, after being stabilised on the ward, he is discharged on salbutamol and beclometasone inhalers (same as on admission) plus a leukotriene antagonist.

1a What is asthma?
1b How does early childhood asthma often present?
1c What are the common symptoms?
1d What class of drug is used for the initial pharmacological management of asthma and how do they work?
1e What route of administration is usually used initially and why?
1f What are the main side-effects of this class of drugs?
2a What are the classes of the drugs being used here to treat the severe asthma attack and how will they help?
2b What side-effect do they all have in common which can be exacerbated by hypoxia, a common feature of severe asthma?
3a What step of the British Thoracic Society guidelines is the boy now on?
3b What is the role of the leukotriene antagonist?
3c What preparations are available and which would probably be most suitable for this 3-year-old boy?
4a What is the most suitable way to administer the beclometasone to this 3-year-old and why?
4b How should the administration device be cared for and why?
4c What are the other main devices used to administer medication in asthma?
5a With a patient with severe asthma such as this, is there any advice that the family can follow at home if an acute asthma attack starts again?
5b Can you suggest a way that the family can monitor response to therapy?

General references

British Thoracic Society (BTS) and Scottish Intercollegiate Guidelines Network (SIGN) (2003) British guidelines on the management of asthma. *Thorax* 58 (Suppl 1): i1–i94. BTS and SIGN (updated May 2008). Available at www.brit-thoracic.org.uk.

Joint Formulary Committee (2008) *BNF for Children*. London: British Medical Association and Royal Pharmaceutical Society of Great Britain.

Answers

Case study level 1 – Croup – see page 391

1   What is croup?

Croup is most commonly caused by the parainfluenza virus and presents with night time symptoms of a barking cough. Hoarseness, inspiratory stridor and respiratory depression may be present in varying degrees of severity. Although both upper and lower airways may be affected it is primarily related to the upper airway.

The small reductions in the subglottic region of the airways secondary to mucosal oedema causes significant changes to airflow. It is this change that results in the bark-like cough and respiratory distress.

2   Should steam therapy be recommended by the community pharmacist?

If a community pharmacist believes that a child may have croup they should refer them immediately to the hospital. While many croup patients can recover with no treatment, it can get worse very quickly. There is no definitive treatment for viral croup and therapy is based on maintaining airways and hydration.

While inhalation has been used for many years there are no randomised controlled trials performed on its use. Menthol and eucalyptus may help ease congestion and thus assist breathing, but there is limited evidence. Boiling water for inhalation should never be recommended due to the risks of burns.

3   What is the first-line treatment of mild to moderate croup?

Glucocorticoids are the first-line treatment for mild to moderate croup. They are effective via many routes (inhaled, oral, parenteral), but dexamethasone given orally as one single dose or in two divided doses has been shown to be as effective as the same dose given via the parenteral route and superior in efficacy to nebulised budesonide.

4   Are there side-effects related to the use of glucocorticoids?

Giving dexamethasone as a stat dose to treat croup is very unlikely to cause any side-effects as many steroid adverse events are related to prolonged use.

However even as a stat dose some biochemistry markers can be significantly affected, such as the potassium and blood glucose. Other longer term side-effects might include immunosuppression, bone demineralisation and Cushingoid symptoms, but these would not be seen after this one dose.

5a   What other treatment has been shown to be effective in severe croup?

Nebulised adrenaline should be considered for infants with moderate to severe symptoms of croup.

5b   How does this treatment work?

There are several actions which adrenaline performs when administered directly into the lungs. By stimulating alpha-adrenergic receptors there is a resultant constriction of the arterioles, resorption of the interstitial fluid and decrease of the oedema in the infraglottic region.

Case study level 2 – Fever – see page 392

1   What is a normal temperature and how should it be recorded?

Normal oral temperature is 37°C (98.6°F), plus or minus one degree. Central temperature follows a circadian rhythm. The temperature falls by about 0.8 degrees during sleep and then rises just before waking and the highest temperature is attained at approximately 6 pm. Peripheral temperatures are about 0.5 degrees lower than central temperatures.

Rectal temperature is the most accurate at about 37°C. However this is not usually practical and thus oral or underarm temperatures are often taken. There are electronic tympanic devices available which take the temperature from the ear. These read in both centigrade (°C) and Fahrenheit (°F) and are placed in the ear for a few seconds (depending on device) and produce a good level of accuracy if used correctly. These are commonly used in hospitals and can be bought over the counter. Also available over the counter are disposable temperature strips; these are popular as they are easy to use but relatively inaccurate.

In most cases a parent/carer will diagnose fever. Placing a hand on a child's head is a good way of assessing fever and a method that carers frequently use. Children may also be 'off colour' and factors such as these are important indicators when evaluating whether a child is unwell. A child maybe irritable or inconsolable, for example, off his or her food or need a greater amount of parental attention than their normal behavioural patterns would indicate.

There may be other more tangible symptoms present, such as cold, cough, sore throat, earache, diarrhoea, drowsiness, convulsions, pains and headaches.

2   What physiological process causes a fever?

Body temperature is a very important clinical marker as slight alterations in temperature can alter cell function and in extreme events cause death. Cell metabolism results in the generation of heat energy; this is lost from the body via radiation, evaporation, conduction and convection. The hypothalamus is responsible for controlling body temperature.

Fever occurs as a result of the presence of pyrogens. These are generally produced as a response to infection, inflammation or an immune response. Pyrogens affect the cells in the hypothalamus and the subsequent response is vasodilatation to get rid of the excess heat. This produces the characteristic 'flushed' appearance of a feverish child.

3   What basic (non-drug) advice would you give to the family?

As the child is older than 1 year and there is a probable focus for the fever (i.e. the cough – probably a viral infection) then there is no need to refer.

■   Advise lots of cool drinks, this prevents dehydration and helps lower the temperature
■   Parents sometimes manage a fever by wrapping a child up. This should be discouraged.
■   Sponging or tepid baths may also be helpful. Tepid water is better than cold water as cold water can cause vasoconstriction and a subsequent further increase in temperature.
■   Do not advise the use of fans as this may cause the air to become cold.

4a   What medication could be offered to reduce the fever? Discuss available products and issues of use.

Paracetamol is available in liquid, soluble tablet, sachet and melt tablet form. The liquid tends to be the most popular, however this varies between children. There are different brands available and flavour can influence how popular these are. Some products contain additional antihistamines. Note: Paracetamol is only indicated for children over three months of age when sold over the counter.

Ibuprofen is available in liquid, sachet, capsule, melt and tablet form. The licensed age range for ibuprofen depends on the product formulation. Ibuprofen is only indicated for children over six months of age over the counter. It has additional anti-inflammatory properties which may be helpful in conditions such as otitis media. Ibuprofen has the potential to cause gastrointestinal disturbances, although if given with food this is unlikely. Note: Caution if using in a child with history of severe asthma or renal disease.

4b   Should medication be used individually or in combination?

Paracetamol and ibuprofen can both be used to reduce temperature. There is limited evidence to support using either alternating drug dosing or giving ibuprofen and paracetamol at the same time. However, single agent cover is generally adequate and generally causes less confusion and decreases potential for error.

4c   Will the medication reduce the chance of the child having febrile convulsions?

There is no evidence that reducing the temperature with antipyretics reduces the chances of having a febrile convulsion. Reducing the temperature makes the child feel more comfortable, but has little clinical benefit apart from that.

5a   Are the parents right to be concerned about the additional risk of febrile convulsions due to the given family history?

Febrile convulsions generally occur between six months and 3 years of age. A family history of epilepsy is not definitely associated with an increased risk of febrile convulsions, but if they happen they are more likely to recur. The younger the age group the higher the risk of recurrence (especially <1 year). By the age of 8 years only 3% of children who have had a febrile convulsion will have developed epilepsy and the two events seem unrelated.

5b   Is there any treatment that can be offered as prophylaxis against febrile convulsions?

No. Antipyretics may make the child feel more comfortable, but there is no evidence that they reduce the incidence or severity of febrile convulsions. Anticonvulsants certainly have no role to play. If a febrile convulsion does happen they are generally tonic or tonic–clonic and last just a couple of minutes. If they were to continue for longer than 5 minutes then conventional treatment for status epilepticus should be used (rectal diazepam or buccal midazolam).

Case study level 3 – Diabetes – see page 393

1a   Describe the presenting symptoms that led to a diagnosis of type 1 diabetes. Explain the mechanism behind each symptom.

Her presenting symptoms include abdominal pain, weight loss, enuresis, thirst, elevated blood glucose and ketones in the urine.

 The onset of type 1 diabetes is often preceded by an acute viral illness which can cause an autoimmune destructive response in the pancreas leading to impaired insulin production. Her weight loss is the product of several of her presenting symptoms. When glucose levels in blood exceed the renal threshold, excess glucose is excreted into the urine, accompanied by water in the process of osmotic diuresis. This leads to loss of calories and fluid, leading to symptoms of thirst, polyuria, enuresis, weight loss and also fatigue. Her ongoing viral illness, plus the abdominal symptoms associated with ketoacidosis may also be reducing her appetite.

1b   How do these symptoms compare to a classic presentation of the disease? Could there have been a misdiagnosis? Consider specifically what is happening at her school.

Her symptoms are classic, but in children such symptoms may initially be associated with urinary tract infection, failure to thrive, gastroenteritis or psychological problems. Polyuria and bed wetting in children are often linked to urinary tract infection. This diagnosis may be further supported by the symptom of abdominal pain. The gastrointestinal upset seen can be caused by the presenting ketoacidosis which is often accompanied by weight loss due to lack of eating and vomiting, together with higher urine output. This in turn leads to symptoms of fatigue and irritability and consequently may frequently lead to concurrent problems at school which may be picked up by the parents or teachers. These behavioural problems at school may then be blamed for symptoms such as bed-wetting and emotional instability, thus leading to an initial misdiagnosis.

2   What are the aims of treatment for DP?

The Diabetes Control and Complications Trial (DCCT) Group (1994) demonstrated that tight control and management of blood glucose levels decreases the risks of complications both in terms of microvascular (retinopathy and renal failure) and macrovascular (stroke, angina, myocardial infarction) complications.

3   How should DP be advised and taught to monitor her regimen?

Testing blood glucose levels is the most reliable assessment of day-to-day control of diabetes. Patients or parents of younger children are taught to conduct a finger prick test to obtain a sample of capillary blood, then place the blood on a test strip and check it using a meter. This provides a current reading of blood glucose. Providing that the test has been conducted in accordance with instructions and the meter has been calibrated for accuracy, the test will provide reliable readings which patients/parents can interpret.

Testing may be required 3–4 times daily 7 days per week for children as their blood sugars are notoriously hard to control due to variety in daily activity and lack of compliance to regular eating patterns. Overall, it is important to encourage tight glucose control and praise children when progress has been made, rather than condemn for being outside a specified range.

Longer term glucose control is assessed using haemaglobin A1c (HbA1c). This is considered the gold standard test for the assessment of glycaemic control and reflects levels of control over the previous 2–3 months. Glucose binds the haemoglobin to form glycosylated haemoglobin. The more glucose in the blood, the more will be taken up to form glycosylated haemoglobin. The test reflects the fraction of haemoglobin that has become irreversibly bound to glucose. Normal levels in non-diabetic children are around 4.5–5% of the circulating haemoglobin. The target for children with type 1 diabetes would be to achieve <7.5%. Aiming for HbA1c levels of around 4% is likely to produce greater incidence of hypoglycaemia. Levels greater than 8.0% are associated with an increased incidence of long-term complications.

4   How should she and her carers be taught to inject her insulin?

Patients are normally advised to inject insulin into the subcutaneous tissue of the abdomen, thighs and buttocks in rotation; however, younger children are often reluctant to inject into their abdomen. It is important that no one site is overused as this may lead to lipohypertrophy and poor insulin absorption, resulting in erratic blood glucose concentrations.

The site of injection also influences the speed of absorption, with the abdomen and arms providing quickest absorption and the thighs and buttocks the slowest. More rapid absorption will be caused by exercise or heat (from a bath for example) following the injection.

Practical instructions for the patient/carer could be as follows:

- Insulin should be given by subcutaneous injection, i.e. into the fat beneath the skin, not into the muscle. To avoid injecting into the muscle, it is important to lift a skin fold with the thumb and index finger ('two-finger pinch-up') and insert the needle at a 45° angle. Lifting a skin fold is important, even if you are using an 8 mm needle. With 5–6 mm needles, injections can be given without lifting a skin fold if there is enough subcutaneous fat (at least 8 mm as skin layers may be compressed when injecting perpendicularly). Lean boys, however, usually have less fat, especially on the thigh.
- Wiggle the needle slightly before injecting. If the tip feels 'stuck' you have probably reached the muscle. If this is the case, withdraw the needle a little before injecting. You can also inject insulin into your buttocks where there is usually a layer of subcutaneous fat that is thick enough to insert the needle perpendicularly without lifting a skin fold.

5   What should her carers be told about her first few months of treatment?

Her parents should be warned that she might experience a 'honeymoon' period in the first few months after diagnosis, which means that her insulin requirements could temporarily drop off dramatically. Around a quarter of all patients who get type 1 diabetes develop a honeymoon period within days or weeks of the onset of treatment. It is as if the patient has gone into remission and this can be confusing for the patient/carer as it would appear that the condition has corrected itself. Some patients actually require no insulin during this phase which may last for weeks or months; however, it is usually best to keep treating with insulin even if the requirements are negligible to avoid possible insulin allergy upon re-exposure and also to maintain a treatment regimen, thus not giving false hope to the patient.

6   Discuss the insulin and devise options for treating type 1 diabetes.

There are a number of indications when a standard two times daily injection regimen is not suitable. These include when irregular eating or fluctuating exercise regimen leads to hypoglycaemia between meals. In such situations multiple injection regimens (so called basal bolus therapy) can be tried. This normally involves the injection of short-acting insulin before meals and an injection of intermediate or long-acting insulin before bedtime. If soluble insulins are used this again requires the discipline of injection 30 minutes before eating. Basal bolus therapy does give greater flexibility to the patient and removes the need to eat every 2–3 hours.

Insulin analogues such as insulin lispro (Humalog) or insulin aspart (Novo Rapid) are alternatives to traditional soluble insulin. They have the advantage of a more rapid action which means that they can be given after meals. This can be important when dealing with food fads and irregular eating habits in children and teenagers. The rapid action and short duration also means lower insulin levels overnight and a reduction in the risk of nocturnal hypoglycaemia. Long-acting analogues such as insulin glargine and detemir have also been developed to give a basal insulin requirement similar to those that would normally be present in the body.

Case study level Ma – Gastro-oesophageal reflux – see page 395

1   What is gastro-oesophageal reflux and what are the main symptoms?

The spontaneous regurgitation of gastric contents into the oesophagus is defined as gastro-oesophageal reflux. It is in fact a normal physiological phenomenon, happening due to relaxation of the lower oesophageal sphincter and not associated with swallowing. When reflux leads to recurrent regurgitation or vomiting problems start to arise, irritability and abnormal posturing may also become common. If the reflux is purely physiological it will normally resolve after the first year of life. Failure to thrive due to decreased food intake may become a problem and prolonged reflux can also result in oesophagitis.

2a   What is the rationale behind the ranitidine treatment already started?

Ranitidine is a H_2 blocker used to reduce gastric acid. The use of such an agent may have benefit for two reasons. First, the more neutral the refluxing gastric content is the less likely it is for oesophagitis to occur. Second, the pressure on the lower oesophageal sphincter may be reduced if the content of the stomach is more neutral, decreasing the likelihood of reflux.

2b   What alternative class of drug may work in the same way as ranitidine, but be more effective?

The proton pump inhibitors block the acid production more completely than ranitidine and thus may achieve even greater acid control.

2c   What are the practical problems of using this second class of medicine in an infant?

Proton pump inhibitors do not come as syrups and thus are much harder to administer to an infant. If the tablets or capsule content are crushed to make a suspension the acid protection on each granule is lost and the active drug is denatured in the stomach before it gets to the duodenum where it should be absorbed. Various methods of administration have been tried: many involving mixing the granules with sodium bicarbonate in order to try and protect the active ingredient.

3a   Name three prokinetic agents which could be added to the regimen at this stage.

The following are prokinetic agents:

■   domperidone
■   metoclopramide
■   erythromycin.

3b   What is the rationale of use of these products?

By increasing the speed of transit of stomach contents through the digestive track, there should be less chance of reflux in the other direction.

3c   Briefly mention the potential issues surrounding the use of each product.

■   *Domperidone* – widely used despite little evidence of effect. Unlikely to cause central nervous system side-effects as it does not cross the blood–brain barrier.
■   *Metoclopramide* – known to be an effective prokinetic. Main disadvantage is the possibility of central side-effects due to ability to cross the blood–brain barrier.
■   *Erythromycin* – no good evidence base, but known to increase peristalsis through the gut. Concerns about using low doses of antibiotics and leading to longer term resistance.

4   What is the problem of using metronidazole suspension when the gastric content is acid suppressed?

The suspension (unlike the tablets) is made up of metronidazole benzoate. The benzoate must be cleaved by acid in order for the active metronidazole to be absorbed. Thus in neutral acid conditions the metronidazole suspension is likely to be less effective.

5   What is the other potential risk of using metronidazole alongside ranitidine suspension?

Ranitidine suspension is formulated with alcohol as an excipient (along with many other suspensions). Metronidazole may react with the alcohol in the blood to cause a disulfiram-like reaction leading to flushing and tachycardia.

Case study level Mb – Asthma – see page 396

1a   What is asthma?

Asthma is a chronic inflammatory disease affecting the airways. Inflammatory mediators such as prostaglandins and histamines cause inflammatory cells to damage the bronchial epithelium and cause bronchial constriction.

1b   How does early childhood asthma often present?

Coughing at night

1c   What are the common symptoms?

Common symptoms include:

- shortness of breath – a peak expiratory flow rate (PEFR) of <50% of the norm would suggest severe asthma
- cough
- wheeze
- tight chest.

1d   What class of drug is used for the initial pharmacological management of asthma and how do they work?

Beta$_2$-agonists – work by causing bronchial dilation.

1e   What route of administration is usually used initially and why?

Beta$_2$-agonists are usually inhaled so that the medicine goes straight to the lungs reducing the amount entering the systemic circulation and thus reducing side-effects.

1f   What are the main side-effects of this class of drugs?

Tremor, nervous tension, headache, peripheral dilation, palpitation and tachycardia. High doses are associated with hypokalaemia.

2a   What are the classes of the drugs being used here to treat the severe asthma attack and how will they help?

- Salbutamol is a beta$_2$-agonist – causes bronchial dilation.
- Aminophylline is a methylxanthine – causes bronchial dilation and stimulates respiration.
- Prednisolone is a corticosteroid – decreases inflammation.

2b   What side-effect do they all have in common which can be exacerbated by hypoxia, a common feature of severe asthma?

Hypokalaemia.

3a   What step of the British Thoracic Society guidelines is the boy now on?

Step 3.

3b   What is the role of the leukotriene antagonist?

Leukotrienes form part of the inflammatory process; their effect can be antagonised using cysteinyl leukotriene antagonists such as montelukast.

3c   What preparations are available and which would probably be most suitable for this 3-year-old boy?

Both montelukast and zafirlukast come as tablets. However montelukast also comes as chewable tablets and granules. The granules may be most suitable in this case as they may be mixed with a spoonful of food and taken immediately.

4a   What is the most suitable way to administer the beclometasone to this 3-year-old and why?

Steroids are best delivered via a spacer device. Use of a spacer helps with the following:

- Less need for coordination of the inhaler device and patient inhalation.
- Less deposition of the steroid to the back of the throat which can lead to hoarseness and oral candidiasis.
- Increased deposition of the drug into the lungs.

4b   How should the administration device be cared for and why?

The spacer device should be washed on a weekly basis in warm soapy water. It must then be left to dry naturally. If wiped with a cloth, the static created will pull all the medicine to stick to the inside of the spacer and prevent it from being inhaled.

4c   What are the other main devices used to administer medication in asthma?

- Metered dose inhalers – with or without spacers.
- Dry powder devices – turbohalers, accuhalers
- Breath-actuated metered dose inhalers – evohalers
- Nebulisers.

5a   With a patient with severe asthma such as this, is there any advice that the family can follow at home if an acute asthma attack starts again?

If an acute attack happens at home, the beta$_2$-agonist may be given in much higher doses. Up to 10 puffs may be administered with one puff every 15–30 seconds. This can be as effective as using nebulised beta$_2$-agonists. Oral steroids may also be given in high dose. These measures may be enough to prevent hospitalisation.

5b   Can you suggest a way that the family can monitor response to therapy?

Peak flow meters should be encouraged for self-management at home. When the child is well a PEFR should be taken as a baseline. Regular monitoring should then be carried out and recorded on a chart. This will detect deterioration and thus allow increases in treatment without a severe attack happening.

17

Care of older people case studies

Chris Cairns and Nina Barnett

Case study level 1 – It is important to be regular: constipation and the older person

> **Learning outcomes**
>
> Level 1 case study: You will be able to:
>
> - describe the risk factors
> - describe the disease
> - describe the pharmacology of the drug
> - outline the formulation, including drug molecule, excipients, etc. for the medicines
> - summarise basic social pharmacy issues (e.g. opening containers, large labels).

Mrs HB comes to your pharmacy and asks to speak to you. She requests a treatment for constipation that has emerged over the past few weeks. You remember that she visited your pharmacy about a month ago when she collected a new prescription for regular co-dydramol to treat her acute exacerbation of osteoarthritis of the knee.

1a What is the definition of constipation?
1b What are the main risk factors for developing constipation?
2a What risk factors for constipation apply to Mrs HB at this point in time?
2b What is the most likely reason for this acute episode?

3a   What classes of drugs are available to treat constipation and how do they work?
3b   Give the main indications for one drug from each group: lactulose, senna, ispaghula husk and docusate.
3c   What would be your choice of agent for Mrs HB, and why?
4a   You decide that senna is appropriate for short-term treatment. Which formulations are available as over-the-counter (P and GSL) medicines
4b   What are the functions of the components of the tablets?
5a   What factors would you take into account when helping Mrs HB to choose the most appropriate product?
5b   What side-effects/cautions/contraindications would you discuss with Mrs HB when you supply her with the medicine?
5c   What lifestyle advice would you give Mrs HB and how would you follow-up her progress.

General references

Assessment and treatment of older patients with constipation. *The Nursing Standard* 46 November 1 (21) 8. Available at http://www.nursing-standard.co.uk/archives/ns/vol21-08/pdfs/v21n08p4146.pdf [Accessed 27 July 2008]

Clinical Knowledge Summary (CKS, formerly PRODIGY), Constipation. (2008) Scenario: Constipation in adults: Last revised in January 2008. Available at: http://cks.library.nhs.uk/constipation [Accessed 27 July 2008]

How to deal with constipation. (2007) *The Pharmaceutical Journal* 7 (279) 23-26. Available at http://www.pjonline.com/pdf/cpd/pj_20070707_constipation.pdf [Accessed 27 July 2008]

NPC nurse prescribing bulletin. (1999) *Prescribing Nurse Bulletin* 1: 6. Available at http://www.npc.co.uk/nurse_prescribing/pdfs/constipationvol1no6%20.pdf [Accessed 27 July 2008]

Petticrew M, Watt I, Sheldon T (1997) Systematic review of the effectiveness of laxatives in the elderly. *Health Technology Assessment* 1997; 1(13).

The management of constipation. MeReC Bulletin (14) 6. Avaialble at http://www.npc.co.uk/MeReC_Bulletins/2003Volumes/Vol14no6.pdf [Accessed 27 July 2008]

Case study level 2 - Puffing away makes you lose your puff: treatment of chronic obstructive pulmonary disease

Learning outcomes

Level 2 case study: You will be able to:

- interpret relevant lab and clinical data
- identify monitoring and referral criteria
- explain treatment choices
- describe goals of therapy, including monitoring and the role of the pharmacist/clinician
- describe issues – counselling points, adverse drug reactions, drug interactions, complementary/alternative therapies and lifestyle advice.

Scenario

Mr PM, aged 82, is admitted to hospital on a Friday evening with a chest infection, via a GP referral. You see him in your ward for the first time on Monday morning. He lives with his wife in a house and they enjoy an active social life. He has smoked since the age of 14 and currently smokes about 40 cigarettes daily. He has tried to give up smoking in the last month and failed. This is his third admission in one year for a chest infection.

Questions

1a What is COPD?
1b What are the main risk factors for COPD?
2a What are the symptoms of COPD?
2b What tests would you look for and why?
3a What classes of drugs are available to treat COPD?
3b Give the main indications for one drug in each group.
3c Mr PM's exacerbation is treated with intravenous antibiotics, nebulised bronchodilators and high-dose oral corticosteroids. What is the rationale for use of steroids in this situation?
4a Mr PM's condition has improved. His FEV_1/FVC is now 44%. He is now able to use inhaled medication. What does NICE guidance recommend?
4b What are the key advantages and disadvantages of a metered dose inhaler, dry powder inhaler and spacers?
5a What factors would you take into account when helping Mr PM to choose the most appropriate product?

5b What side-effects would you discuss with Mr PM if you supplied tiotropium (Spiriva)?

5c How would you follow-up his progress?

Reference

NICE (National Institute for Health and Clinical Excellence) (2004) Chronic obstructive pulmonary disease. Available at http://guidance.nice.org.uk/CG12/niceguidance/pdf/English [Accessed 4 July 2008].

Case study level 3 – 'Not what you first thought': multiple morbidity in older people – acute confusional state, dehydration and Parkinson's disease

Learning outcomes

Level 3 case study: You will be able to:

- interpret clinical signs and symptoms
- evaluate laboratory data
- evaluate treatment options
- state goals of therapy
- describe a pharmaceutical care plan to include advice to a clinician
- describe the prognosis and long-term complications
- describe the social pharmacy issues which could include supply (e.g. complex treatments at home, concordance and compliance) and lifestyle issues.

Scenario

Mr DM, a 79-year-old man who lives alone, is brought into A&E suffering from dehydration, which appears to be the result of prolonged (>24 hours) nausea and vomiting. He is shaking, confused, incoherent and unable to provide a lucid history. His basic laboratory values are:

Na$^+$	152 mmol/L (137–145 mmol/L)
K$^+$	3.1 mmol/L (3.6–5.0 mmol/L)
Bicarbonate	29 mmol/L (22–30 mmol/L)
Urea	7.3 mmol/L (2.5–7.5 mmol/L)
Creatinine	115 micromol/L (62–133 micromol/L)
White blood count	8.4×10^9 /L (4–11×10^9 /L)

He has an intravenous cannula inserted and rehydration commenced with sodium chloride 0.9% w/v infusion.

Mr DM continues to retch and vomit. He is administered 10 mg metoclo-pramide by i.v. injection and promptly suffers an oculogyric crisis. This is reversed by the administration of i.v. procyclidine.

Twelve hours later Mr DM is conscious and lucid but now has a pro-nounced tremor, characteristic of Parkinson's disease. He reports he was initially diagnosed about a year ago by his GP. His GP has been prescribing Sinemet-110 (co-careldopa) tablets, (the initial dose was titrated) but Mr DM did not take any as the tremor did not really bother him until earlier this week. He decided to start taking the Sinemet but as the tremor was troublesome he started at the dose of 1 tablet t.d.s.

Questions

1   Briefly outline the epidemiology, pathophysiology and clinical features of Parkinson's disease.
2a   Outline the pharmacological basis of the nausea and vomiting caused by the Sinemet.
2b   Outline the pharmacological basis of the adverse effect, oculogyric crisis, Mr DM suffered.
2c   Briefly discuss the alternative options that could have been considered for managing Mr DM's nausea and vomiting, with relative advantages and disadvantages.

Contact with the GP confirmed the history of Parkinson's disease and the pre-scription history. Mr DM was re-titrated but at three times a day dosage his symptoms were still not controlled. The dose was increased to five times a day.

3a   What is the logic behind the use of Sinemet, which is a combined product of levodopa and carbidopa?
3b   Briefly outline the rationale for reducing the dosage interval rather than increasing the dosage.
3c   The on/off syndrome and end-of-dose deterioration are both features of treated Parkinson's disease. What are they, and are there any risk factors?
4   In addition to levodopa therapy, what other options are available to treat Parkinson's disease and what is their place in therapy?

Mr DM is to be discharged on the following prescription:

- Sinemet-110 (co-careldopa) tablets five times a day
- senna tablets 2 p.r.n.
- lactulose liquid 15 mL b.d. p.r.n.
- domperidone 10 mg tablets t.d.s. p.r.n.

5   Mr DM is concerned that he is likely to forget the five times daily dosage regimen and/or find it difficult to maintain a regular dosage interval. Is there anything you could do to help him?

General references

Clinical Knowledge Summary (CKS, formerly PRODIGY), Constipation. (2008) Scenario: Constipation in adults: Last revised in January 2008. Available at: http://cks.library. nhs.uk/constipation [Accessed 27 July 2008]

How to deal with constipation. (2007) *The Pharmaceutical Journal* 7 (279) 23-26. Available at http://www.pjonline.com/pdf/cpd/pj_20070707_constipation.pdf [Accessed 27 July 2008]

Joint Formulary Committee (2008) *British National Formulary 55*. London: British Medical Association and Royal Pharmaceutical Society of Great Britain, March.

The management of constipation. MeReC Bulletin (14) 6. Avaialble at http://www. npc.co.uk/MeReC_Bulletins/2003Volumes/Vol14no6.pdf [Accessed 27 July 2008]

Case study level Ma – Eating is not the only problem: treatment of stroke and its complications in the older person

Learning outcomes

Level M case study: You will be able to:

- interpret clinical signs and symptoms
- evaluate laboratory data
- critically appraise treatment options
- state goals of therapy
- describe a pharmaceutical care plan to include advice to a clinician
- describe the prognosis and long-term complications
- describe the social pharmacy issues which could include supply (e.g. complex treatments at home, concordance and compliance) and lifestyle issues
- describe the monitoring of therapy.

Scenario

Mrs SL, aged 75, is admitted to hospital unable to speak, swallow or move her right arm and leg, having collapsed when out to dinner with her son. She has an urgent CT scan which reveals an ischaemic stroke of the partial anterior circulation (PAC) type. She had a transient ischaemic attack (TIA) two weeks ago and her son says she has had them infrequently for the last year. She has been treated for hypertension and high cholesterol for the past 2 years and has been taking aspirin.

1a   What are the key features of stroke that distinguish it from a TIA?
1b   What are the modifiable risk factors for stroke?
1c   Why do you need to know if the stroke is ischaemic or haemorrhagic?

You see Mrs SL on the ward, 2 days after admission – she is still unable to swallow and has a nasogastric tube inserted.

2a   What are the acute treatments goals for stroke?
2b   What therapies can be used to treat acute acute stroke and what would you use for Mrs SL?

After two weeks, Mrs SL regains some movement in her right arm but cannot grip with her hand. Her swallowing has partially returned and she is permitted a soft, puréed diet. She has been restarted on her old medications including:

- simvastatin 10 mg o.d.
- amlodipine 5 mg o.d.
- irbesartan 150 mg o.d.
- aspirin 75 mg o.d.
- lactulose 10 mL b.d.
- senna 2 tablets o.n.
- latanoprost eye drops 1 drop o.n.
- dorzolamide eye drops 1 drop b.d.

3a   What concordance issues do you think the patient might have with the above medication?
3b   What monitoring would you undertake to ensure maximal efficacy of treatment (including compliance)?

The next day you visit the ward to find that Mrs SL had a grand mal seizure during the night. She was given lorazepam to treat the fit acutely. You attend the ward round and are asked for advice.

4a   What would you use to treat the epilepsy to prevent recurrence? Give reasons for your choice.
4b   What are the differences between the formulations of phenytoin, carbamazepine and sodium valproate and what factors do you need to take into consideration according to Mrs SL's current and future needs?
4c   You have chosen sodium valproate. What monitoring would you undertake and recommend to monitor therapy?
5   What would you do to support her recovery outside hospital, focusing on potential medication-related issues after discharge?

References

ESPRIT Study Group; Halkes PH, van Gijn J, Kappelle LJ *et al.* (2006) Aspirin plus dipyridamole versus aspirin alone after cerebral ischaemia of arterial origin (ESPRIT): randomised controlled trial. *Lancet* 20 May, 367: 1665–1673.
Royal College of Physicians (2004) National clinical guidelines for stroke, 2nd edn.
Available at http://www.rcplondon.ac.uk/pubs/books/stroke/stroke_guidelines_
2ed.pdf [Accessed 4 July 2008].

General Reference

NICE (National Institute for Health and Clinical Excellence) (2008) Stroke Guideline.
Available at http://www.nice.org.uk/nicemedia/pdf/CG68FullGuideline.pdf.

Care Study Level Mb – Hearts and bones

Learning outcomes

Level Mb case study: You will be able to:

- interpret clinical signs and symptoms
- evaluate laboratory data
- critically appraise treatment options
- state goals of therapy
- describe a pharmaceutical care plan to include advice to a clinician
- describe the prognosis and long term complications
- describe the social pharmacy issues which could include supply (e.g. complex treatments at home, concordance and compliance) and lifestyle issues
- describe the monitoring of therapy.

Scenario

Mrs GG, an 81-year-old lady is admitted through A&E following a fall. She reports that she felt dizzy all of a sudden and 'just went over'. She also felt a 'jump in her chest'. As a result of her fall she has a Colles fracture of her right wrist and extensive bruising on her face, right arm and right leg. She says she feels lucky that she did not do more damage to herself, especially as she lives alone, and she knows that falls are dangerous in older people.

She has a 4 month history of chronic atrial fibrillation (AF) and is attending her local community pharmacy anticoagulant clinic. Her current prescription is:

- warfarin as per INR
- digoxin 125 micrograms daily

Her arm is in a sling and she will have no effective use of her right arm and hand for the coming 6–8 weeks.

Questions

1a Falls are common in older people and as Mrs GG points out can be very dangerous. What are the risk factors; pharmacological and non pharmacological, for falls in older people?

1b Briefly discuss those risk factors which apply specifically to Mrs GG.

1c Outline how Mrs GG's risk factors can be reduced.

2a There are a number of sources of 'best practice' to provide advice for treating Mrs GG's atrial fibrillation (AF). Identify four common sources and provide the current references and/or URL for the management of AF.

2b Briefly summarise the advice for managing Mrs GG's chronic AF from each of these sources. Highlight any significant differences between the sources of advice.

3 A risk factor for fracture following a fall in older people is osteoporosis. Is there any best practice advice? If so what is the source and provide a brief summary of that advice.

4a Increasing or preventing further loss of bone density will minimise the risk of fracture following a fall. What specific risk factors does Mrs GG have that may increase her likelihood of having decreased bone density?

4b What are the treatment options available to reduce or halt the reduction in Mrs GG's bone density?

4c What would you recommend for Mrs GG and why?

4d The multidisciplinary team decide to recommend treatment with a bisphosphonate for Mrs GG. What issues need to be taken into consideration both before prescribing and for counselling once prescribed

5a The benefits of bisphosphonate treatment are explained to Mrs GG. She accepts that they will be of benefit and are the best treatment currently available but tells you firmly that she will not take a bisphosphonate under any circumstances. Her best friend was on alendronate and suffered intolerable gastric discomfort. She also doesn't fancy the idea of standing or sitting upright for up to an hour after taking the tablets. Using the 4 key ethical principles of beneficence, malevolence, autonomy and justice discuss how you would address this dilemma.

5b Discuss alternative medication or other strategies that may be less effective but more acceptable to the patient.

General references

American College of Cardiology. ACC/AHA/ESC 2006 Guidelines for the Management of patients with Atrial Fibrillation. Available at http://acc.org/qualityandscience/clinical/guidelines/atrial_fib/pdfs/AF_Full_Text.pdf [Accessed 8 October 2008].

Centre for Change & Innovation, Cardiology: palpitations/suspected clinically significant arrhythmia patient pathway. NHS Scotland, 2005. Available at www.pathways.scot.nhs.uk [Accessed 8 October 2008].

Clinical Knowledge Summaries. Atrial fibrillation. (2007). Available at http://cks.library.
nhs.uk/ atrial_fibrillation# [Accessed 8 October 2008].

Clinical Knowledge Summaries. Atrial fibrillation. The management of atrial fibrillation
(2006). Available at http://www.nice.org.uk/nicemedia/pdf/CG036niceguideline.
pdf [Accessed 8 October 2008].

Clinical Knowledge Summaries. Osteoporosis (2006). Available at http://cks.library.
nhs.uk/osteoporosis_treatment [Accessed 8 October 2008].

De Denus, S., Sanoski, C.A., Carlsson, J. et al. (2005) Rate vs rhythm control in patients
with atrial fibrillation: a meta-analysis. Archives of Internal Medicine 165(3):
258–262.

Joint Formulary Committee (2008) British National Formulary 55. London: British Medical
Association and Royal Pharmaceutical Society of Great Britain, March.

Medicines and Healthcare products Regulatory Agency, 2005. MHRA Latest data on HRT
from the UK Million Women Study. Available at http://www.mhra.gov.uk/home/
groups/comms-po/documents/news/con002085.pdf [Accessed 08 October 2008].

National Collaborating Centre for Chronic Conditions (2006) Atrial fibrillation. National
clinical guideline for management in primary and secondary care (full NICE guideline). Royal College of Physicians.

National Institute for Health and Clinical Excellence (2008) NICE Technology appraisal
161, Osteoporosis – secondary prevention, including strontium ranelate. Alendronate, etidronate, risedronate, raloxifene, strontium ranelate and teriparatide for
secondary prevention of osteoporotic fractures in post menopausal women. Available at http://www.nice.org.uk/Guidance/TA161 [Accessed 18 November 2008].

National Institute for Health and Clinical Excellence (NICE) (June 2006) Clinical Guideline
36, The management of Atrial fibrillation. Available at http://www.nice.org.uk/
nicemedia/pdf/CG036niceguideline.pdf [Accessed 8 October 2008].

Royal College of Physicians of Edinburgh, 1999, The Sir James MacKenzie Consensus
Conference: atrial fibrillation in hospital and general practice. Proceedings of the
Royal College of Physicians of Edinburgh. 29 (Suppl 6), 1–34.

Scottish Intercollegiate Guidelines Network, 2003. Management of osteoporosis.
Available at http://www.sign.ac.uk/pdf/sign71.pdf [accessed 8 October 2008].

Answers

Case study level 1 – see page 409

1a   What is the definition of constipation?

Although there is no one definition for constipation, it is usually described as infrequent defecation, which is often accompanied by straining as well as the passage of hard, uncomfortable stool.

1b   What are the main risk factors for developing constipation?

Risk factors include:

- immobility
- female gender
- increasing age

- low-fibre diet
- dehydration
- disease (e.g. Parkinson's disease)
- drugs (e.g. anticholinergics, opioid analgesics, many psychotropics, etc.).

2a   What risk factors for constipation apply to Mrs HB at this point in time?

She has immobility from osteoporosis, she is a female older person, and she is taking drugs that could cause constipation.

2b   What is the most likely reason for this acute episode?

The recently prescribed co-dydramol is the most likely cause as it contains an opiate, dihydrocodeine, which can cause constipation.

3a   What classes of drugs are available to treat constipation and how do they work?

- Osmotic laxatives – increase the amount of water in the large bowel (either by drawing water from the body or by retaining the water that the laxative was given with).
- Stimulant laxatives – stimulation of smooth muscle of the gastrointestinal tract increasing intestinal motility causing muscle contraction and thus defecation.
- Bulk-forming laxatives – increase the volume of the stool to stimulate peristalsis.
- Stool softener laxatives – increase the amount of fluid penetrating the stool and decrease surface tension.

3b   Give the main indications for one drug from each group: lactulose, senna, ispaghula husk and docusate.

Lactulose

- Treatment of constipation.
- Treatment of hepatic encephalopathy (portal systemic encephalopathy); hepatic coma.

Senna

- Relief of occasional constipation.

Ispaghula husk

- For the treatment of patients requiring a high-fibre regimen: for example, for the relief of constipation, including constipation in pregnancy and the maintenance of regularity; for the management of bowel function in patients with colostomy, ileostomy, haemorrhoids, anal fissure, chronic diarrhoea associated with diverticular disease, irritable bowel syndrome and ulcerative colitis.

Docusate

- To prevent and treat chronic constipation by softening hard, dry stools in order to ease defecation and reduce straining at stool; and in the presence of haemorrhoids and anal fissure, to prevent hard, dry stools and reduce straining.
- As an adjunct in abdominal radiological procedures.

3c   What would be your choice of agent for Mrs HB, and why?

A stimulant such as bisacodyl or senna because it is for occasional use. This group is also pharmacologically appropriate as they improve gut motility, which is currently reduced by the opiate in co-dydramol. Docusate can be used as it has both stimulant and softener actions. Note: As these medications may be purchased over the counter, docusate is a more expensive choice.

4a   You decide that senna is appropriate for short-term treatment. Which formulations are available as over-the-counter (P and GSL) medicines?

Senna is available in the form of tablets, chewable tablets, granules or liquid (oral solution).

4b   What are the functions of the components of the tablets?

The ingredients and their functions for two senna formulations are listed in Table A17.1.

Table A17.1 Ingredients and their functions for two senna formulations

Ingredient	Function
Boots senna tablets	
Senna	Active ingredient
Tricalcium phosphate 118	Dispersant
Magnesium stearate	Lubricant and filler
Maize starch	Binder
Senokot tablets (Britannia Pharmaceuticals)	
Senna	Active ingredient
Calcium phosphate	Dispersant
Magnesium stearate	Lubricant
Maize starch	Binder
DC lactose	Filler

5a   What factors would you take into account when helping Mrs HB to choose the most appropriate product?

Factors to take into account include:

- palatability
- swallowing
- personal preference (taste, preference for specific dosage form – tablet, liquid)
- previous experience
- side-effects.

5b   What side-effects/cautions/contraindications would you discuss with Mrs HB when you supply her with the medicine?

Side-effects

Senna may cause abdominal cramps and diarrhoea. Prolonged use of senna may produce watery diarrhoea with excessive loss of fluid and electrolytes, particularly potassium, muscular weakness and weight loss. Changes in the intestinal musculature associated with malabsorption and dilation of the bowel, similar to ulcerative colitis and to megacolon, may also occur. Cardiac and renal symptoms have been reported. Melanosis coli and a red or yellow discoloration of the urine and faeces may also occur.

Cautions

Use should be reviewed after a week. Senna should not be used for prolonged periods since it may decrease the sensitivity of the intestinal mucous membranes, so larger doses have to be taken and the bowel fails to respond to normal stimuli.

Contraindications

Mrs HB should stop taking senna if she has severe abdominal pain, feels sick or vomits. If these occur Mrs HB should see her doctor. In general, laxatives should not be taken where there is severe abdominal pain or used regularly for prolonged periods, except on medical advice. Over-the-counter senna should not be used when abdominal pain, intestinal obstruction, nausea or vomiting is - present.

5c   What lifestyle advice would you give Mrs HB and how would you follow-up her progress.

Increase dietary intake of fibre, only if 1.5–2.0 L daily fluid intake is possible. Add 30 g unprocessed bran to food or fruit juice, especially if stools are small and hard. Encourage establishment of regular bowel habits. Explain the importance of adopting good positioning (sitting with knees above hips, feet on the floor/well supported) to facilitate bowel movement if it is possible for Mrs HB to do this. Encourage regular exercise within her ability.

Recommend that she contacts you in a few days and discusses the efficacy of the product. Discuss the need for discontinuing the senna if she no longer needs the co-dydramol. It would be worth discussing whether Mrs HB can step down her analgesia to paracetamol alone which should lead to resolution of the constipation.

Case study level 2 – see page 411

1a   What is COPD?

Chronic obstructive pulmonary disease, as defined by the World Health Organization, is an umbrella term for a disease state characterised by airflow limitation that is not fully reversible. It includes chronic bronchitis and emphysema.

1b   What are the main risk factors for COPD?

Smoking is the main risk factor (about 1 in 4 smokers who smoke 40 cigarettes per day develop COPD if they continue to smoke); non-smokers very rarely suffer from COPD. Other environmental factors include exposure to occupational dusts, inhaled chemicals and air pollution. Some rare genetic conditions are risk factors.

2a   What are the symptoms of COPD?

Chronic cough, regular sputum production, breathlessness causing decreased activity and mobility, wheeze and frequent winter bronchitis.

2b   What tests would you look for and why?

- Temperature, pulse, respiratory rate – infection and respiratory function.
- WBC, U+Es, FBC, inflammatory markers – monitoring for infection, dehydration, etc.
- Blood gases – respiratory acidosis, oxygen saturation.
- Spirometry FEV_1/FVC – measure of how badly his lung function has been affected.
- Peak expiratory flow (PEF) – to support spirometry in monitoring changes in airway flow as a result of infection/inflammation (however use for COPD not supported by British Thoracic Society guidelines).

3a   What classes of drugs are available to treat COPD?

The following classes of drugs can be used to treat COPD:

- beta$_2$-agonists
- anticholinergics
- corticosteroids
- methylxanthines.

3b Give the main indications for one drug in each group.

- Salbutamol (Ventolin Accuhaler) – management of asthma, bronchospasm and/or reversible airways obstruction (also terbutaline, formoterol, salmeterol, etc.).
- Ipratropium (Atrovent Inhaler) – regular treatment of reversible bronchospasm associated with COPD and chronic asthma (also tiotropium).
- Beclometasone – note two formulations with different indications:

    – Becotide Inhaler is indicated in the prophylactic management of mild, moderate, or severe asthma in adults or children.
    – Filair 100 Inhaler is indicated for the prophylactic treatment of chronic reversible obstructive airways disease (also budesonide, fluticasone – unlicensed, though Seretide Accuhaler is licensed).

- Theophylline (Uniphyllin) treatment and prophylaxis of bronchospasm associated with asthma, chronic obstructive pulmonary disease and chronic bronchitis. Also indicated for the treatment of left ventricular and congestive cardiac failure.

3c Mr PM's exacerbation is treated with intravenous antibiotics, nebulised bronchodilators and high-dose oral corticosteroids. What is the rationale for use of steroids in this situation?

The steroids will reduce inflammation in the bronchial tree and lungs; this treatment has only been shown to be effective consistently in acute exacerbations.

4a Mr PM's condition has improved. His FEV_1/FVC is now 44%. He is now able to use inhaled medication. What does NICE guidance recommend?

The following is from the NICE guidelines (2004):

> Long-acting inhaled bronchodilators (beta$_2$-agonists or anticholinergics) should be used to control symptoms and improve exercise capacity in patients who continue to experience problems despite the use of short-acting drugs.
>
> Inhaled corticosteroids should be added to long-acting bronchodilators to decrease exacerbation frequency in patients with an FEV_1 less than or equal to 50% predicted who have had two or more exacerbations requiring treatment with antibiotics or oral corticosteroids in a 12-month period – not effective for all patients (steroid trial).
>
> Treat breathlessness and exercise limitation initially with short-acting bronchodilators (beta$_2$-agonists or anticholinergics) as needed. If this does not control symptoms, prescribe a long-acting bronchodilator. Also prescribe a long-acting bronchodilator if the patient has two or more exacerbations a year.

Inhaled corticosteroids should be prescribed for patients with an FEV_1 of 50% predicted or less, who have two or more exacerbations needing treatment with antibiotics or oral corticosteroids a year. Warn patients about the possible risk of osteoporosis and other side effects of high-dose inhaled corticosteroids. None of the inhaled corticosteroids currently available is licensed alone for use in COPD.

Drug combinations can increase clinical benefits. Examples include:

- beta$_2$-agonist and anticholinergic
- beta$_2$-agonist and theophylline
- anticholinergic and theophylline
- long-acting beta$_2$-agonist and inhaled corticosteroid.

4b What are the key advantages and disadvantages of a metered dose inhaler, dry powder inhaler and spacers?

The key features of metered dose inhalers, dry powder inhalers and spacers are listed in Table A17.2.

Table A17.2 Key features of metered dose inhalers, dry powder inhalers and spacers

Formulation	Key features
Inhalers	• Most patients, whatever their age, can learn how to use an inhaler unless they have significant cognitive impairment • Hand-held devices are usually best, with a spacer if appropriate • If a patient cannot use a particular device, try another • Teach technique before prescribing an inhaler, and check regularly • Titrate the dose against response for each patient
Dry powder	• Higher dose needed as lower bioavailability • Choice often dictated by drug available and patient preference/ability to use device • Many devices available in 'patient-friendly' designs • May cause paradoxical bronchospasm
Spacers	• Ensure the spacer is compatible with the patient's inhaler • Patients should make single actuations of the inhaler into the spacer, and inhale as soon as possible, repeating as needed • Tidal breathing is as effective as single breaths

5a What factors would you take into account when helping Mr PM to choose the most appropriate product?

Factors to take into account include:

- product availability
- ability to use the device, given age and home circumstances
- personal preference

- previous experience
- side-effects.

5b What side-effects would you discuss with Mr PM if you supplied tiotropium (Spiriva)?

Side-effects are classified according to EU guidelines as: very common ($\geq 1/10$), common ($\geq 1/100$ and $<1/10$), uncommon ($\geq 1/1000$ and $<1/100$), rare ($\geq 1/10\,000$ and $<1/1000$) or very rare ($<1/10\,000$), including isolated reports. The side-effects of tiotropium that should be discussed with Mr PM are as follows:

- very common: dry mouth
- common: constipation
- uncommon: palpitations, tachycardia. urinary retention.

Note: In common with all other inhalations, tiotropium may cause inhalation-induced bronchospasm.

5c How would you follow-up his progress?

Recommend that he discusses his progress with the practice nurse or community pharmacist a few days after discharge from hospital. His GP should monitor effectiveness of inhaled steroids after discharge. Monitor for oral candidiasis if inhaled steroids prescribed.

Case study level 3 – see page 412

1 Briefly outline the epidemiology, pathophysiology and clinical features of Parkinson's disease.

Parkinson's disease is primarily a disease of older people, although it can result as a consequence of brain injury or viral infection. Environmental exposure to some toxins may also be a cause. Incidence increases with age from very low in 60-year-olds to around 50% of people in their nineties. The incidence of Parkinson's disease is approximately 1:1000 in the general population, rising to 1:100 over the age 65 and 1:50 over the age of 80. There are more than 120 000 people with Parkinson's disease in the UK and it is common in all parts of the world.

Parkinson's disease is a progressive disease with no cure. There are no recognised specific risk factors. It is characterised by a loss of dopamine from cells in the brain, particularly in corpus striatum.

The common clinical features are tremor, restlessness, rigidity, a characteristic gait, a characteristic featureless expression and involuntary movements. As the disease progresses, if untreated these symptoms deteriorate and worsen. Depression and constipation are commonly associated with Parkinson's disease. In the later stages aphagia can occur. Symptoms can be both debilitating and disabling.

2a   Outline the pharmacological basis of the nausea and vomiting caused by the Sinemet.

Levodopa is peripherally metabolised to dopamine and high peripheral levels of dopamine cause nausea and vomiting. Levodopa also causes nausea and vomiting due to irritation of the gastrointestinal tract.

2b   Outline the pharmacological basis of the adverse effect, oculogyric crisis, Mr DM suffered.

Metoclopramide is a centrally acting dopamine antagonist. Although this should be an advantage in the management of dopamine-induced vomiting, in patients with Parkinson's disease it antagonises the already depleted dopamine in the brain so causing deterioration in parkinsonian symptoms. An oculogyric crisis is an extreme form of extrapyramidal adverse effect.

2c   Briefly discuss the alternative options that could have been considered for managing Mr DM's nausea and vomiting, with relative advantages and disadvantages.

Domperidone is a dopamine antagonist, it does not pass the blood–brain barrier. Therefore it is a good choice as it will treat non-central dopamine-induced nausea and vomiting. Unlike metoclopramide it does not cross the blood–brain barrier and block dopamine centrally, thus worsening the parkinsonian symptoms. However, domperidone is not available in an injectable form due to unacceptable cardiovascular adverse effects, so it is limited to oral and rectal forms. Although a suppository formulation is available, it is not really suitable for emergency use. However, given orally it would be a good choice for maintenance treatment once nausea and vomiting is under control.

Phenothiazines and other psychotropic agents (e.g. prochlorperazine and haloperidol) are contraindicated because they cause extrapyramidal symptoms despite being potentially efficacious.

$5HT_3$ antagonists (e.g. ondansetron and granisetron) are useful and efficacious both orally and by injection. They do not adversely affect parkinsonian symptoms as they do not affect dopamine. They are expensive.

Anticholinergics (e.g. cyclizine and cinnarizine) are useful and efficacious but can cause drowsiness, which limits long-term use in the elderly. They also cause classic anticholinergic symptoms of dry mouth, blurred vision, constipation, etc., which can be troublesome in the elderly in general. In addition, constipation is commonly associated with Parkinson's disease, and unsteadiness due to Parkinson's disease will be compounded by drowsiness caused by anti-cholinergic drugs. Therefore they are not a good choice for long-term use in Parkinson's disease. The mode of action, however, does not adversely affect parkinsonian symptoms, therefore they are a good choice in managing acute vomiting. As cyclizine is available in an i.v. form it can be used in an emergency and would be an appropriate choice in this patient for his acute vomiting.

3a What is the logic behind the use of Sinemet, which is a combined product of levodopa and carbidopa?

It is not possible to administer dopamine as it has a very short biological half-life and is not active orally. Therefore the precursor of dopamine, levodopa, is used instead. Levodopa is extensively metabolised peripherally to dopamine by the enzyme dopa decarboxylase. Therefore, to achieve adequate brain levels large doses are required. These large doses lead to nausea and hypotension, often limiting treatment. The co-administration of carbidopa (or benserazide), a peripheral dopa decarboxylase inhibitor, will considerably decrease this metabolism, permitting smaller doses of levodopa to be given. These inhibitors cannot cross the blood–brain barrier and so do not affect central metabolism. Levodopa combined with carbidopa is called co-careldopa and combined with benserazide is called co-beneldopa. There are a large number of forms of both these drugs, which should help dose titration.

3b Briefly outline the rationale for reducing the dosage interval rather than increasing the dosage.

Achieving adequate dopamine levels while avoiding excessive fluctuation in those levels produces better control of symptoms. Therefore, frequent dosing is preferred to long intervals between higher doses.

3c The on/off syndrome and end-of-dose deterioration are both features of treated Parkinson's disease. What are they, and are there any risk factors?

Levodopa treatment is associated with the development of potentially trouble-some motor complications, including large fluctuations in response and dys-kinesias. This is known as the on/off syndrome. During the 'on' period normal function occurs but there is weakness and restricted mobility during the 'off' period.

Frequently end-of-dose deterioration occurs when the duration of benefit after each dose becomes progressively shorter. In addition to frequent dosing, modified release levodopa preparations may be of benefit to help with end-of-dose deterioration and nocturnal immobility and rigidity.

The main risk factors for the on/off syndrome are time, typically appearing after six months and the fact that the Parkinson's disease is treated. End-of-dose deterioration is also associated with treatment and again there are no specific risk factors.

4   In addition to levodopa therapy, what other options are available to treat Parkinson's disease and what is their place in therapy?

Dopamine agonists include bromocriptine, cabergoline, lysuride, pergolide, apomorphine, pramipexole and ropinirole. These drugs are not converted into dopamine but have a direct effect on dopamine receptors in the brain. Dopamine agonists are used both as adjuncts to co-careldopa and co-beneldopa therapy and also initially in early Parkinson's disease, especially in younger adults.

Dopamine agonists are used in newly diagnosed patients but also have a place in the treatment of more advanced disease. Apomorphine is only used in advanced disease.

When used alone, dopamine agonists are less likely to cause involuntary movements but their effect on improving motor performance is slightly less. They are also more likely to cause hallucinations or sleepiness.

Apomorphine is a potent dopamine agonist, which is sometimes useful in advanced Parkinson's disease for patients with severe unpredictable 'off' periods on treatment. It is only available as a subcutaneous injection or infusion and thus requires significant patient and/or carer involvement in treatment. It is highly emetogenic so patients must receive domperidone, starting at least 2 days before apomorphine treatment.

Monoamine-oxidase B inhibitors, such as selegiline and rasagiline, have a use alone in the management of early disease. Early treatment with selegiline alone has been shown to delay the need for levodopa therapy for some months, but other more effective drugs are preferred. Both drugs can be used in conjunction with levodopa preparations to reduce end-of-dose deterioration in advanced disease.

Entacapone and tolcapone are peripheral inhibitors of catechol-O-methyl-transferase (COMT). COMT metabolises levodopa to an inactive product so their use enables greater amounts of levodopa to reach the brain. They are licensed for use as an adjunct to co-beneldopa and co-careldopa for patients who experience end-of-dose deterioration and cannot be stabilised on the combined preparations alone.

Tolcapone should only be prescribed under specialist supervision when other COMT inhibitors are ineffective. This is due to the risk of hepatotoxicity.

Amantadine has a modest antiparkinsonian effect. It improves mild bradykinetic symptoms as well as tremor and rigidity. Tolerance may occur.

Anticholinerigics such as orphenadrine, procyclidine and trihexyphenidyl (benzhexol) block the effect of acetylcholine, which has the opposite effect to dopamine so ameliorating symptoms. They have limiting side-effects due to their peripheral anticholinergic effects, which are troublesome and include constipation, sedation and blurred vision, all of which can worsen the effects of Parkinson's disease. They are little used nowadays.

5   Mr DM is concerned that he is likely to forget the five times daily dosage
regimen and/or find it difficult to maintain a regular dosage interval. Is there
anything you could do to help him?

Compliance with awkward regimens such as five times a day may be problematic as usual reference points such as meals are less useful. Mr DM has a combination of regular and 'when required' medication which would make the use of a monitored dosing system (MDS) a challenge. However, symptomatic treatment of nausea, which is usually self-limiting, and constipation are likely to be less of a problem.

Simple measures such as assessment of ability to use and open conventional and child-resistant containers, handle large bottles of liquids (lactulose) should be made before discharge and appropriate steps taken to deal with any problems.

The use of an MDS for the Sinemet may be of use but there are a variety of products available. The disadvantages as well as the advantages of using an MDS must be assessed for Mr DM before discussing with him those which may be of use and testing his ability to use before choosing a device. If a device is chosen then Mr DM must not be discharged before it is confirmed that he is able to manage it. Continuity of supply of the device needs to be confirmed with Mr DM's usual community pharmacist. A change of MDS device will invalidate any previous assessment work.

The potential disadvantages of MDS for patients with Parkinson's disease are that:

- few have facility for five dosing times,
- none hold liquids, and
- many are small and require intricate manipulative skills, which can be a limiting factor in patients with Parkinson's disease.

Simple aids such as medication charts or a medication diary should also be considered. Mr DM is generally lucid and aware of his condition so a simple reminder may suffice.

Case study level Ma – see page 414

1a   What are the key features of stroke that distinguish it from a TIA?

A TIA usually lasts less than 24 hours and there is full recovery of pre-TIA function. Symptoms may include facial or limb weakness, dysphagia and dysphasia as well as collapse.

A stroke results in numbness or weakness down one side; facial weakness; problems with balance/coordination, dysphagia, dysphasia and dysarthria; and loss of consciousness (in severe stroke).

1b   What are the modifiable risk factors for stroke?

The modifiable risk factors are:

- hypertension
- high cholesterol
- diabetes
- lack of exercise
- obesity
- smoking
- alcohol consumption.

1c   Why do you need to know if the stroke is ischaemic or haemorrhagic?

Ischaemic and haemorrhagic strokes are identified by CT scan within 24–48 hours of a stroke, not by clinical signs and symptoms. However, seizures, nausea, vomiting and headache may increase the clinical likehood of haemorrhagic stroke. Haemorrhagic strokes must not be treated with any anticoagulants (e.g. aspirin) in the acute phase, whereas this is recommended for patients with ischaemic stroke.

2a   What are the acute treatments goals for stroke?

The acute treatment goals are:

- to prevent further stroke damage,
- to confirm diagnosis to ensure prevention and treatment are optimised, and
- to identify the extent of stroke damage and manage sequelae of stroke.

2b   What therapies can be used to treat acute acute stroke and what would you use for Mrs SL?

Thrombolysis can be considered for ischaemic stroke but ideally needs to be given within 3 hours of the stroke. There are strict guidelines which must be adhered to to maximise benefit and minimise harm from this intervention (e.g. haemorrhagic stroke must be excluded). Aspirin 300 mg orally or rectally should be given as soon as possible after the diagnosis of ischaemic stroke has been made. Many centres reduce this dose to 75 mg daily after two weeks. However, aspirin treatment should be not be initiated until 24 hours after thrombolysis (Royal College of Physicians, 2004).

Mrs SL should be given aspirin 300 mg rectally daily from admission, once ischaemic stroke has been diagnosed. Dipyridamole SR 200 mg b.d. may be added when Mrs SL can swallow, following recommendations for secondary prevention of stroke (ESPRIT Study Group, 2006).

3a   What concordance issues do you think the patient might have with the above medication?

Mrs SL might have difficulty with:

- swallowing solid dose forms
- use of eye drops – coordination
- use of lactulose – manipulation of bottle
- timing of doses
- remembering all her medicines.

3b   What monitoring would you undertake to ensure maximal efficacy of treatment (including compliance)?

Mrs SL should be monitored for the following:

- cholesterol levels – total cholesterol, HDL, LDL, ratios.
- blood pressure
- bowel function
- liver function (six monthly LFTs)
- glaucoma (regular visits to optician/ophthalmologist)
- muscle pain, especially if simvastatin dose is required to be increased.

4a   What would you use to treat the epilepsy to prevent recurrence? Give reasons for your choice.

Consider the difference in response to drugs between older and younger people. Treatment should reflect biological age (rather than chronological). Pharmacokinetics, pharmacodynamics, tolerability, adverse reactions, economy and patient choice will all influence therapy chosen. Most commonly, carbamazepine or sodium valproate are chosen for older people as their effects in older people are well documented. Both show a favourable balance of safety, efficacy and economy. Phenytoin is less preferable because of drug interactions, adverse effects and potential for toxicity (zero order kinetics).

4b   What are the differences between the formulations of phenytoin, carbamazepine and sodium valproate and what factors do you need to take into consideration according to Mrs SL's current and future needs?

The formulations of phenytoin, carbamazepine and sodium valproate are compared in Table A17.3 overleaf.

4c   You have chosen sodium valproate. What monitoring would you undertake and recommend to monitor therapy?

The following should be monitored:

- LFTs baseline and six monthly,
- full blood count and ensure no undue potential for bleeding, and
- blood levels if poor compliance suspected, lack of effect, toxicity suspected. Routine monitoring is not recommended as there is a poor correlation between plasma levels and therapeutic efficacy.

Adverse effects should be discussed with the patient, especially sedation, signs and symptoms of pancreatitis (e.g. abdominal pain, nausea and vomiting).

Table A17.3 Comparison of formulations of phenytoin, carbamazepine and sodium valproate

Formulation	Key features
Phenytoin	
Tablet	Bioavailability different to capsules, discussion about generic equivalence has led to patient being prescribed branded products
Capsule	Biovailability different to tablets. Brand prescribing occurs
Liquid	Strength of liquid can cause confusion (30 mg in 5 mL as base; oral solid formulations are the salt except Infatabs, which is base)
i.v.	Cardiac adverse effects can occur, requiring ECG monitoring during infusion, rate of administration must be less than 50 mg/min, high pH causes local irritation
i.m.	Not recommended as may precipitate once administered. Bioavailability is only 50% of oral. May accumulate – not to be given for more than one week via this route. Not to be used in status epilepticus due to erratic absorption
Carbamazepine	
Tablet	Retard formulation has 15% lower bioavailability than standard release. Dose adjustment may be needed. Benefit is less fluctuation of levels. Retard is given as twice daily dosing (rather than three times day for standard). Chewable tablets reach peak plasma concentration more slowly than syrup (6 hours vs. 2 hours)
Liquid	Suitable for long-term use. No clinically relevant difference between oral dose forms. No dose adjustments between oral formulations
Suppository	Bioavailability is 25% lower than with oral formulations. Licensed only for short-term use. Unlikely to be suitable for use at home
Sodium valproate	
Tablet	Chrono to be given once or twice a day, not sucked or chewed. Reduces fluctuations of plasma level compared to standard release. Tablets may be given twice a day
Liquid	Dose as tablets, twice a day
i.v.	No dosage adjustment. Given as slow i.v. bolus or infusion. Not to be mixed with other i.v. drugs in the same line

5 What would you do to support her recovery outside hospital, focusing on potential medication-related issues after discharge?

You should:

■   ensure that Mrs SL's GP, primary care nursing and community pharmacist are aware of her new medication and compliance needs, including formulation choices;

■ spend time with the patient, practising administration of medicines;

■ discuss the patient's concerns with managing medicines prior to discharge, review and optimise medication accordingly well before discharge; and

■ communicate all changes and rationale to primary care health professionals and care workers if appropriate.

Case study level Mb – see page 416

1a Falls are common in older people and as Mrs GG points out can be very dangerous. What are the risk factors; pharmacological and non pharmacological, for falls in older people?

Pharmacological

Prescribed medicines such as:

■ sedatives – phenothiazines, benzodiazepines, older antidepressants
■ diuretics
■ hypotensive agents – ACE inhibitors, calcium antagonists, alpha blockers
■ antihistamines – chlorphenamine, cyclizine, cinnarizine, alimemazine, clemastine, hydroxyzine, promethazine
■ narcotic analgesics
■ eye drops
■ digoxin
■ laxatives
■ alcohol
■ non prescription medicines
■ abuse of non-prescription drugs

Non pharmacological

Disease and pathology:

■ Parkinson's disease
■ Meniere's disease
■ infection
■ dehydration
■ stroke
■ arthritis – rheumatoid and osteoarthritis, other rheumatic diseases
■ poor sight
■ arrhythmias including atrial fibrillation
■ dementia/Alzheimer's disease
■ epilepsy
■ post surgery, especially knee and hip surgery

Home environment:

- loose carpets
- clutter
- lack of hand rails, etc.
- poor fitting shoes, etc.
- living alone
- poor lighting

Age in general:

- infirmity & frailty

1b Briefly discuss those risk factors which apply specifically to Mrs GG.

Mrs GG is elderly and as such is more likely to be frail and in general more likely to fall.

Mrs GG has atrial fibrillation which if not controlled can cause temporary loss of cardiac output resulting in a drop of blood pressure. Mrs GG's description of suddenly going dizzy associated with a 'jump in the chest' suggest that her fall was probably caused by this. Her sudden dizziness is consistent with an arrhythmia and not some other acute cause such as epilepsy.

Digoxin at high levels can cause confusion and sedation in the elderly but Mrs GG does not present with confusion. Also digoxin toxicity can cause arrhythmias or bradycardia which can result in a drop in cardiac output leading to a fall. Again she does not presently exhibit any symptoms of digoxin toxicity so this is unlikely. A digoxin serum level may be useful to confirm this.

Nothing is known about Mrs GG's home circumstances apart from the fact that she lives alone. However, there may be factors in her home environment that may increase her risks of a fall.

1c Outline how Mrs GG's risk factors can be reduced.

Her age and frailty cannot be altered but the consequences of any fall can be minimised by optimising her bone density.

Optimising Mrs GG's digoxin therapy should reduce the incidence of dizzy spells. A digoxin level should be taken and appropriate dosage adjustment made if the level is subtherapeutic. The level should also rule out digoxin toxicity, although the clinical picture appears to rule this out. She should also be asked about compliance with her digoxin to rule out missing of doses. This is also important for pharmacokinetically based dosage adjustment based on levels.

The overall management plan for her atrial fibrillation should be reviewed to see if defibrillation is indicated.

If defibrillation is to be considered the warfarin therapy must be optimised as the risk of a thrombotic event is increased if anticoagulant control is poor pre-defibrillation.

A home assessment would be beneficial to reduce and/or remove any risks in her home environment.

2a   There are a number of sources of 'best practice' to provide advice for treating Mrs GG's atrial fibrillation (AF). Identify four common sources and provide the current references and/or URL for the management of AF.

■   *British National Formulary* – BNF
    url: http://bnf.org/bnf/bnf/current/2409.htm
■   National Institute for Health and Clinical Excellence – NICE,
    url: http://guidance.nice.org.uk/CG36/quickrefguide/pdf/English
    http://www.nice.org.uk/nicemedia/pdf/CG036niceguideline.pdf
■   NHS Clinical Knowledge Summaries (CKS) formerly known as Prodigy,
    http://www.prodigy.nhs.uk/atrial_fibrillation/view_whole_guidance
    http://cks.library.nhs.uk/atrial_fibrillation
■   American College of Cardiology – ACC
    http://www.acc.org/qualityandscience/clinical/guidelines/atrial_fib/pdfs/
    AF_Full_Text.pdf

2b   Briefly summarise the advice for managing Mrs GG's chronic AF from each of these sources. Highlight any significant differences between the sources of advice.

BNF

The heart rate can be controlled with a beta-blocker or diltiazem (unlicensed indication) or verapamil. If control of heart rate is inadequate during normal activities then digoxin can be added. For patients who require additional control during exercise a combination of diltiazem or verapamil with digoxin should be used. Care is needed using these combinations if ventricular function is diminished. Digoxin is usually effective for controlling heart rate at rest; it is usually appropriate if AF is accompanied by congestive heart failure. Digoxin monotherapy should only be used in predominantly sedentary patients.

Anticoagulants are indicated in the elderly. In the very elderly the overall benefit and risks need careful assessment. Aspirin is less effective than warfarin at preventing emboli but may be appropriate if there are no other risk factors for stroke. Aspirin 75 mg once daily may be used.

NICE

Mrs GG is over 65 and has persistent or permanent AF so should be considered for rate control of her AF. She is also over 75 but does not have additional risk factors such as hypertension, diabetes or vascular disease so should be considered for aspirin therapy before warfarin therapy. If she is considered for cardioversion then warfarin would be appropriate.

NICE recommends a beta-blocker or a rate limiting calcium antagonist treatment in the first instance. If the rate is not controlled then digoxin should be added. If the loss of rate control is associated with exercise then a calcium antagonist should be given with digoxin. If this does not work specialist referral is recommended. NICE does not recommend the use of digoxin as monotherapy in predominantly sedentary patients. Mrs GG is normally active so digoxin could be considered for monotherapy. Mrs GG is currently on digoxin but it does not seem to be controlling her symptoms effectively.

NICE provides very good treatment algorithms for rhythm control, rate control, management of the various types of AF and assessing stroke risk to determine appropriate antithrombotic therapy that aid treatment decisions.

Clinical Knowledge Summaries (CKS) (formerly known as Prodigy)

Clinical Knowledge Summaries are designed to provide health care providers, particularly those in primary care with answers on managing common conditions encountered in primary care. They are a reliable source of evidence-based information and practical 'know how' about these conditions. CKS provides advice on which patients should be referred to hospital for management (Centre for Change and Innovation, 2005).

CKS effectively mirrors NICE guidance with some additional information and evidence. The basic treatment goal is usually to keep the ventricular rate less than 90/minute at rest and 180/minute on exercise (Royal College of Physicians of Edinburgh, 1999).

The recommended first-line treatment in General Practice is a beta-blocker or a rate-limiting calcium channel blocker. If rate control is not achieved despite adequate monotherapy, then consider combining digoxin with a beta-blocker or verapamil, or consider referral. Verapamil must not be combined with a beta-blocker, owing to the risk of bradycardia and reduced cardiac output.

Rhythm control is not recommended as first line treatment in older people with persistent AF and all patients with permanent AF, as rate control would be the preferred treatment. If a patient requires rhythm control, referral to a specialist is recommended rather than commencing in primary care. At least one meta-analysis has shown that, in people with atrial fibrillation at moderate to high risk of stroke, survival rates were similar for rate control or rhythm control.

Cardioversion

Cardioversion is an option in patients with persistent atrial fibrillation and has an initial success rate of 70 – 90% in selected people. Success is more likely in recent-onset AF and in younger people.

CKS recommends that antithrombotic treatment is indicated in all people with atrial fibrillation (AF). The choice of treatment should be determined by the person's risk of stroke. CKS uses the risk stratification recommended by NICE see Table A17.4.

Table A17.4 Stroke risk stratification guide (from CKS [3])

High risk	Moderate risk	Low risk
Previous ischaemic stroke/ transient ischaemic attack or thromboembolic event	Age > 65 years with no high risk factors	Age less than 65 years with no moderate or high risk factors
Age ≥ 75 years with hypertension, diabetes, or vascular disease (coronary artery disease or peripheral artery disease)	Age < 75 years with hypertension, diabetes, or vascular disease (coronary artery disease or peripheral artery disease)	
Clinical evidence of valve disease or heart failure, or impaired LV function on echocardiography*		

*Echocardiogram is not needed for routine assessment, but refines clinical risk stratification in the case of moderate or severe left ventricular dysfunction and valve disease but not needed.

Mrs GG is at moderate risk of stroke because of her age. The choice of anti-thrombotic agent is between warfarin and aspirin. Warfarin is more effective but aspirin has a wider margin of safety. Clear-cut evidence is lacking, therefore a decision should be made on an individual basis, balancing the risks and benefits of warfarin versus aspirin. The patient's preferences should be taken into account in this decision. Risk factors are cumulative, therefore the presence of two or more moderate risk factors may favour the use of warfarin. However, Mrs GG's only risk factor is her age (National Collaborating Centre for Chronic Conditions, 2006).

ACC

The ACC guidance is similar to NICE and CKS.

There are no major differences between any of the sources of guidance although CKS has a primary care focus.

3   A risk factor for fracture following a fall in older people is osteoporosis. Is there any best practice advice? If so what is the source and provide a brief summary of that advice.

There is best practice advice available from CKS, NICE guidance and SIGN guidance. Both the NICE and SIGN guidance are incorporated into the CKS guidance.

CKS Guidance

In women aged 75 years and older, treatment is recommended without the need for prior dual energy X-ray absorptiometry (DXA) scanning. Bisphosphonates, strontium ranelate, and raloxifene are all suitable for initiation in primary care. However both SIGN (2003) and NICE (2008) recommend that a bisphosphonate (alendronate, etidronate, risedronate, ibandronate) should be used first-line.

Alendronate and risedronate reduce the incidence of both vertebral and non-vertebral fractures in women with established osteoporosis. Etidronate reduces the incidence of vertebral fractures but the evidence is weaker for its effect on non-vertebral fractures.

Alendronate and risedronate are both available as once-daily and once-weekly preparations, whereas etidronate is given in 90 day cycles (etidronate for 14 days followed by calcium carbonate for the remaining 76 days). Ibandronate taken monthly may be considered as an alternative to the other daily and weekly bisphosphonate preparations. However CKS notes that there is currently very limited experience with prescribing ibandronate and more established bisphosphonates may be preferred

Raloxifene is recommended in patients (NICE, 2008) in whom bisphosphonates are contraindicated, those who cannot comply with the requirements needed to take bisphosphonates, or who have had an unsatisfactory response or are intolerant of bisphosphonates. Strontium ranelate is a suitable alternative if a bisphosphonate cannot be taken. However, NICE guidelines on secondary prevention of osteoporosis does not currently recommend the use of strontium ranelate.

Ibandronate 150 mg taken monthly is a relatively recently licensed bisphosphonate (September 2005) that may be considered as an alternative to the other daily and weekly bisphosphonate preparations. Only monthly treatment is available in the UK.

Intranasal calcitonin (salmon calcitonin) reduces the incidence of vertebral fractures, but evidence is lacking on whether it reduces the incidence of non-vertebral fractures.

Hormone replacement therapy (HRT), including tibolone, is not recommended for postmenopausal women over the age of 50 years unless other treatments for osteoporosis are contraindicated or not tolerated (MHRA, 2005).

Specialist use

Teriparatide (a recombinant human parathyroid hormone) stimulates bone formation and is given daily by subcutaneous injection. There is evidence that teriparatide reduces vertebral and non-vertebral fractures. NICE recommends that it should be considered for the secondary prevention of osteoporotic fragility fractures in women aged 65 years and over who are intolerant of bisphosphonates or who have had an unsatisfactory response to bisphosphonates *and* who have severe osteoporosis (NICE, 2008).

Adjunctive treatment with calcium + vitamin D should be considered. Once treatment for osteoporosis is started, it is likely that this will need to be continued indefinitely (Scottish Intercollegiate Guidelines Network, 2003).

4a   Increasing or preventing further loss of bone density will minimise the risk of fracture following a fall. What specific risk factors does Mrs GG have that may increase her likelihood of having decreased bone density?

Mrs GG is elderly and a post menopausal female, which are risk factors. These are risk factors that cannot be altered.

4b   What are the treatment options available to reduce or halt the reduction in Mrs GG's bone density?

A bisphosphonate (alendronate, etidronate, risedronate, ibandronate) should be used first-line (Scottish Intercollegiate Guidelines Network, 2003, NICE 2008).

Strontium ranelate is a suitable alternative if a bisphosphonate cannot be taken.

Raloxifene can be considered if both a bisphosphonate and strontium ranelate cannot be given.

- Intranasal calcitonin (salmon calcitonin)
- Teriparatide (a recombinant human parathyroid hormone)
- Hormone replacement therapy (HRT)
- Adjunctive treatment with calcium + vitamin D should be considered no matter what treatment is considered.

4c   What would you recommend for Mrs GG and why?

A bisphosphonate would appear to be a suitable first choice as all current guidance recommends this as first line therapy. Alendronate and risendronate can be given once daily or once weekly, while etidronate has a more complex dosing regimen. Ibandronate could be prescribed monthly but CKS guidance suggests a more established bisphosphonate should be considered first. Current BNF prices (Joint Formulary Committee, 2008) would suggest that alendronate is the cheaper option and should be considered initially.

4d   The multidisciplinary team decide to recommend treatment with a bisphosphonate for Mrs GG. What issues need to be taken into consideration both before prescribing and for counselling once prescribed?

There are a range of drugs available. The regimen that suits Mrs GG best should be discussed; there are currently formulations for daily, weekly and monthly administration with the likelihood of an annual dose preparation being possibly available. Weekly and monthly administration may improve compliance but they may also possibly reduce compliance due to them being forgotten. Etidronate has a complex dosage regimen in comparison to the other bisphosphonates. They are toxic to the oesophagus and must be swallowed with a large amount of water and the patient must remain in an upright position for an hour afterwards. They need to be taken on an empty stomach for optimal absorption but this can lead to uncomfortable and sometimes severe gastric irritation and sometimes bleeding. As Mrs GG is on warfarin this could be dangerous.

The bisphosphonates are involved in a number of drug interactions, although not with warfarin or digoxin.

5a The benefits of bisphosphonate treatment are explained to Mrs GG. She accepts that they will be of benefit and are the best treatment currently available but tells you firmly that she will not take a bisphosphonate under any circumstances. Her best friend was on alendronate and suffered intolerable gastric discomfort. She also doesn't fancy the idea of standing or sitting upright for up to an hour after taking the tablets. Using the 4 key ethical principles of beneficence, malevolence, autonomy and justice discuss how you would address this dilemma.

Although the patient's best interests are at the heart of any ethical discussion, it is important to consider the interests of all the major stakeholders, in this case the health care team looking after Mrs GG and the local health economy as well as Mrs GG herself.

Beneficence: do benefit, act to do good

Mrs GG will benefit by having the best available treatment to reduce her chances of suffering a fracture if she suffers a further fall.

The personal cost of a fracture to Mrs GG could be great and could even lead to her death, avoiding this is a prime aim of treatment.

The health care team's prime aim is to benefit Mrs GG by providing her with the best treatment.

No treatment will save the money that would have been spent on the drugs.

Malevolence: avoid harm

Mrs GG may suffer a severe adverse effect, i.e. severe gastric intolerance and possibly bleeding.

She also feels that it is an unacceptable imposition to remain in an upright position for a prolonged period after taking the drug.

The healthcare team caring from Mrs GG may feel that they have failed her by her refusal to accept the best available treatment.

The cost to the health economy of managing a fall with a major fracture such as neck of femur is great.

Bisphosphonates are relatively expensive choices in the treatment of osteoporosis.

Autonomy: respect individuals choices

Mrs GG's opinion must be respected as her decision has been made lucidly and logically with the benefit of her own appraisal of the evidence she has available to her.

This evidence has been provided to her both by the healthcare team and her own experience.

Mrs GG has the right to make her own decisions.

The healthcare team are right to advocate the treatment they consider to be the best.

Justice: treat all involved fairly

The healthcare team have provided Mrs GG with the available information to reach a decision.

5b   Discuss alternative medication or other strategies that may be less effective but more acceptable to the patient.

Although Mrs GG may not wish to take a bisphosphonate she may be persuaded to take calcium with or without vitamin D which is effective although less effective than a bisphosphonate. It is a cheaper and less toxic option. Other options such as teriparatide and strontium ranelate are more expensive and there is less experience in their use but they should be discussed with Mrs GG.

Non pharmacological management such as the use of hip protectors could be considered, even if a bisphosphonate was to be used. Weight-bearing exercise is useful and just because Mrs GG is elderly does not mean that she can not undertake appropriate exercise.

Index